GIARDIASIS

Human Parasitic Diseases

Volume 3

Series Editors

E.J. RUITENBERG
(Bilthoven, RIM)

and

A.J. MacINNIS
(Los Angeles, UCLA)

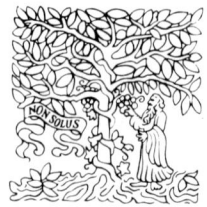

ELSEVIER
AMSTERDAM • NEW YORK • OXFORD

Giardiasis

Edited by

E.A. MEYER

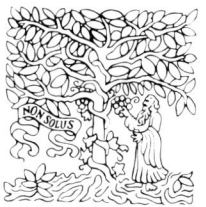

1990
ELSEVIER
AMSTERDAM • NEW YORK • OXFORD

© 1990 Elsevier Science Publishers B.V. (Biomedical Division)

All rights reserved. No part of this publication may be reproduced, stored in a retrieval system or transmitted in any form or by any means, electronic, mechanical, photocopying, recording or otherwise without the prior written permission of the Publisher, Elsevier Science Publishers B.V. (Biomedical Division), P.O. Box 1527, 1000 BV Amsterdam, The Netherlands.

No responsibility is assumed by the Publisher for any injury and/or damage to persons or property as a matter of products liability, negligence or otherwise, or from any use or operation of any methods, products, instructions or ideas contained in the material herein. Because of the rapid advances in the medical sciences, the Publisher recommends that independent verification of diagnoses and drug dosages should be made.

Special regulations for readers in the U.S.A.:
This publication has been registered with the Copyright Clearance Center Inc. (CCC), Salem, Massachusetts. Information can be obtained from the CCC about conditions under which the photocopying of parts of this publication may be made in the U.S.A. All other copyright questions, including photocopying outside the U.S.A., should be referred to the publisher.

ISBN Volume: 0-444-81258-X (Hardback)
ISSN Series: 0169-3727

This book is printed on acid-free paper.

Published by:
Elsevier Science Publishers B.V. (Biomedical Division)
P.O. Box 211
1000 AE Amsterdam
The Netherlands

Sole distributors for the U.S.A. and Canada:
Elsevier Science Publishing Company, Inc.
52 Vanderbilt Avenue
New York, NY 10017
U.S.A.

Library of Congress Cataloging in Publication Data
Giardiasis / edited by E.A. Meyer.
p. cm. – (Human parasitic diseases; v. 3)
Includes bibliographical references.
ISBN 0-444-81258-X (U.S.: alk. paper)
1. Giardiasis. I. Meyer, Ernest A. (Ernest Alan) II. Series.
[DNLM: 1. Giardiasis. W1 HU457 v. 3 / WC.700 G4359]
QR201.G45G54 1990
616.9'62- -dc20
DNLM/DLC
for Library of Congress 90–2708
CIP

PRINTED IN THE NETHERLANDS

Preface

During the working lives of clinicians presently active, the status of *Giardia* has changed from that of (i) a harmless commensal to (ii) a potential pathogen to (iii) one of the 10 major parasites of humans. One factor which contributed to this change has been the reduction of other serious diseases. Other factors are those advances which have made it possible to study the organism and the disease it causes: these include the introduction of anti-*Giardia* agents, and the development of culture methods for *Giardia*.

We now know that giardiasis is ubiquitous and is found all over the world. The causative agent(s) may be enzootic as well. Although always transmitted fecal-orally, the precise means of transmission varies in different parts of the world. And decisions regarding the treatment of the *Giardia*-infected individual vary in different parts of the world. For these reasons, it is appropriate that a well-rounded treatment of the subject reflect these diverse views. The authors of this volume reflect that world-wide view. Each contributor is a *Giardia* authority in her/his own right. I thank all of them for their cooperation and patience.

Many papers on *Giardia* and giardiasis have appeared since the publication in 1984 of a monograph on the subject. The present volume focuses on developments in the last decade. I have tried to make it comprehensive and up-to-date, a single-source reference useful for a broad readership including the researcher, the teacher, the clinician and the public health administrator. Some readers may not peruse every chapter. Those who do will detect minor intentional redundancy.

If this volume helps to promote research on *Giardia* and thereby decreases the world-wide impact of giardiasis, it will have served its purpose.

I thank the series editor, Professor Austin J. MacInnis, for his guidance in the preparation of this volume.

Ernest Alan Meyer
Portland, Oregon, February, 1990

Editor's note: Consensus does not exist regarding the nomenclature of the *Giardia*. The parasitic protozoa responsible for human giardiasis can be found described in the literature by various genus (e.g., *Giardia, Lamblia*) and species (e.g., *duodenalis, enterica, intestinalis, lamblia*) names. In an attempt to reduce confusion, in this volume they are referred to either as *Giardia duodenalis* or human source *Giardia*. The subject is discussed in Chapter 2.

List of Contributors

M. BELOSEVIC
Department of Zoology, Biological Sciences Building, University of Alberta, Edmonton, Alberta T6G 2E1, Canada.

G.F. CRAUN
U.S. Environmental Protection Agency, 26 West Saint Clair, Cincinatti, OH 45268, U.S.A.

S. DAS
Department of Pathology, H811F, University of California, San Diego Medical Center, 225 Dickinson Street, San Diego, CA 92103, U.S.A.

R.A. DAVIDSON
Department of General Medicine, University of Florida College of Medicine, Gainesville, FL 32610, U.S.A.

P.G. ENGELKIRK
Program in Medical Technology/Cytogenetics, Freeman Building, Room 1.704, University of Texas Health Science Center, Houston, TX 77225, U.S.A.

S.L. ERLANDSEN
Department of Cell Biology and Neuroanatomy, University of Minnesota Medical School, Minneapolis, MN 55455, U.SA.

G.M. FAUBERT
Institute of Parasitology of McGill University, Macdonald College, 21, 111 Lakeshore Road, Ste-Anne de Bellevue, Québec H9X 1C0, Canada.

D.E. FEELY
Department of Oral Biology and Basic Science, College of Dentistry, University of Nebraska Medical Center, Lincoln, NE 68583, U.S.A.

A. FERGUSON
Western General Hospital, University of Edinburgh, Crewe Road, Edinburgh EH4 2XU, U.K.

F.D. GILLIN
Department of Pathology, H811F, University of California, San Diego Medical Center, 225 Dickinson Street, San Diego, CA 92103, U.S.A.

J. GILLON
Western General Hospital, University of Edinburgh, Crewe Road, Edinburgh EH4 2XU, U.K.

G.R. HEALY
905 Vistavia Circle, Decatur, GA 30033, U.S.A.

D.V. HOLBERTON
Department of Zoology, The University of Hull, Hull HU6 7RX, U.K.

A. ISLAM
International Centre for Disease Research, GPO Box 128, Dhaka 1000, Bangladesh.

W. JAKUBOWSKI
Health Effects Research Laboratory, U.S. Environmental Protection Agency, Cincinnati, OH 45268, U.S.A.

E.N. JANOFF
NIH-IMI, Building 30, Room 324, Bethesda, MD 20892, U.S.A.

E.L. JARROLL
Department of Biology, Cleveland State University, 1983 E. 24th Street, Cleveland, OH 44115, U.S.A.

A.M.M. JOKIPII
University of Helsinki, Haartmaninkatu 3 B, 00290 Helsinki, Finland.

L. JOKIPII
University of Helsinki, Haartmaninkatu 3 B, 00290 Helsinki, Finland.

D.G. LINDMARK
Department of Biology, Cleveland State University, 1983 E. 24th Street, Cleveland, OH 44115, U.S.A.

E.A. MEYER
Department of Microbiology and Immunology, Oregon Health Sciences University, 3181 S.W. Sam Jackson Park Road, Portland, OR 97201–3098, U.S.A.

G. MUNRO
Western General Hospital, University of Edinburgh, Crewe Road, Edinburgh EX4 2XU, U.K.

L.K. PICKERING
Program in Infectious Diseases and Clinical Microbiology, Department of Pediatrics, University of Texas Medical School at Houston, 6431 Fannin Street, Houston, TX 77030, U.S.A.

S. RADULESCU
Cantacuzino Institute, 113 Splaiul Independentei, Bucharest, Romania.

D.S. REINER
Department of Pathology, H811F, University of California, San Diego Medical Center, 225 Dickinson Street, San Diego, CA 92103, U.S.A.

F.W. SCHAEFER, III
Health Effects Research Laboratory, United States Environmental Protection Agency, 26 West Martin Luther King Drive, Cincinnati, OH 45268, U.S.A.

D.G. SCHUPP
Department of Cell Biology and Neuroanatomy, University of Minnesota Medical School, Minneapolis, MN 55455, U.S.A.

P.D. SMITH
Cellular Immunology Section, Laboratory of Immunology, National Institute of Dental Research, National Institutes of Health, Bethesda, MD 20892, U.S.A.

D.P. STEVENS
Department of Medicine, Case Western Reserve University, School of Medicine, University Hospitals of Cleveland, Cleveland, OH 44106, U.S.A.

M.S. WOLFE
Tropical Medicine Unit, Office of Medical Services, Department of State, Washington, DC 20520, U.S.A.

Contents

Preface and Editor's note   v
List of Contributors   vii

Introduction
   E.A. Meyer   1
1. The biology of *Giardia*
   D.E. Feely, D.V. Holberton and S.L. Erlandsen   11
2. Taxonomy and nomenclature
   E.A. Meyer   51
3. *Giardia* metabolism
   E.L. Jarroll and D.G. Lindmark   61
4. Animal models for *Giardia duodenalis* type organisms
   G.M. Faubert and M. Belosevic   77
5. Animal model of *Giardia muris* in the mouse
   D.P. Stevens   91
6. In vitro cultivation of *Giardia* trophozoites
   S. Radulescu and E.A. Meyer   99
7. Methods for excystation of *Giardia*
   F.W. Schaefer, III   111
8. In vitro encystation of *Giardia*
   D.G. Schupp, D.S. Reiner, F.D. Gillin and S.L. Erlandsen   137
9. Pathology and pathogenesis of the intestinal mucosal damage in giardiasis
   A. Ferguson, J. Gillon and G. Munro   155
10. Clinical symptoms and diagnosis by traditional methods
   M.S. Wolfe   175
11. Detection of *Giardia* by immunologic methods
   P.G. Engelkirk and L.K. Pickering   187
12. Nonspecific defenses against human *Giardia*
   F.D. Gillin, S. Das and D.S. Reiner   199
13. The role of immunity in *Giardia* infections
   E.N. Janoff and P.D. Smith   215

14. Giardiasis in developing countries
    A. Islam — 235
15. Waterborne giardiasis
    G.F. Craun — 267
16. *Giardia* among children in day care
    L.K. Pickering and P.G. Engelkirk — 295
17. Giardiasis in perspective: the evidence of animals as a source of human *Giardia* infections
    G.R. Healy — 305
18. Nitroimidazole treatment of giardiasis
    L. Jokipii and A.M.M. Jokipii — 315
19. Treatment of giardiasis: the North American perspective
    R.A. Davidson — 325
20. The control of *Giardia* in water supplies
    W. Jakubowski — 335
21. Prospects and future goals
    E.A. Meyer — 355

Subject Index — 359

Giardiasis (E.A. Meyer, ed.)
© *1990 Elsevier Science Publishers B.V. (Biomedical Division)*

Introduction

ERNEST A. MEYER

Department of Microbiology and Immunology, Oregon Health Sciences University, Portland, OR 97201, U.S.A.

1. Historical background	1
1.1. Pathogenesis	3
1.2. Host specificity	4
1.3. Taxonomy	4
1.4. In vitro culture	6
1.5. Animal models	7
1.6. Chemotherapy	7
References	8

1. Historical background

Although we can speculate that the human intestinal disease giardiasis existed millennia ago, we can *only* speculate: none of the symptoms of this disease are so distinctive as to separate giardiasis from any of a number of other gastrointestinal ailments. The association of *Giardia* with disease symptoms occurred largely in this century. On the other hand, most parasitologists are aware of the evidence that *Giardia* trophozoites were the first intestinal protozoa to be seen and described.

   A literature search for the first description of the *Giardia* organism inevitably leads to two remarkable individuals: Antony van Leeuwenhoek (1632-1723) and Clifford Dobell (1886-1949). Most scientists believe that Leeuwenhoek was the first to see and to provide a written description of the protozoan. Dobell, more than two centuries later, translated van Leeuwenhoek's letters with the eyes of a parasitologist, and published his conclusions.

   Clifford Dobell wrote (1932) that his interest in trying to learn something about Leeuwenhoek dated to about 1907. Subsequently, he taught himself modern Dutch, then 17th century Dutch, and translated a number of Leeuwenhoek's writings from Dutch and Latin. In the process he became convinced that Leeuwenhoek, in a letter dated 4 November 1681, had described *Giardia* trophozoites from his own diarrheic stool. Dobell's translation (1932) of part of that letter follows:

'I weigh about 160 pound, and have been of very nigh the same weight for some 30 years[1], and I have ordinarily of a morning a well-formed stool; but now and then hitherto I have had a looseness, at intervals of 2, 3, or 4 weeks, when I went to stool some 2, 3, or 4 times a day[2]. But this summer[3] this befell me very often, and especially when I partook of hot smoked beef, that was a bit fat[4], or ham, which food I'm very fond of; indeed, it persisted once for three days running, and whatever food I took, I kept in my body not much[5] above 4 hours; and I imagined (for divers reasons) that I could get myself well again by drinking uncommon hot tea, as hath happened[6] many a time before.

My excrement being so thin[7], I was at divers times persuaded to examine it[8]; and each time[9] I kept in mind what food I had eaten and what drink I had drunk, and what I found afterwards[10]: but to tell all my observations here would make all too long a story. I will only say that I have generally seen, in my excrement, many irregular particles of sundry sizes, most of then tending to a round figure which are very clear and of a yellow colour[11]: these were the ones that make the whole material[12] look yellow to our eye. And there were also, besides, such like particles that were very bright and clear without one being able to discern any colour in them[13].

All the particles aforesaid lay in a clear transparent medium, wherein I have sometimes also seen animalcules[14] a-moving very prettily; some of 'em a bit bigger, others a bit less, than a blood-globule, but all of one and the same make. Their bodies were somewhat longer than broad, and their belly which was flatlike, furnisht with sundry little paws, wherewith they made such a stir in the clear medium and among the globules, that you might e'en fancy you saw a pissabed[15] running up against a wall; and albeit they made a quick motion with their paws, yet for all that they made but slow progress. Of these animalcules I saw at one time only one in a particle of matter as big as a sand-grain; and anon, at other times some 4, 5 or even 6 or 8. I have also once seen animalcules of the same bigness, but of a different figure[16].

---

[1] When he wrote this, Leeuwenhoek was 49 years old.

[2] The Latin version of this passage is somewhat ambiguous, and has apparently led some readers to suppose that L. frequently suffered from diarrhoea lasting for 2-4 weeks. It has even, indeed, given rise to the belief that he suffered from chronic dysentery for 30 years. His own words do not countenance any such conclusions. Cf. Dobell (1920).

[3] *i.e.*, anno 1681.

[4] *dat een weynig vet was*. These words are in the printed version but not in the original MS. A similar remark is made by L. much later in *Send-brief* XXXIX, 13 July 1717, to J.G. Kerkherdere.

[5] *veel* is here in the printed letter, but not in the MS.

[6] *is gelukt* [= succeeded] MS. *is geschied* [= befell] printed version.

[7] *i.e.*, dilute or watery.

[8] *i.e.*, with the microscope.

[9] *soo nu en dan* MS. *soo nu als dan* printed version.

[10] This word is not in the originals. I add it to preserve the sense.

[11] Probably incompletely digested remains of meat (striated muscle).

[12] *i.e.*, the faeces *en masse*.

[13] Probably fat-droplets.

[14] The following description – as I have elsewhere tried to show (Dobell, 1920) – is a graphic account of the flagellate *Giardia* (= *Lamblia*) *intestinalis*.

[15] The woodlouse or sow-bug (*Onicus asellus*). The Latin translation of this passage has given rise to many curious misunderstandings. Cf. Dobell (1920), where 'pissabeds' are more fully discussed.

[16] As no other details are given, it is impossible to identify these organisms. Possibly they were *Trichomonas* or *Chilomastix*.

During the first two decades of this century, Vilem Lambl (1824-1895), a Czech physician, was credited with the discovery in 1859 of this flagellate; the name *Lamblia*, in fact, had been applied to the genus by Blanchard in 1888. Dobell wanted to set the record straight. In a paper published in 1920, Dobell translates the Leeuwenhoek letter in point, painstakingly considers all of the possibilities, and concludes 'the honour of discovering this protozoon belongs in reality not to Lambl and Austria, but to Holland and the Father of Protozoology'. Dobell's writings on Leeuwenhoek make interesting reading.

Although Leeuwenhoek probably, and Lambl certainly, saw and described the organism we presently know as *Giardia* (and Lambl described its habitat in the intestine), there is no evidence that either man saw or recognized the cyst form of the parasite. The cysts of this organism were first noted by Grassi, who, in 1879, thought they might possibly be coccidia. Later (1881, 1888), he associated them with the flagellated form of the organism.

1.1. Pathogenesis

Can *Giardia* cause human disease, or is it merely a commensal? The answer to that question was long in coming, partly because asymptomatic *Giardia* infection is so common. Koch's postulates, the ground rules for proving that an organism causes disease, can be applied in those cases where the organism consistently causes disease. *Giardia* does not always cause disease. Small wonder that, in the absence of compelling evidence, the scientific jury was out so long on the issue of *Giardia's* pathogenicity.

In 1921, Dobell and O'Connor considered the question of the pathogenicity of intestinal flagellates and concluded 'in our opinion, there is as yet no good evidence to prove that any intestinal flagellate found in man is pathogenic, but there is very considerable evidence to show that most and probably all of them are harmless'.

The experiments of Robert Rendtorff, reported in 1954, involved feeding *Giardia* cysts from human donors to uninfected prison volunteers. Rendtorff later wrote (1979) that at the time of these experiments, interest was mainly focused on amebiasis, and because it was considered improper to expose prisoners to *E. histolytica*, nonpathogenic amoebae and *Giardia* were used. In the 1950s, most people considered *Giardia* a nonpathogen. The results of these experiments convinced Rendtorff (1979) that the *Giardia* they were studying were nonpathogenic.

In the quarter century after Rendtorff's (1954) publication, considerable information regarding *Giardia* pathogenicity had accumulated. Kulda and Nohnykova reconsidered the question of *Giardia* pathogenicity in 1978 and concluded, on the basis of disease symptoms, malabsorption, and histopathology, that 'there is no doubt that the organism is capable of causing disease in man'. The World Health Organization (1981) agrees. Detailed evidence that *Giardia* is a pathogen is presented in this volume in Chapter 9.

1.2. Host specificity

An aspect of *Giardia* epidemiology that has long fascinated – and divided – workers in the field, has been the host specificity of these organisms. Two schools of thought emerged. One school espouses the notion that, with rare exceptions, the *Giardia* of mammals are rigidly host specific. Robert Hegner (1926), a proponent of this idea, also contended that such *Giardia*, which he considered species, were distinct morphologically.

The other school holds that *Giardia* are not highly host specific, and bases this belief on demonstration of the apparent transfer of *Giardia* infection between different animal species. Meyer and Radulescu (1979) lists a number of such reports. Most such cross-transmission studies have been criticized (see, e.g., Bemrick, 1984) on the grounds that sufficient care was not taken to prove that the recipient animals were free of their own *Giardia* at the outset of, and did not acquire extraneous infection during, the experiment. Although to date no such experiments have escaped criticism, two (Grant and Woo, 1979; Hewlett et al., 1982) recent papers would seem to suggest that the distinct possibility exists that some *Giardia* strains are capable of infecting more than one vertebrate host species, while others may be host specific. Definitive experiments of this type need to be done if we are to fully understand the epidemiology of giardiasis.

1.3. Taxonomy

The rediscovery by Lambl in 1859 of *Giardia* was followed by the description of similar organisms from the rabbit in 1875 (Davaine), from the mouse in 1879 (Grassi), and from the tadpole in 1882 (Kunstler). In the present century interest increased in this group of protozoa, and *Giardia* were described from a number of vertebrates including mammals, birds, and amphibia. By 1978, Kulda and Nohynkova were able to list 40 *Giardia* 'species' from different animal hosts, although the authors recognized the problem of defining a species in this genus. A common criterion for assigning names to *Giardia* species has been the animal host species from which the organism was obtained; *Giardia* species continue to be described from new animal hosts.

The taxonomy and nomenclature of organisms in this protozoan group have presented problems since the last century. Early, two different generic names were applied to these protozoa. Organisms from the tadpole were classified as *Giardia* (Kunstler, 1882) and those from mammals as *Lamblia* (Blanchard, 1888). Hegner (1922) compared these two groups and concluded that differences between them were not sufficient to place them in separate genera. Most workers now affix the genus name *Giardia* to all representatives of this group, and use the word giardiasis to describe the disease caused by these organisms. *Lamblia*, and lambliasis, to describe the same genus of flagellates and the disease they cause, respectively, can still be found in some of the literature from the Soviet Union and Eastern Europe.

The criteria for designating a species in this genus continue to be a problem. Filice made this the subject of his research, published in 1952. This monograph had a profound influence on the thinking of subsequent protozoologists interested in the problem.

Filice noted that three criteria had been used primarily to differentiate species of *Giardia*: (1) host specificity, (2) various body dimensions, and (3) variations in structure. After a critical review of the literature and of the results of his own experiments, he rejected the first two criteria and believed that *Giardia* species should be named on more evidence than species of host, and size of the flagellate.

What about the third criterion – structural variation – among the *Giardia*? Filice noted that Nieschulz in 1924 had divided all the then known 'species' of *Giardia* into three groups primarily on the basis of the morphology of organelles within the trophozoites, which have come to be known as median bodies. (The function of these microtubular structures is still not clear.) The three identified groups derived from such structural criteria were (1) amphibian *Giardia* (represented by a single organism, *G. agilis*), which had long teardrop-shaped median bodies, (2) the 'muris' group, with two small rounded median bodies, and (3) the 'intestinalis' group, in which the single or double median bodies resemble the claw of a claw hammer and lie transversely across the trophozoite. Organisms with 'muris' type median bodies have been described from rodents and birds; 'intestinalis' type organisms have been reported as parasites of a variety of mammals, including humans and rodents, as well as birds and reptiles.

Nieschulz proposed assigning these three groups the rank of subgenera. Filice instead suggested that the type species of each of the three of Nieschulz's groups be recognized as species, and that morphologically indistinguishable *Giardia* from other hosts be assigned a nontaxonomic status, such as race. New species in this genus would be named as new forms were recognized that could be consistently distinguished from existing species by morphologic and/or biologic differences. The type species of these three groups were *G. agilis*, *G. muris*, and, because it was the first reported *Giardia* of its type, *G. duodenalis* (Davaine, 1875). The species name *intestinalis* was not available, having been assigned to another organism earlier.

Filice's proposal is logical. It assigns species names on the basis of those characteristics that are distinctive and constant. It avoids associating a name of a *Giardia* species with any particular animal host. And the proposal is provident, because it permits the addition of new species, as they are discovered, that are different morphologically or biologically from those already recognized. The reader will note, in Chapter 1, this volume, that a morphologically different *Giardia* has recently been demonstrated, for which a new species name, *G. psittaci*, has been proposed (Erlandsen and Bemrick, 1987). Furthermore, chemotaxonomic studies presently under way give promise that biologic differences in this group may also ultimately contribute to their distinction as species.

The protozoan described from humans by Lambl has been assigned a number of names over the years, and to this day there is no general agreement as to its most appropriate name. In the years after 1888 it was called *Lamblia intestinalis* (*intestinalis* after Lambl's suggestion in 1859, *Lamblia* after Blanchard's in 1888). Subsequently that genus name became invalid when it was acknowledged to be a synonym of, and preempted by, *Giardia*. The validity of the species name *intestinalis* was also called into question, and *Giardia enterica* (Corradetti, 1935) and *Giardia lamblia* (Kofoid and Christiansen, 1915) were proposed instead. The latter name has been used particularly in the United States. Despite disagreement as to the validity of the names *intestinalis* and *lamblia*, both continue to be used to describe this organism.

What system of *Giardia* nomenclature should be used in this volume? I have decided to follow Filice's (1952) lead: *Giardia duodenalis* and *Giardia* of the *duodenalis* type will be used as synonyms, which will be followed, where necessary for clarity, by the name of the animal from which the organisms were obtained.

1.4. In vitro culture

Of the common intestinal protozoa, *Giardia* have proven among the most difficult to cultivate in vitro. Media capable of supporting the non-axenic growth of most of the parasitic flagellates of the alimentary canal were available as early as 1921. Axenic culture of some of the trichomonads was reported by 1939; the introduction of antimicrobial agents facilitated these efforts.

By 1960, despite several early unsubstantiated reports, none of the *Giardia* had been cultured in vitro. In that year, two workers in Japan (Iwata and Araki) reported that they had kept *Giardia* trophozoites from a human alive in a complex medium for 12 days. A breakthrough came when Karapetyan (1960) in the Soviet Union described the in vitro culture of *Giardia* trophozoites from a human for seven months. Karapetyan used a complex medium that included chick fibroblasts and fungi in the genus *Candida*. Later (1962), he modified the system by deleting *Candida* and fibroblasts and adding living *Saccharomyces cerevisiae*; *Giardia* from the rabbit and human lived up to five months in this medium. His efforts to axenize these cultures were unsuccessful.

In 1965, Meyer and Pope reported culture of rabbit and chinchilla *Giardia* monoxenically with *S. cerevisiae* using a modification of Karapetyan's method. Axenic cultures of *Giardia* from the rabbit, chinchilla and cat were reported by Meyer in 1970. In 1976, Meyer described axenic cultivation of trophozoites from humans, and Fortess and Meyer axenically cultured guinea pig *Giardia*. Human serum was one ingredient of the complex culture media employed by Meyer.

Subsequently, the *Giardia* strains in culture were adapted to growth in media devised for *Entamoeba histolytica*. Visvesvara in 1980 adapted human *Giardia* trophozoites to grow in Diamond's TPS-1 medium, which contains bovine serum. A year later, Gillin and Diamond (1981) succeeded in growing this same organism in filter-sterilized TYI-S-33 medium; L-cysteine proved to be an essential ingredient. Although other workers have since reported successful isolation of *Giardia* of the *duodenalis* type, the establishment of these cultures is by no means routine. In 1983, two groups of workers (Keister, and Farthing et al.) noted that bile, added to TYI-S-33 medium, promoted the growth of *Giardia* trophozoites. To date, all of the *Giardia* obtained in culture have been of the *duodenalis* type; *Giardia* of the *agilis* and *muris* types thus far have resisted all efforts at in vitro cultivation.

Bingham and Meyer demonstrated in 1979 that *Giardia* excystation was pH dependent, and that, after suitable exposure at pH 2.0, *Giardia* could be induced to excyst. These excysted trophozoites then could be used as inocula to initiate cultures.

It has proven more difficult to elucidate the factors involved in the encystation of *Giardia* trophozoites. The findings of several groups of workers on this problem will be presented and discussed in this volume.

1.5. Animal models

Two animal models have been introduced recently for studying *Giardia* infections. Roberts-Thomson et al. (1976) pioneered the use of certain strains of mice for studying infections caused by *Giardia* of the *muris* type. In 1983, Belosevic et al. described the use of the Mongolian gerbil for studying infections caused by organisms of the *duodenalis* type. Not only do these animal models offer a valuable means of studying the host-parasite relationship; they serve as a source of trophozoites and cysts as well.

1.6. Chemotherapy

If the number of published papers on the treatment of giardiasis is any indication, numerous early clinicians were convinced that *Giardia* is involved in human intestinal disease. Starting in 1917, a great variety of compounds were tested in individuals with giardiasis; Lucian, in a 1971 monograph in Romanian, summarizes the chemotherapeutic agents, the dietetic treatments, and other diverse substances that were early used.

The presently accepted armamentarium for treating *Giardia* infections includes the following: (1) quinacrine, (2) several nitroimidazole derivatives, and (3) a nitrofuran, furazolidone. Details of the use of these agents will be found in later chapters of this volume. The effectiveness of quinacrine in treating giardiasis was first noted separately by two workers (Brumpt and Galli-Vallerio) in 1937. Metronidazole, an imidazole derivative, was reported useful in treating this disease in 1961 by Schneider; a related compound, tinidazole, was introduced for this purpose in 1972 and has been widely used in Europe. The first report of the use of the agent furazolidone in treating giardiasis was by Webster in 1960.

Interest in *Giardia* has accelerated in recent years. Part of this interest has resulted from the recognition, by the scientific community generally and by the World Health Organization specifically, that *Giardia* is an important cause of human disease. And part of this interest has been generated by the relatively recent availability of axenic cultures of these organisms, as well as the development of animal models. These serve as sources of trophozoites and cysts and provide a means of studying the host-parasite relationship. The increasing evidence that at least some *Giardia* from lower animals may infect humans indicates that it is appropriate to classify giardiasis as a zoonosis, and thus a disease which may occur unexpectedly, sometimes in epidemic form, in communities in which the incidence of *Giardia* in humans, and the chance of person to person transmission, is low.

Sargeaunt and Williams recently reported (1979) that biochemical markers can be used to distinguish pathogenic and nonpathogenic strains of *Entamoeba histolytica*. This raises the inevitable questions whether (1) pathogenic and nonpathogenic strains of *Giardia* exist, and, if so, (2) whether they can be distinguished biochemically. In any event, the biochemical characterization of the *Giardia* will be a valuable addition to our understanding of this group.

It is the purpose of this volume to bring the reader up to date on the status of *Giardia* and giardiasis, through an accounting by the investigators themselves of recent developments and of the many problems which remain to be solved in this field.

References

Belosevic, M., Faubert, G.M., MacLean, J.D., Law, C. and Croll, N.A. (1983) *Giardia lamblia* infections in Mongolian gerbils: an animal model. J. Infect. Dis. 143, 222-226.

Bemrick, W.J. (1984) Some perspectives on the transmission of giardiasis. In: S.L. Erlandsen and E.A. Meyer (Eds), *Giardia* and Giardiasis, pp. 379-400. Plenum Press, New York.

Bingham, A. and Meyer, E.A. (1979) Giardia excystation can be induced in vitro in acidic solutions. Nature (London) 277, 301-302.

Blanchard, R. (1888) Remarques sur le Mégastome intestinal. Bull. Soc. Zool. France 30, 18-19.

Brumpt, L. (1937) Traitement expérimental de la lambliase. C. R. Seances Soc. Biol. 124, 1040-1042.

Corradetti, A. (1935) *Giardia enterica* (Grassi, 1881), the correct name for the *Giardia* of man. J. Parasitol. 21, 1-2.

Davaine, C. (1875) Monadiens. In: Dictionnaire Encyclopédique des Sciences Médicales, ser. 2, vol. 9. P. Asselin and G. Masson, Place de L'Ecole de Medicine, Paris.

Dobell, C. (1920) The discovery of the intestinal protozoa of man. Proc. R. Soc. Med. 13, 1-15.

Dobell, C. (1932) Antony van Leeuwenhoek and his 'Little Animals'. Constable and Company Limited, London.

Dobell, C. and O'Connor, F.W. (1921) The Intestinal Protozoa of Man. William Wood & Co., New York.

Erlandsen, S.L. and Bemrick, W.J. (1987) SEM evidence for a new species, *Giardia psittaci*. J. Parasitol. 73, 623–629.

Farthing, M.J.G., Varon, S.R. and Keusch, G.T. (1983) Mammalian bile promotes growth of *Giardia lamblia* in axenic culture. Trans. R. Soc. Trop. Med. Hyg. 77, 467-469.

Filice, F.P. (1952) Studies on the cytology and life history of a *Giardia* from the laboratory rat. Univ. Calif. Publ. Zool. 57, 53-146.

Fortess, E. and Meyer, E.A. (1976) Isolation and axenic cultivation of *Giardia* trophozoites from the guinea pig. J. Parasitol. 62, 689.

Galli-Valerio, B. (1937) La lambliase et son traitement par l'atebrine. Schweiz. Med. Wochenschr. 67, 1181-1182.

Gillin, F.D. and Diamond, L.S. (1981) *Entamoeba histolytica* and *Giardia lamblia*: growth responses to reducing agents. Exp. Parasitol. 51, 382-391.

Grant, D.R. and Woo, P.T.K. (1978) Comparative studies of *Giardia* spp. in small mammals in southern Ontario. II. Host specificity and infectivity of stored cysts. Can. J. Zool. 56, 1360-1366.

Grassi, B. (1879) Interno a speciali corpuscoli (Psorospermi) dell'uomo. Rendiconti R. 1st. Lombardo (Milano), XII, (2) 632.

Grassi, B. (1881) Interno ad alcuni protisti endoparassitici ed appartenenti alle classi dei Flagellati, Lobosi, Sporozoi e Ciliati. Atti Soc. Ital. Sci. Nat., XXIV, 135.

Grassi, B. (1888) Morfologia e sistematica di alcuni protozoi parassiti. Atti R. Accad. Lince 1 Rendiconti, (4 ser.) IV, (I sem.) 5.

Hegner, R.W. (1922) The systemic relationship of *Giardia lamblia* Stiles, 1915, from man and *Giardia agilis* Kunstler, 1982, from the tadpole. Am. J. Hyg. 5, 250-257.

Hegner, R.W. (1926) The biology of host-parasite relationships among protozoa living in man. Q. Rev. Biol. 1, 393-418.

Hewlett, E.L., Andrews, J.S., Ruiffier, J. and Schaefer, F.W. (1982) Experimental infection of mongrel dogs with *Giardia lamblia* cysts and cultured trophozoites. J. Infect. Dis. 145, 89-93.

Iwata, S. and Araki, T. (1960) Studies on giardiasis. Bull. Osaka Med. Sch. 6, 92-106.

Karapetyan, A.E. (1960) Methods of *Lamblia* cultivation. Tsitologiia 2, 379-384.

Karapetyan, A.E. (1962) In vitro cultivation of *Giardia duodenalis*. J. Parasit. 48, 337-340.

Keister, D.B. (1983) Axenic culture of *Giardia lamblia* in TYI-S-33 medium supplemented with bile. Trans. R. Soc. Trop. Med. Hyg. 77, 487-488.

Kofoid, C.A. and Christiansen, E.B. (1915) On *Giardia microti* sp. nov., from the meadow mouse. Univ. Calif. Zool. 16, 23-29.

Kulda, J. and Nohynkova, E. (1978) Flagellates of the human intestine and of intestines of other species. In: J.P. Kreier (Ed.), Protozoa of Veterinary and Medical Interest, Vol. II, pp. 69-104. Academic Press, New York, London.

Kunstler, J. (1882) Sur cinq protozoaires parasites nouveaus. C. R. Seances Soc. Biol. 95, 347-349.

Lambl, W. (1859) Mikroskopische Untersuchungen der Darmexcrete. Vierteljahrsschr. Prakt. Heilk. (Prague) 61, 1-58.

Lucian, O. (1971) Lambliaza, pp. 1-248. Editura Academiei Republicii Socialiste, Bucharest, Romania.

Meyer, E.A. (1970) Isolation and axenic cultivation of *Giardia* trophozoites from the rabbit, chinchilla, and cat. Exp. Parasitol. 27, 179-183.

Meyer, E.A. (1976) *Giardia lamblia*: isolation and axenic cultivation. Exp. Parasitol. 39, 101-105.

Meyer, E.A. and Pope, B.L. (1965) Culture in vitro of *Giardia* trophozoites from the rabbit and chinchilla. Nature (London) 207, 1417-1418.

Meyer, E.A. and Radulescu, S. (1979) *Giardia* and giardiasis. Adv. Parasitol. 17, 1–14.

Nieschulz, O. (1924) Ueber den Bau von *Giardia* caprae mihi. Arch. Protistenk. 49, 278-286.

Rendtorff, R. (1954) The experimental transmission of human intestinal protozoan parasites. II. *Giardia lamblia* cysts given in capsules. Am. J. Hyg. 59, 209-220.

Rendtorff, R.C. (1979) The experimental transmission of *Giardia lamblia* among volunteer subjects. In: W. Jakubowski and J.C. Hoff (Eds), Waterborne Transmission of Giardiasis, U.S. Environmental Protection Agency 600/9-79-001, Cincinnati, 64-81.

Roberts-Thomson, I.C., Stevens, D.P., Mahmoud, A.A.F. and Warren, K.S. (1976) Giardiasis in the mouse: an animal model. Gastroenterology 71, 57-61.

Sargeaunt, P.G. and Williams, J.E. (1979) Electrophoretic isoenzyme patterns of the pathogenic and non-pathogenic intestinal amoebae of man. Trans. R. Soc. Trop. Med. Hyg. 73, 255-227.

Schneider, J. (1961) Traitement de les giardiase (lambliase) par le metronidazole. Bull. Soc. Pathol. Exot. 54, 84-95.

Visvesvara, G. (1980) Axenic growth of *Giardia lamblia* in Diamond's TPS-1 medium. Trans. R. Soc. Trop. Med. Hyg. 74, 213-215.

Webster, B.H. (1960) Furazolidone in the treatment of Giardiasis. Am. J. Digest. Dis. 5, 618-622.

WHO Expert Committee (1981) Intestinal protozoan and helminthic infections. WHO Technical Report Series 666, World Health Organization, Geneva.

Giardiasis (E.A. Meyer, ed.)
© 1990 Elsevier Science Publishers B.V. (Biomedical Division)

1

The biology of *Giardia*

DENNIS E. FEELY[1], DAVID V. HOLBERTON[2] and STANLEY L. ERLANDSEN[3]

[1]*Department of Oral Biology and Basic Science, College of Dentistry, University of Nebraska Medical Center, Lincoln, NE 68583, U.S.A. and* [2]*Department of Zoology, The University of Hull, Hull HU6 7RX, U.K. and* [3]*Department of Cell Biology and Neuroanatomy, University of Minnesota, Minneapolis, MN 55455, U.S.A.*

1. Introduction	11
2. Life cycle and morphology	12
3. Ultrastructure	17
3.1. Trophozoite	17
3.1.1. The ventral disc	17
3.1.1.1. The disc cytoskeleton	17
3.1.1.2. The ventrolateral flange	20
3.2. Cytoskeletal proteins	21
3.2.1. Dorsal ribbons	21
3.2.2. Ribbon proteins	23
3.2.3. Microtubules and tubulin	26
3.3. Flagella	30
3.4. The plasma membrane	32
3.5. The vacuolar system	33
3.6. Cyst	34
4. Microbial symbionts of *Giardia*	38
5. Attachment to substrates	43
References	47

1. Introduction

Giardia duodenalis has been familiar to parasitologists and protozoologists for approximately one hundred years. This curious flagellate was considered to be a commensal of the small intestine, but experience during the past twenty years has firmly established its role as a significant pathogen of man. Interest in the organism has increased not only among scientists and physicians, but among the public as well due to coverage of giardiasis outbreaks by the press. Backpackers and campers in montainous regions are now well aware of the potential of contracting giardiasis (also known as backpacker's diarrhea or beaver fever) by drinking untreated water. Commercial firms are now producing portable filtration devices for the purpose of eliminating *Giardia* cysts from water on camping trips. This once obscure flagellate is recognized as a potential hazard to the general population, children in day care centers, and individuals with acquired immunodeficiency syndrome.

2. Life cycle and morphology

Giardia has a simple, direct life cycle similar to that of the intestinal amoebae. The trophozoite, or intestinal dwelling stage, attaches to the epithelium of the host villi (Fig. 1A) by the ventral disc or attachment organelle. The attachment is intimate and firm and may result in the production of an impression of the ventral surface of the trophozoite on the microvillous border. Attached trophozoites may remain in place or detach from the surface. It is assumed that the trophozoites must detach from the epithelium which is replaced every 72 h and sloughed off the tip of the villus. The trophozoites undergo mitotic division within the intestinal lumen, but a certain number become encysted within a protective wall and pass from the host in the feces (Fig. 1B). The cysts are transmitted to a new host through contaminated water or ingestion of food contaminated with feces. Cysts can remain viable for several months if they remain wet and cool but cannot withstand desiccation. After gaining entrance into a new host, the organism emerges from the cyst (Fig. 1C) in the duodenum. The newly excysted organism then completes an arrested mitotic division (Fig. 1D) resulting in mature trophozoites which through continued proliferation establish the new infection.

The morphology of *Giardia* at the light microscopic level has been studied traditionally by use of the iron-hematoxylin stain. This stain renders to the trophozoite the face-like appearance familiar to students of protozoology and parasitology (Fig. 2A). Several excellent reviews have been published on the morphology of the trophozoite and cyst based on this stain (Simon, 1921; Filice, 1952; Ansari, 1952). The trophozoite, so prepared, measures approximately 12-15 μm in length and 5-9 μm wide and resembles a pear cut in half lengthwise with the flattened side representing the ventral surface. The pair of nuclei are found in the anterior half of the organism. The axonemes of the four symmetrically placed flagella originate from basal bodies at the anterior pole of the nuclei and the axonemes of the three posterior directed flagella run between the nuclei (Fig. 2A). A prominent, dark staining structure, the median body, is found in the posterior half of the organism. This structure is described as 'claw-hammer' in shape in *Giardia duodenalis* and is of use in taxonomy. This structure has been incorrectly called a parabasal body but is in fact a bundle of microtubules and bears no resemblance to

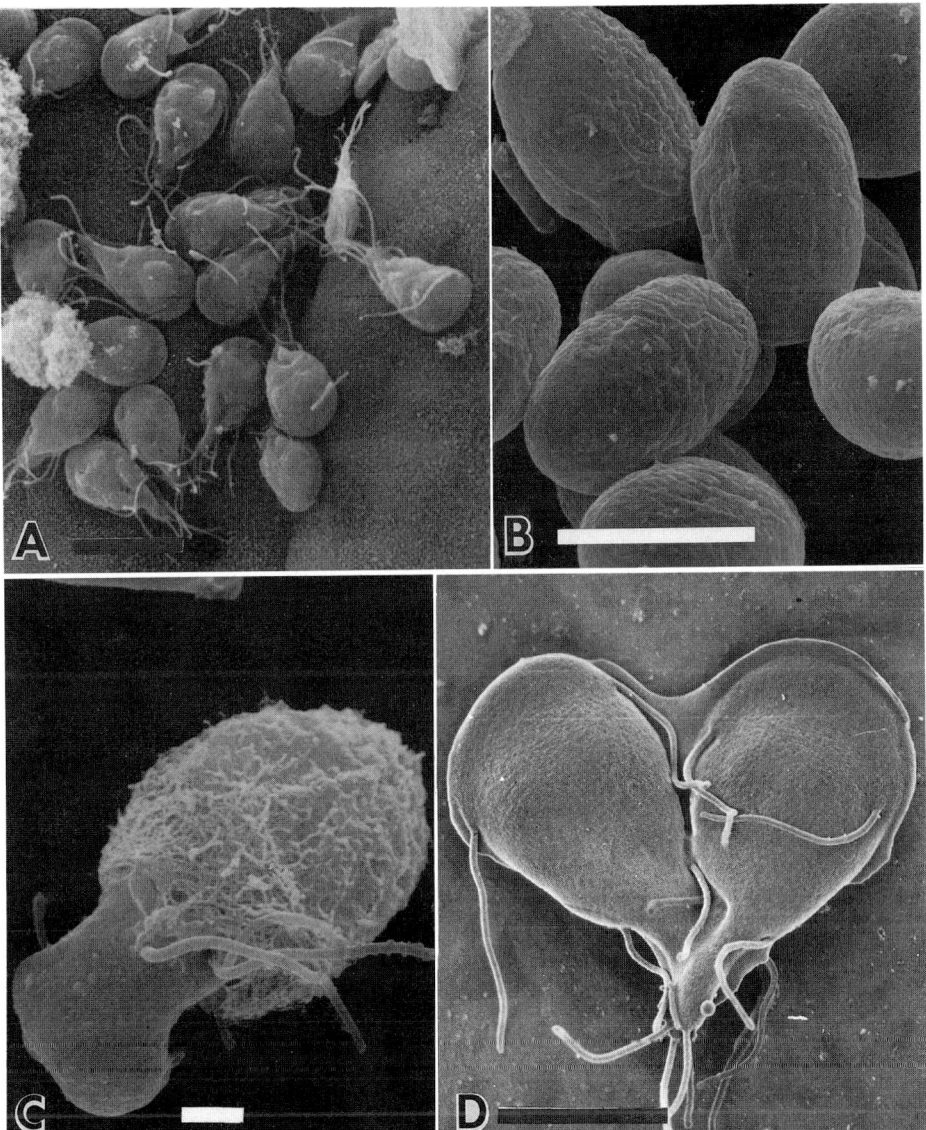

Fig. 1. Panels A-D show the stages of the life cycle by SEM. (A) The trophozoites of human source *Giardia* are seen here attached experimentally to a mouse villus. Note that a number of organisms are attached by their ventral surface. The tips of the intestinal microvilli are also evident. Bar = 10 μm. (B) The cysts of *G. muris* shown here, are similar to those of *G. duodenalis*. The organism is secure within the cyst wall. Little detail is evident on the cyst wall. Bar = 5 μm. (C) Within the duodenum of the host, the organism excysts from one end of the cyst. This excysting *G. muris* emerges from one end and is accompanied by two flagella. Note the coarse fibrous appearance of the surface of the cyst wall. Bar = 1 μm. (D) After emergence from the cyst, the organism completes binary fission and forms two daughter trophozoites. (High resolution low voltage SEM.) Bar = 5 μm.

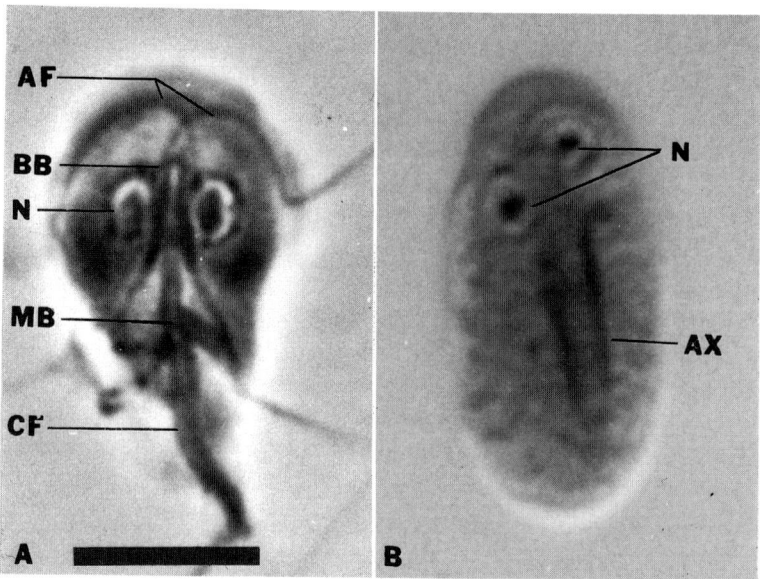

Fig. 2. (A) This light micrograph of an iron-hematoxylin stained trophozoite shows the features commonly described in textbooks of parasitology. The anterior flagella (AF) are seen originating from the basal bodies (BB) which lie between the anterior poles of the nuclei (N). The median body (MB) is clearly seen as are the axonemes of the caudal flagella (CF). Bar = 5 μm. (B) Fewer structures are visible in the cyst. Nuclei (N), either two or four, and axonemes of flagella (AX) are easily detected. Often, crescent-shaped fragments of the ventral disc are also seen.

a Janicki-type parabasal body (Filice, 1952). Four pair of flagella originate from basal granules at the anterior pole of the nuclei.

The cyst bears only slight resemblance to the trophozoite in iron-hematoxylin stained preparations (Fig. 2B). Cysts are somewhat resistant to the environment and may remain viable for days to months if kept wet and cold. They are elliptical in shape and are approximately 6-10 μm long. A few internal structures may be recognized. There may be two or four nuclei in the cyst depending on whether cell division has commenced. Axonemes of the flagella are often seen and crescent-shaped fragments of the ventral disc, heavily stained by iron-hematoxylin, are common but have often been labeled parabasal bodies in older literature. The cyst wall is easily detected by light microscopy but little of its structure can be seen.

Scanning electron microscopy (SEM) of *Giardia* has demonstrated greater detail of the surface structures of this organism (Fig. 3A, B) not detectable by light microscopy. The dorsal surface of the trophozoite has few named structures. It may be slightly roughened in appearance and bear slight depressions or pits related to underlying cytoplasmic vacuoles. Three of the four pairs of flagella can be seen emerging at anterior, posterior, and caudal positions (Fig. 3A). The fourth pair, the ventral flagella, emerge from the crevice between the posterior portion of the ventral disc and the body of the trophozoite (Fig. 3B). The ventrolateral flange (Fig. 3A, B) separates the dorsal surface from the

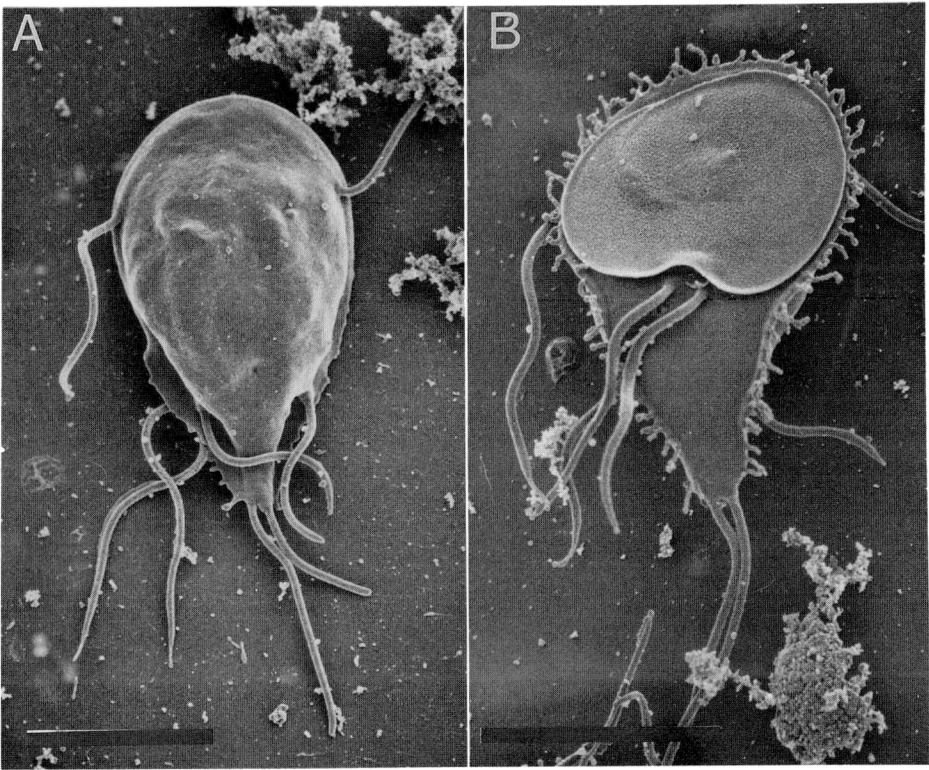

Fig. 3. (A) This dorsal view of a trophozoite shows the specialized membrane surfaces and the relative positions of the three pair of flagella: anterior flagella, posterior flagella and the caudal flagella. Bar = 1 μm. (B) The ventral surface of a trophozoite is shown to advantage in this SEM. The ventral disc is readily seen with its limiting lateral crest. The ventral flagella are seen emerging from the ventral groove. Numerous microvilli-like appendages are found along the lateral margin of the trophozoite. Bar = 1 μm.

ventral surface. The flange often is marked by the presence of short microvilli (Fig. 3B). The ventral disc is the most prominent structure of the ventral surface and is found on the anterior half of the trophozoite. The prominent lateral crest marks the periphery of the disc and produces the characteristic overlapping spiral visible on the surface of the disc (Fig. 3B). The surface of the disc is smooth but depressions, presumably from endocytotic vesicles, may be found in the center of the disc.

16

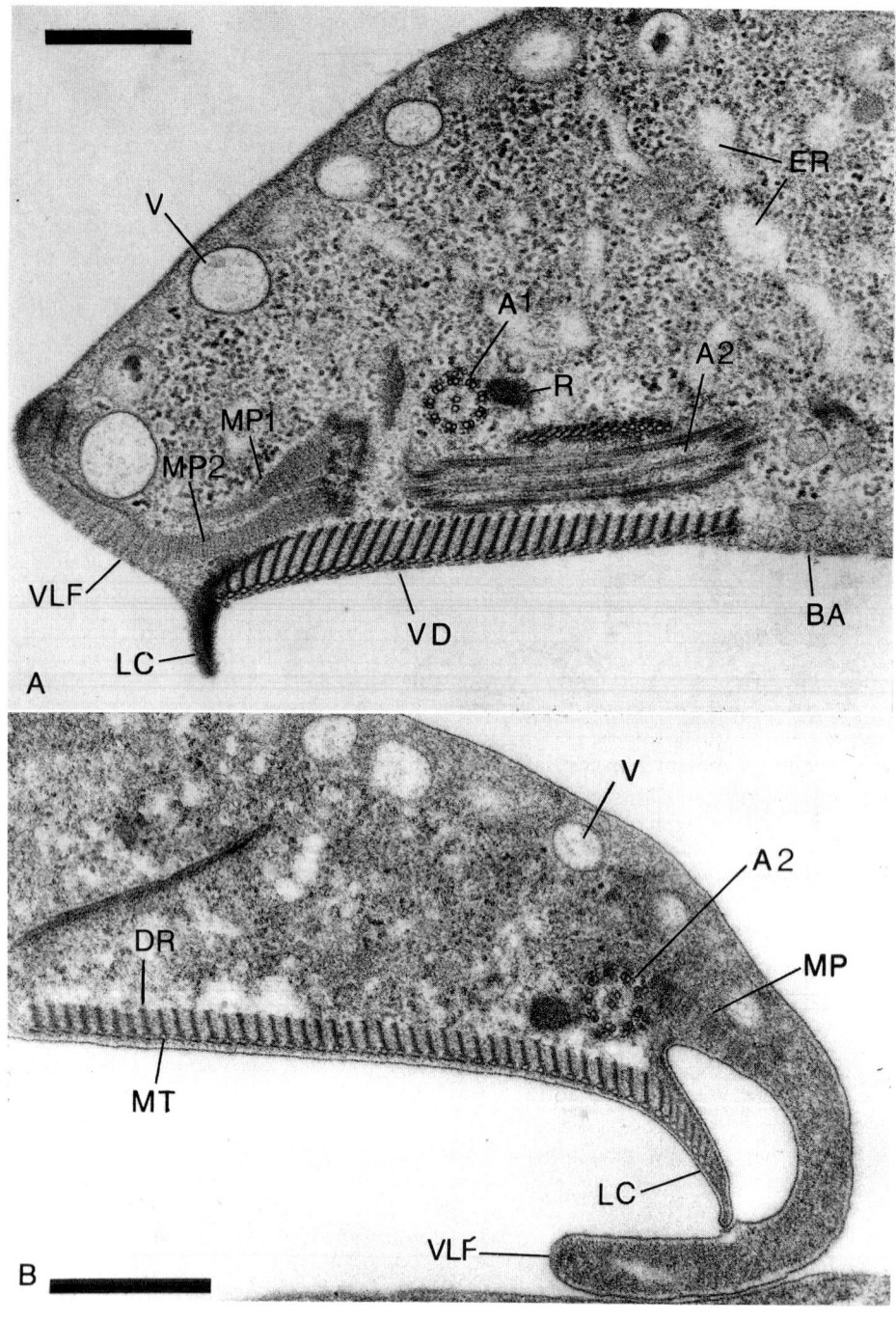

3. Ultrastructure

3.1. Trophozoite

3.1.1. The ventral disc

The disc cytoskeleton. The visible attachment disc of *Giardia* distinguishes this organism from other flagellates. From the earliest electron microscope studies, it was apparent that the cytological counterpart of the surface organelle is a massive structural pontoon, variously called the ridged pellicle (Cheissin, 1964; 1965), striated disc (Friend, 1966) or disc cytoskeleton (Holberton and Ward, 1981). The cytoskeleton is a complicated assembly of filamentous elements and microtubules associated with the cluster of basal bodies that give rise to the eight flagella. Although unique to *Giardia*, it is probable that this elaborate structure has evolved from flagellar rootlet structures seen in other diplozoans (Brugerolle, 1975b) to provide for the unusual mode of attachment of the parasite. The disc apparatus can therefore be viewed as a modified mastigont.

Physically, the disc is a rigid structure with a large number of internal crossbridges between its components and direct attachments to the flagella. For these reasons it is a simple procedure to collect discs and flagellar axonemes into a pellet, after detergent demembranation of trophozoites and dispersal of the cytosol (Holberton and Ward, 1981). In recent years progress has been made in the biochemical characterization of disc-associated proteins, starting with this preparation (Crossley and Holberton, 1983a). These proteins are present in excess in the overall composition of *Giardia*. Recent studies of the serological response of giardiasis patients suggest that cytoskeleton antigens may be strongly immunogenic during infection (Taylor and Wenman, 1987).

The basic structure of the disc in the transmission electron microscope (TEM) has been described in detail by several authors (Friend, 1966; Holberton, 1973; Brugerolle, 1975a), and reviewed recently (Feely et al., 1984). In vertical sections the disc appears as a platform or raft of evenly spaced microtubules, 50-60 nm apart (Fig. 4). The platform is pierced by a wide central hole covered only by the ventral plasma membrane. This unsupported central part of the ventral disc surface has been called the 'bare zone' (Cheissin, 1964; Feely et al., 1984). Vesicles are frequently seen in the adjacent cytoplasm

Fig. 4. (A) TEM cross-sections of *Giardia* trophozoites. The anterior region of *Giardia muris* sectioned at the point of cross-over of the anterior axonemes (A1, A2), above the ventral disc (VD). Note the dense rod (R) accompanying the right axoneme. In the ventrolateral flange (VLF), the striated marginal plates (MP1, MP2) from each side also overlap in this region. The lateral crest (LC) in *G. muris* is electron dense. Some of the cortical vacuoles (V) in the dorsal ectoplasm contain dense aggregates. Small vesicles are present also in the bare area (BA) at the disc center. Endoplasmic reticulum (ER) appears as transparent clefts. Bar equals 500 nm. (B) The lateral region of the ventral disc in cultured *Giardia* sp. Labelling as above. Crossbridges can be seen between the dorsal ribbons (DR) projecting from disc microtubules (MT). The microtubules and ribbons continue into the lateral crest which is more translucent than in *G. muris*. The flexible ventrolateral flange has a thin marginal plate which is most visible where it abuts the anterior axoneme. Bar equals 500 nm.

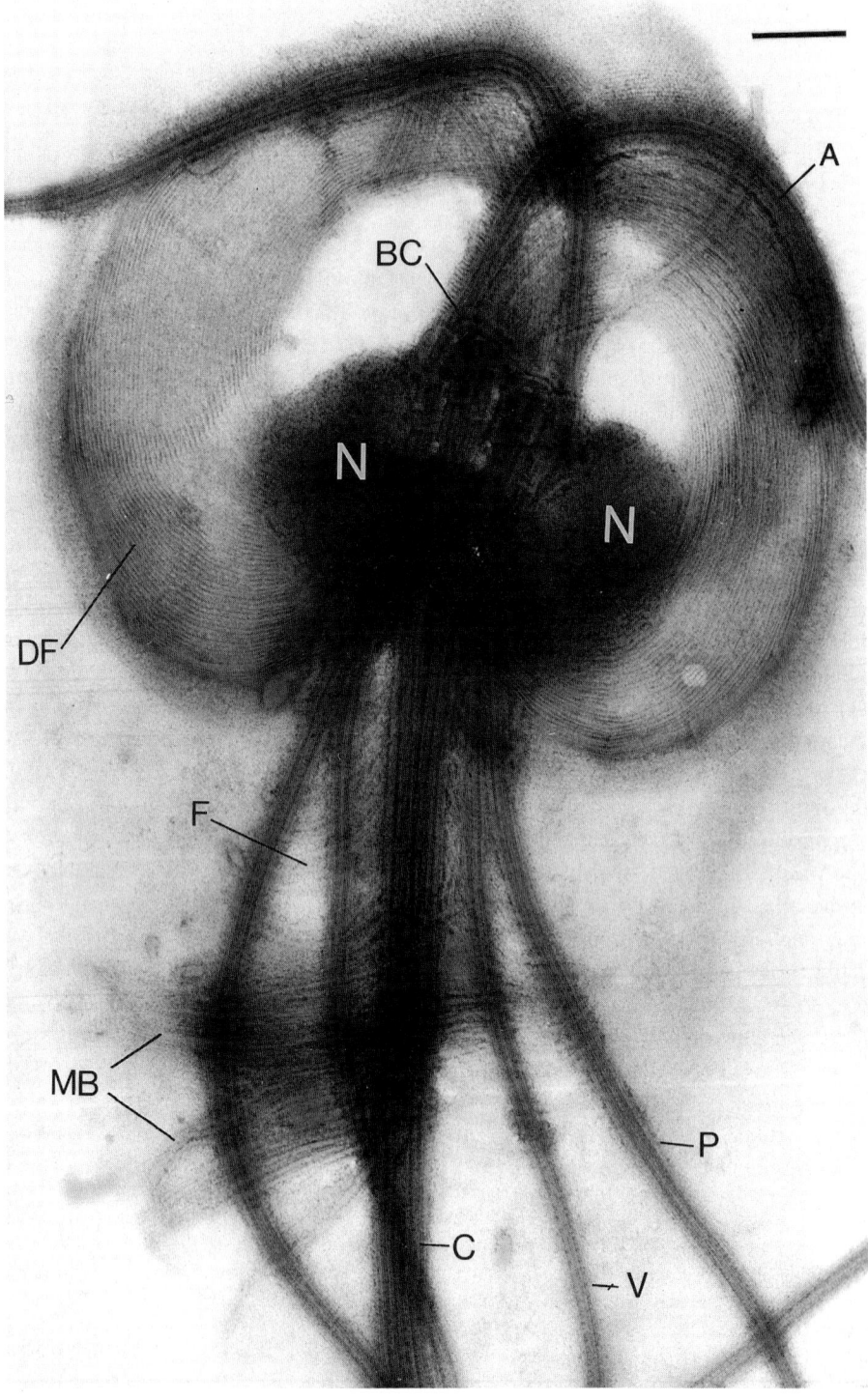

at this point (Fig. 4A). Microtubules at the outer edge of the disc are embedded in the lateral crest, a large electron-dense fiber with a tooth-like profile in cross-section, to which the ventral membrane is tightly applied. The crest forms the projecting rim of the disc which in *Giardia* from the mouse projects strongly downwards and leaves characteristic deep imprints on the surface of the parasitized gut mucosa (Erlandsen and Chase, 1974; Owen et al., 1979). In *Giardia* from humans the rim is less pronounced and appears to be more easily flattened on contact with a cellular substrate, leaving an incomplete impression (Chavez et al., 1986).

The disc microtubules carry ventrally a series of paired arms with a hooked appearance (Fig. 6) that locate into the adjacent face of the plasma membrane (Holberton, 1973). The function of these arms is unknown, but they have a cytochemical reaction for ATPase under conditions which localize dynein ATPase in axonemes in the same sections (J. Marshall, unpublished results). They may have a role in the active propulsion of membrane domains or membrane-associated material. Projecting dorsally from each microtubule is an upright dorsal ribbon. These ribbons are very large and run the full length of microtubules (Fig. 7A). Together, the two structures are often referred to as a 'disc fiber'. Numerous horizontal crossbridges hold adjacent ribbons in a strictly parallel stack, which leads to the striated appearance of the disc at low magnifications. The molecular composition of ribbons is discussed below.

The disc is about 0.4 μm deep at its thickest point. Its unusual geometry is most striking in plain view. The correct shape was deduced originally by Brugerolle (1975a) from serial thin sections through the mouse *Giardia*. It is more completely visible in thick (0.5 μm) sections of *Giardia duodenalis* from the rat, photographed by high voltage electron microscopy (Feely et al., 1984), or in negatively-stained whole mounts (Fig. 5) of cytoskeletons isolated from cultured *Giardia* (Crossley et al., 1986).

In *Giardia* sp., the disc is a flat right-handed helicoid of one and a quarter to one and three-quarter turns, with tapering ends overlapping on the anterior right side (from above). In projection it appears as an annulus indented at the most posterior margin. Individual disc fibers describe a spiral path within this plane. There are approximately 100 concentric fibers in the disc. Of these, only about 40-50 originate together from the 'proximal' end, the end fused to the set of flagellar roots in the left half of the organism (Fig. 5). At this junction a banded or septate collar holds the microtubules together. About two-thirds of the area of a fully-developed disc is therefore composed of fibers that have no direct rootlet connection with the basal bodies (Holberton and Ward, 1981). These fibers start at the inner edge of the disc bordering the central bare zone, and reach the outer edge after about one turn. They are joined to the flagella-associated fibers mainly

---

Fig. 5. Complete cytoskeleton from *Giardia* sp. (Portland-1 strain), isolated from a trophozoite attached to a poly-L-lysine film by washing with 0.5% Triton X-100. Note that, as seen from above, the disc cytoskeleton is a clockwise spiral of disc fibers (DF), anchored proximally to the left group of basal bodies at a banded density or collar (BC). Microtubules of the funis (F) splay out to left and right behind the disc. The median body (MB) is two bundles of microtubules oriented across the axonemes of the caudal (C) and posterior-lateral (P) flagella. A, anterior axoneme; V, ventral axoneme; N, nucleus. Bar equals 1 μm.

by the lateral connections between ribbons and their common insertion into the dense crest at the disc rim. This fact may have important implications for the way a disc is assembled when a trophozoite divides.

The ventrolateral flange. The ventrolateral flange (VLF) around the disc is supported internally by two plates. These marginal plates (Holberton, 1973) are prominent in *Giardia* of the *muris* type, less pronounced in *Giardia* of the *duodenalis* type (Fig. 4). Anteriorly they follow the cytoplasmic axonemes of the anterior flagella and therefore overlap close to the midline where the axonemes cross over. They extend caudally beyond the disc to the margins of the ventral groove where they form the lateral shields. The plates are Triton-soluble and lost from cytoskeleton preparations; therefore their biochemical composition is unknown. They have a filamentous substructure of paracrystalline regularity which appears as a complex hexagonal net in horizontal section, and various striated patterns in different vertical orientations. A dense lamella emerging

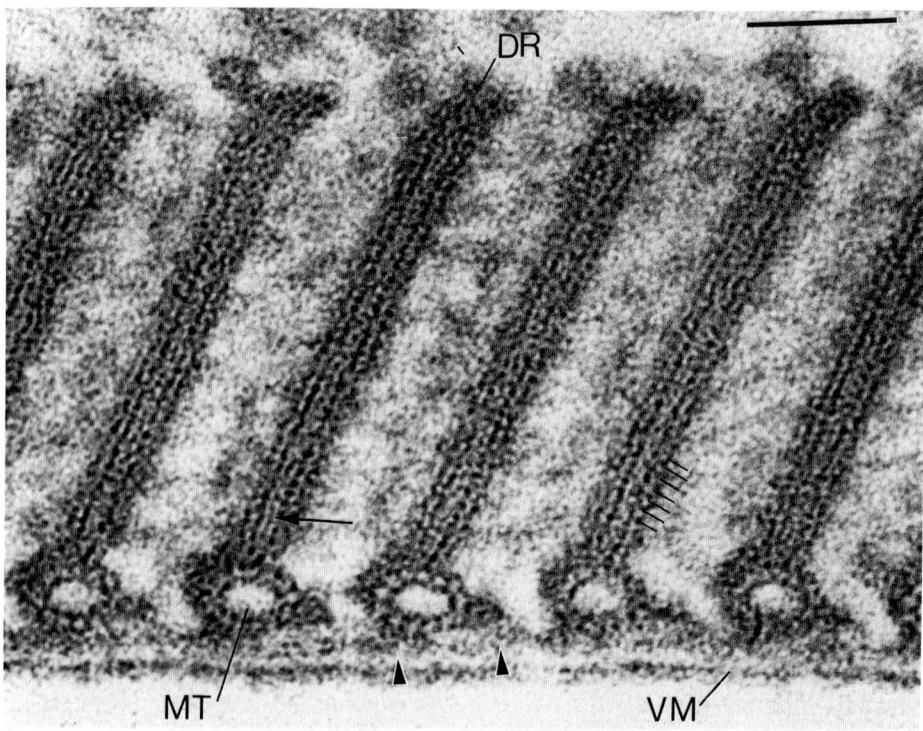

Fig. 6. Vertical section of disc fibers in mouse *Giardia* at high magnification. Fixed in the presence of 8% tannic acid to outline protein subunits. The microtubules (MT) have the normal 13 protofilaments and are linked to the ventral membrane (VM) by paired arms (arrowheads). The large dorsal ribbon (DR) on each microtubule is composed of 4 parallel layers. Features in the outer layers appear as globular subunits (dashed lines). The 2 filamentous sheets making up the core are slightly narrower (arrow). At the bottom, the core layers wrap partly over the surface of the microtubule. Bar equals 50 nm.

from the membrane at the edge of the VLF extends partly over the upper surface of the plates.

The function of these plates is unclear. A contractile role in governing the mobility of the flange lip seems probable from the various upward and downward flexed postures seen in electron microscope profiles of the VLF (Fig. 4). The flange is usually lifted up in front of the ventral disc in trophozoites attached to mouse gut (Holberton, 1973). Motility in the flange was confirmed directly by Erlandsen and Feely (1984). They used interference reflexion microscopy to observe ripples of focal contacts forming a moving seal between the lateral edge of the flange and the substrate. However, the biochemical basis of this contractile system remains uncertain. After some proteins comigrating with myofibrillar proteins were extracted from *Giardia*, immunological probes for actin, α-actinin, tropomyosin and myosin were used in immunofluorescence tests to localize these proteins in trophozoites from rats (Feely et al., 1982). Although fluorescent antibody binding was clear at the rim of the disc in the position of the lateral crest, the flange outside this bright ring was generally unstained.

3.2. Cytoskeleton proteins

3.2.1. Dorsal ribbons
The disc ribbons have been the subject of detailed structural and biochemical studies. Their large size implies that a significant component of protein synthesis in dividing *Giardia* will be to provide ribbon proteins. *In vitro* translation of unfractionated mRNA sequences extracted from trophozoites has confirmed that ribbon proteins are prominent amongst the products (D.A. Baker, unpublished results).

The internal structure of a sectioned ribbon is seen after binding tannic acid to protein subunits (Fig. 6). The ribbon is a sandwich of four sheets. The outer layers contain large, apparently globular, subunits. The two inner layers appear thinner and more filamentous. At the bottom edge of the ribbon they wrap partly over the surface of microtubule, covering 5 or 6 protofilaments on the side facing the perimeter of the disc. The two face layers appear to stop short of the microtubule. Components of the core layers can accordingly be considered the structural scaffold of the ribbon: on the one hand rooted to tubulin subunits in the microtubule, and on the other hand providing surfaces for the adhesion of additional ribbon layers and crossbridges.

Working with isolated discs, Holberton (1981) obtained detailed images of ribbon faces by disrupting crossbridges and other links with ultrasound to allow ribbons to flatten on carbon support films. The original pictures were of *Giardia* from the mouse, and a later series (Crossley and Holberton, 1985) from cultured *Giardia* sp. (Fig. 7A). Ribbons are markedly periodic structures with a dominant orthogonal stripping at distances of approximately 15 nm along the axis. Optical diffraction patterns from these images show that higher orders of this interval are also accentuated because of the precise alignment of submolecular features in ribbon layers, which are essentially paracrystalline. Strongly diffracting lattices of features with the dimensions of tubulin subunits were revealed.

22

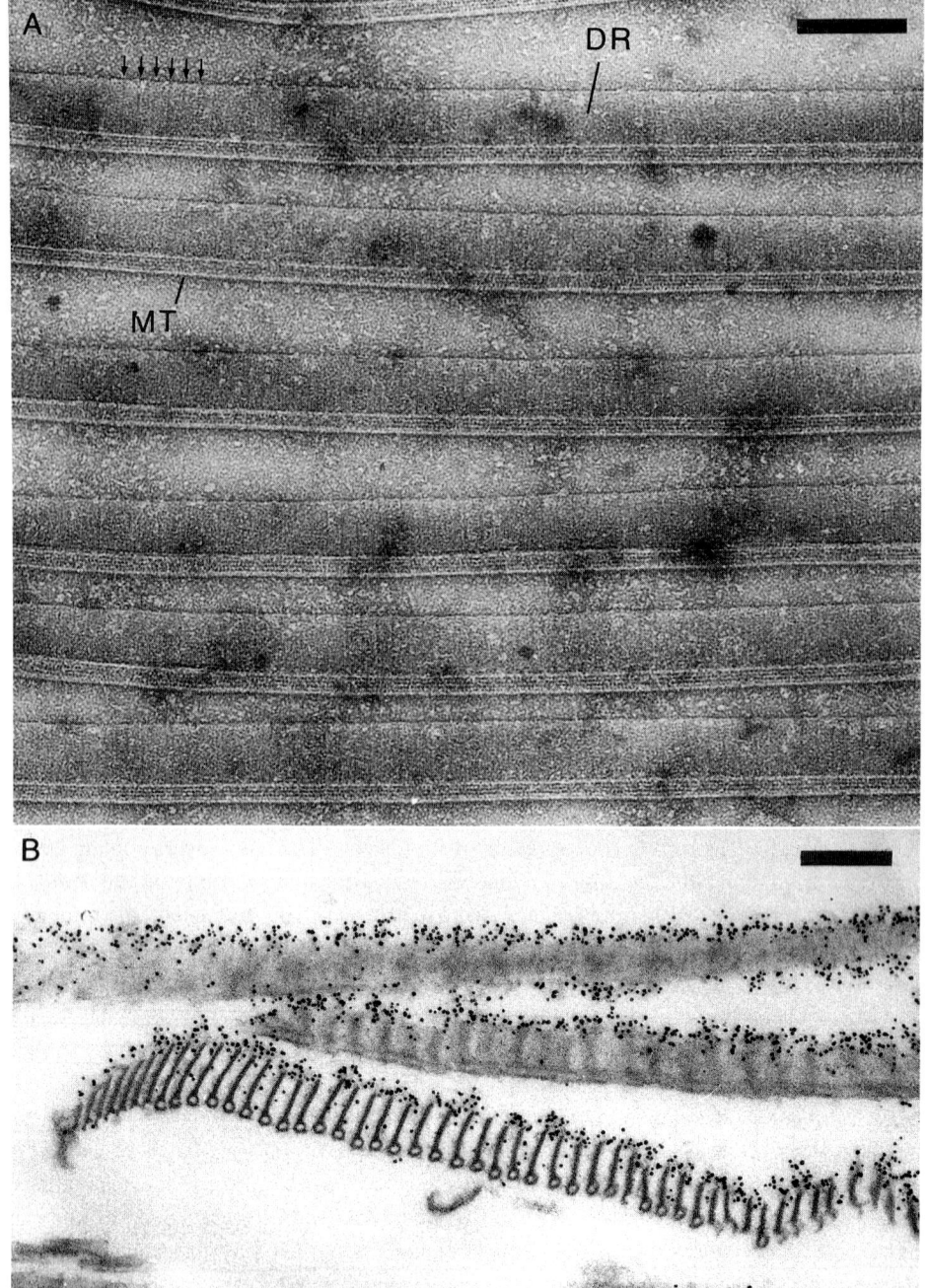

This finding led to the suggestion that the prominently demarcated subunits in ribbon face layers are tubulin protofilaments (Holberton, 1981). There had not yet been a direct test, for example, by antitubulin immunolabelling (Crossley et al., 1986), to confirm this aspect of the ribbon structural model.

3.2.2. Ribbon proteins

Ribbon proteins were identified initially by sodium dodecyl sulfate polyacrylamide gel electrophoresis (SDS-PAGE) of isolated cytoskeletons, and subsequently by their extraction and reconstitution *in vitro* (Crossley and Holberton, 1985). A prominent double band in the electrophoretic separation of cytoskeleton proteins was first noted by Holberton and Ward (1981), and called giardin by Crossley and Holberton (1983a). The giardin bands migrate with relative molecular weights close to 30 000 (30 kDa). On gels, they were accompanied by two fainter bands which might be related chains. Because the giardin chains account for about 20% of cytoskeleton proteins it was thought that they were likely to be major ribbon proteins. Later, a rabbit polyclonal antiserum to giardin bands was found to label discs strongly by immunofluorescence. At the ultrastructural level (Fig. 7B), the antibodies were visualized sticking to the tops of the ribbons where the inner layers were exposed (Crossley et al., 1986).

Denatured giardin chains were purified by column chromatography of disc proteins solubilized in SDS. The purified material contained eight isoforms separable by isoelectric focusing (IEF), all with a net acidic charge. More recently, at least 10 giardin-sized chains have been resolved by two-dimensional gel analysis of cytoskeleton proteins, and a further 4 are associated with purified flagella (see below). Crossley and Holberton (1983a) determined the gross amino acid composition of the giardin column fraction. A high content of helix-forming residues suggested that giardins are extended rod proteins of the α-coiled-coil type.

In keeping with their role in the cell, giardins are relatively insoluble. To extract them from discs without losing their native properties, solubilizing buffers have been developed based on the detergent Sarkosyl (Crossley and Holberton 1983b), or low ionic strength HEPES-EDTA at high pH (Crossley and Holberton, 1985). The dissociation of giardins is reversible. On dialysis back to physiological buffers, soluble giardins in high speed supernatants reassembled into ribbon-like structures and crystalline tactoids (Fig. 8). It was possible to repeat the assembly cycle in order to purify giardins. After two cycles, the two major and one of the minor giardin chains, together with some low molecular weight proteins, remained in the preparation. All of the structures formed from purified giardins came about by lateral aggregation of thin filaments about 2.5 nm wide. Disc

---

Fig. 7. (A) Negatively-stained disc fibers from *Giardia* sp., flattened onto a carbon film by extracting crossbridges with Tris-EDTA buffer at pH 7.7. Protofilaments in the microtubules (MT) are clearly contrasted. Dorsal ribbons (DR) are cross-striated at intervals of about 15 nm (arrowheads). Bar equals 100 nm. (B) Electron immunocytochemical localization of giardins in the dorsal ribbons of isolated washed disc cytoskeletons. Three discs appear in this section. Binding of rabbit antigiardins along the tops of ribbons was visualized with gold-labelled goat anti-rabbit IgG. Bar equals 200 nm.

24

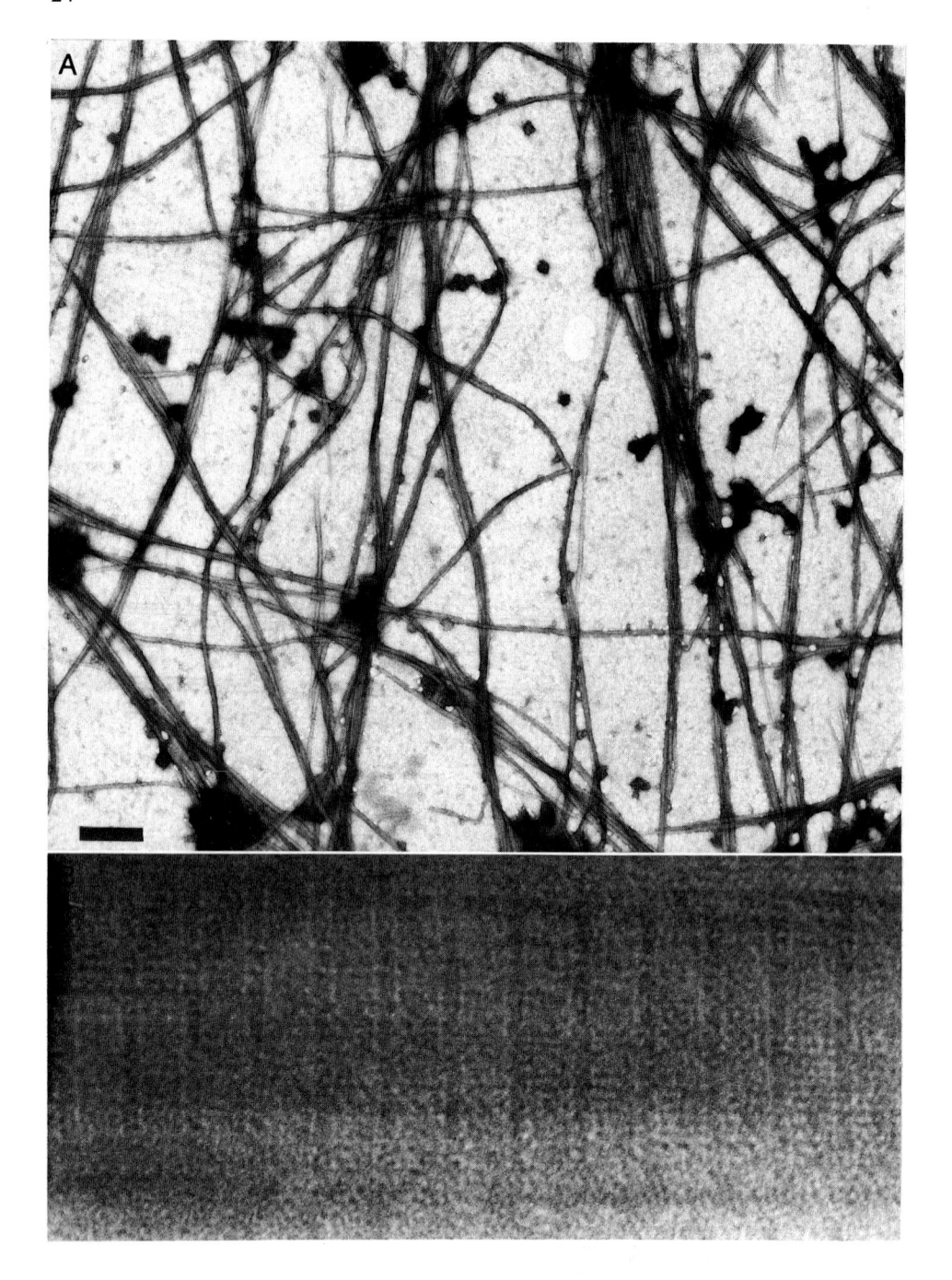

TABLE 1

MET-Asp-Lys-Pro-Asp-Asp-Leu-Thr-Arg-Ser-Ala-Thr-Glu-Thr-Ala-
Val-Lys-Leu-Ser-Asn-Met-Asn-Gln-Arg-Val-Ser-Arg-Phe-His-Asp-
Lys-Met-Glu-Asn-Glu-Ile-Glu-Val-Arg-Arg-Val-Asp-Asp-Asp-Thr-
Arg-Val-Lys-Met-Ile-Lys-Asp-Ala-Ile-Ala-His-Leu-Asp-Arg-Leu-
Ile-Gln-Thr-Glu-Ser-Arg-Lys-Arg-Gln-Ala-Ser-Phe-Glu-Asp-Ile-
Arg-Glu-Glu-Val-Lys-Lys-Ser-Ala-Asp-Asn-Met-Tyr-Leu-Thr-Ile-
Lys-Glu-Glu-Ile-Asp-Thr-Met-Ala-Ala-Asn-Phe-Arg-Lys-Ser-Leu-
Ala-Glu-Met-Gly-Asp-Thr-Leu-Asn-Asn-Val-Glu-Thr-Asn-Leu-Gln-
Asn-Gln-Ile-Ala-Ile-His-Asn-Asp-Ala-Ile-Ala-Ala-Leu-Arg-Lys-
Glu-Ala-Leu-Lys-Ser-Leu-Asn-Asp-Leu-Glu-Thr-Gly-Ile-Ala-Thr-
Glu-Asn-Ala-Glu-Arg-Lys-Lys-Met-Tyr-Asp-Gln-Leu-Asn-Glu-Lys-
Val-Ala-Glu-Gly-Phe-Ala-Arg-Ile-Ser-Ala-Ala-Ile-Glu-Lys-Glu-
Thr-Ile-Ala-Arg-Glu-Arg-Ala-Val-Ser-Ala-Ala-Thr-Thr-Glu-Ala-
Leu-Thr-Asn-Thr-Lys-Leu-Val-Glu-Lys-Cys-Val-Asn-Glu-Gln-Leu-
Glu-Asn-Val-Ala-Ser-Glu-Ile-Arg-Ala-Ile-Gln-Glu-Glu-Ile-Asp-
Arg-Glu-Lys-Ala-Glu-Arg-Lys-Glu-Ala-Glu-Asp-Lys-Ile-Val-Asn-
Thr-Leu-Glu-Asp-Val-Val-Ser-Lys-Ile-Gln-Gly-Gly-Leu-Ser-Met-
Val-Thr-Lys-His

The amino acid sequence of a giardin polypeptide corresponding to the band 14b protein of Crossley and Holberton (1983a). The sequence was determined by D.A. Baker from a cDNA copy of a Giardia mRNA, cloned in λgt11, and selected with specific antigiardins. Only one reading frame of the nucleic acid sequence is open translating to a polypeptide of 259 residues. There is a single proline residue in the aminoterminal tetrapeptide. The sequence as a whole is predicted to form an α-helical rod by the algorithm of Garnier et al. (1978).

ribbons break down to filaments of the same size in the initial stages of extraction. Like native ribbons, the purified giardin paracrystals were strongly cross-banded, confirming that the source of the ribbon periodicity is to be found in an intrinsic alignment of giardin molecules. The dimensions of giardin molecules have been estimated from the behavior of soluble protein on gel filtration columns. Giardins elute in an early position appropriate to an asymmetrical elongated molecule. For a rod containing two parallel chains with a total molecular mass of about 60 000 daltons, hydrodynamic analysis of the elution peak suggests that the molecule is about 2.5 nm wide and somewhat longer than 30 nm (Crossley and Holberton, 1985). To generate the ribbon periodicity, molecules in adjacent filaments would therefore need to be half-staggered. This packing also brings into alignment some regular domains within the giardin molecule which show as light and dark bands in the stained paracrystals (Fig. 8B).

The amino acid sequence of a single giardin chain has now been determined from cloned cDNA copies of a giardin mRNA (Table 1). There are 259 residues in the

Fig. 8. Reassembly of purified giardins into ribbon structures in 150 mM KCl. (A) Long 30-60 nm wide ribbons forming after 2 cycles of dissociation and assembly. SDS-gel electrophoresis showed these ribbons were composed of 3 different giardin polypeptides. (B) The banding pattern on a giardin paracrystal, enhanced by superposition printing. The interval between the dense bands is about 15 nm. Note that the pattern is generated by lateral alignment of filaments running horizontally. The filaments are 2.5 nm wide, which is the dimension of a proposed 2-chain giardin molecule.

polypeptide which gives a chain molecular weight of 29 874 daltons. The sequence has features that help to explain the structural properties of giardins discussed above. For example, there is a pseudo-heptad repeat of hydrophobic residues characteristic of α-helical chains that associate in a two strand coiled-coil structure. Charged residues are concentrated in zones at the ends of the chain which may lead to the rods sticking together in an end-to-end fashion to form filaments. In addition, clusters of hydrophobic residues occur on the surface of the coil at regular intervals of 38-40 residues (approximately 5 nm) along the molecule.

3.2.3. Microtubules and tubulin

The utilization of tubulin in *Giardia* has not yet been studied in detail. Preliminary results from single-dimension IEF have detected a minimum of 5 tubulin isoforms (Crossley and Holberton, 1983a). Two-dimensional gels of cytoskeletal and flagellar proteins indicate that there may be segregation of α-tubulin isoforms in different microtubules (Fig. 9), as occurs in some other flagellates (McKeithan and Rosenbaum, 1981; Russell et al., 1984).

Morphologically, four organelle systems composed of microtubules are present in *Giardia* trophozoites, and these might be differentiated also at a chemical level. The four sets are found in the disc, the axonemes and basal bodies, the median body, and the funis. The term 'funis' was introduced by Kulda and Nohynkova (1978) to describe two longitudinal sheets of extra microtubules, previously called 'paraxonemal fibrils' (Cheissin, 1965), that partly enclose the caudal axonemes. They are seen clearly in

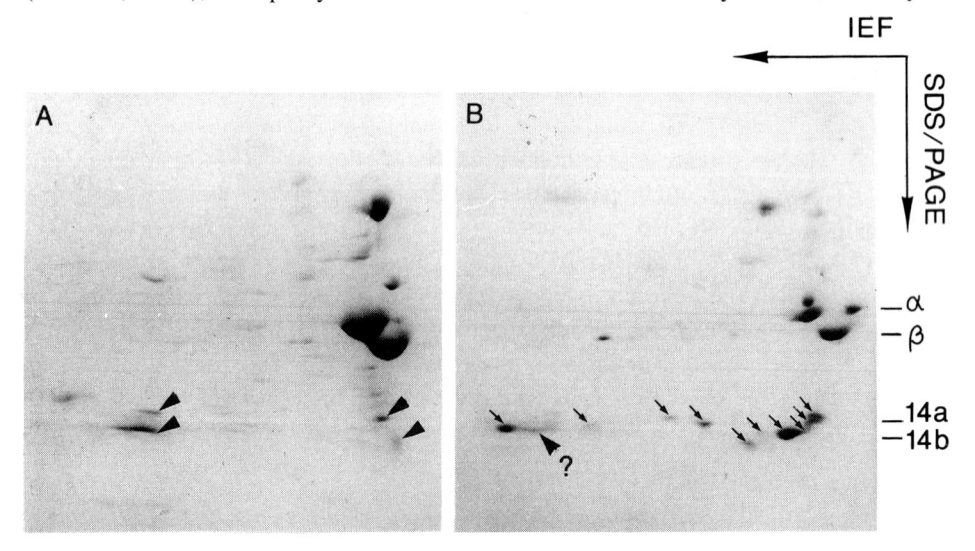

Fig. 9. Two-dimensional gel electrophoresis of proteins from (A) purified flagella, (B) cytoskeletons. Isoelectric focusing was carried out on broad range (pH 3.5-10) gels. Focused proteins were electrophoresed from gel strips into vertical 5-20% acrylamide gradient gels. The positions of tubulin subunits (α,β) and the major giardin chains (band 14a and 14b polypeptides) are indicated. Note the difference in α-tubulin subunit patterns for the two organelles, and in the positions of giardin isoforms (arrows) and flagellar 30 kDa chains (arrowheads). Ten giardin-sized components can be resolved in the cytoskeleton sample. (From Clark, 1985).

transverse sections of *Giardia* in the region between the nuclei (see Fig. 12A). The microtubules arise from dense fibers close to the basal bodies, the 'supranuclear fibers' (Brugerolle, 1975a), and pass into the tail of the organism. At the level of the nucleus the microtubules are connected by short dense bridges. As they emerge beyond the disc, those lying mainly above the right axoneme cross over the midline and fan out on the left side of the ventral groove. The ventral group of microtubules run initially beneath the left caudal axoneme, but on the tail fan out towards the right. The rib-like appearance of funis microtubules behind the disc is seen clearly in whole mounts of trophozoites extracted in Triton after adhering to poly-*l*-lysin films (Fig. 5). In most of these preparations the median body remains attached to funis tubules on the left side. Early electron microscope studies of mouse *Giardia* revealed that the median body is a bundle of microtubules in a zone of moderately dense, inclusion-free cytoplasm (Friend, 1966). Funis tubules pass through the ventral edge of this region. In whole mounts of cultures of *Giardia* sp., the median body usually appears double. The microtubules are crudely aligned like two sheaves of straw.

Monoclonal antibodies to specific epitopes on α-tubulin subunits (Kilmartin et al., 1982) have been used to probe for chemical differentiation of *Giardia* microtubules in unfixed isolated cytoskeletons (Crossley et al., 1986). The monoclonal antibody YL 1/2 binds to the carboxyterminal of α-tubulin only when it is tyrosylated (Wehland et al., 1984). This antibody immunostained basal bodies, axonemal tubules in patches, and the funis. Disc microtubules were unstained except for a ring of fluorescence near the rim. At this point, the end of each tubule is inserted into the lateral crest, and subunits at this site might be chemically modified. A second antibody, YOL 1/34, stained disc microtubules uniformly, but not the funis or axonemal structures. The median body was brightly reactive to both antibodies.

The median body is also immunostained by antigiardins (Crossley et al., 1986), and antiactin and anti α-actinin (Feely et al., 1982). The presence of these cytoskeleton proteins points to an involvement of the median body in forming a second disc during the division cycle. The median body may be a store of materials, or even provide a nucleating template for new disc fibers. The latter possibility is suggested by electron micrographs showing ribbon structures forming on the sides of median body microtubules (Brugerolle, 1975a; Crossley et al., 1986).

The fact that disc fibers and funis microtubules stem from structures linked to axonemes is noteworthy. Attention is drawn to this region as a possible organizing center for microtubule expression in the course of cytoskeleton morphogenesis. In situ, the disc fibers issue from the banded collar attached to the left-hand group of basal bodies. In many interphase cells the smaller collar on the right is also found to sprout a rudimentary sheet of aligned disc fibers, which appears to be the first stage in assembly of a second disc (Fig. 10).

There is some direct evidence that the banded collars have an intrinsic organizing capability. Holberton et al. (1981) found that isolated collars in sonicated disc material dramatically nucleated the assembly of new microtubules when incubated in a solution

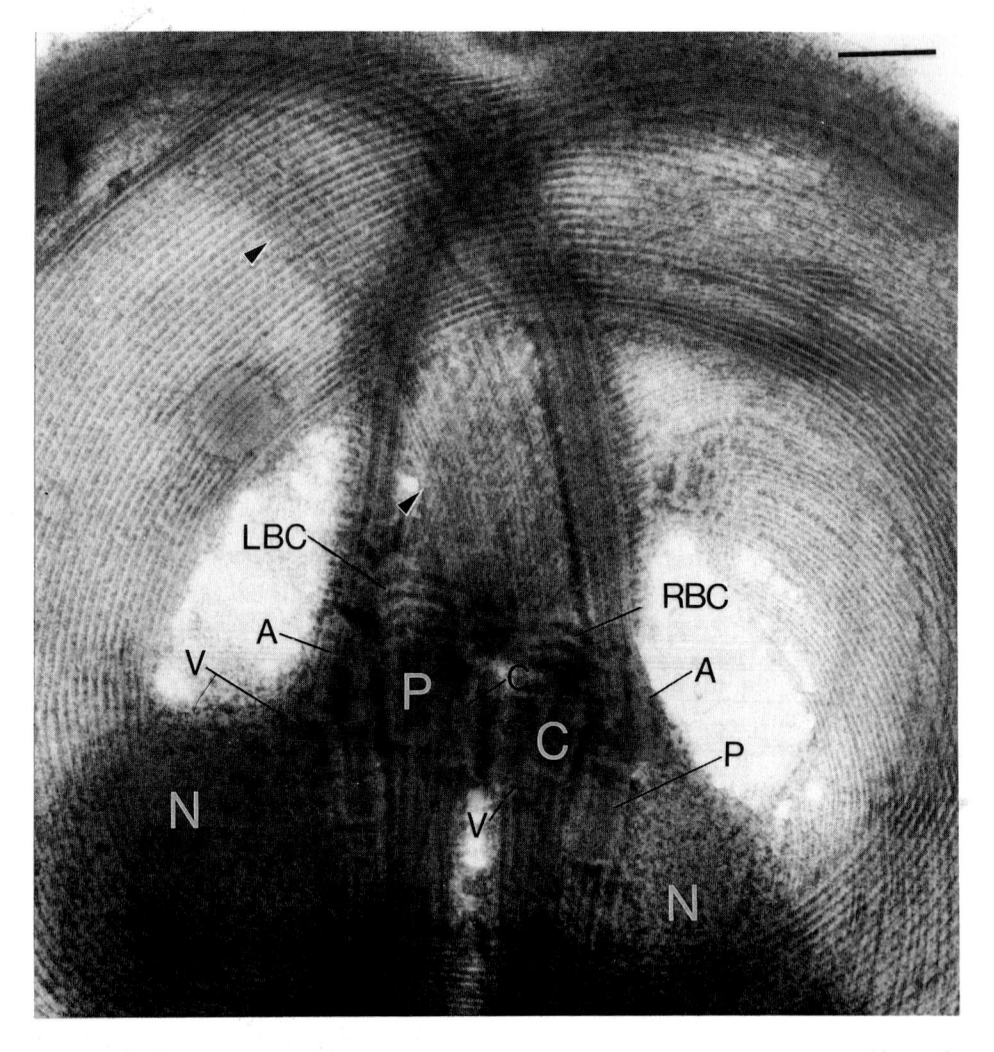

Fig. 10. Structures at the flagellar roots of *Giardia* sp., from above. The basal bodies are arranged in tetrads. Each tetrad is associated with a banded collar and is attached to the anterior pole of a nucleus (N). The left banded collar (LBC) gives rise to microtubules of the disc cytoskeleton. The right banded collar (RBC) is smaller, and produces a similar but rudimentary sheet of microtubules (arrowhead) which curves to the left for a short distance alongside the anterior axoneme. This sheet is seen in section between the axonemes in Fig. 1A. Note that the caudally-directed basal bodies in apparently similar positions in the two halves of the organism do not give rise to equivalent flagella. A, anterior basal body; C, caudal basal body; P, posterior-lateral basal body; V, ventral basal body. Bar equals 500 nm.

of rat brain tubulin (Fig. 11A). Interestingly, in these tubulin nucleation experiments a second site of extensive microtubule growth was the median body (Fig. 11B), which may also have a morphogenetic role.

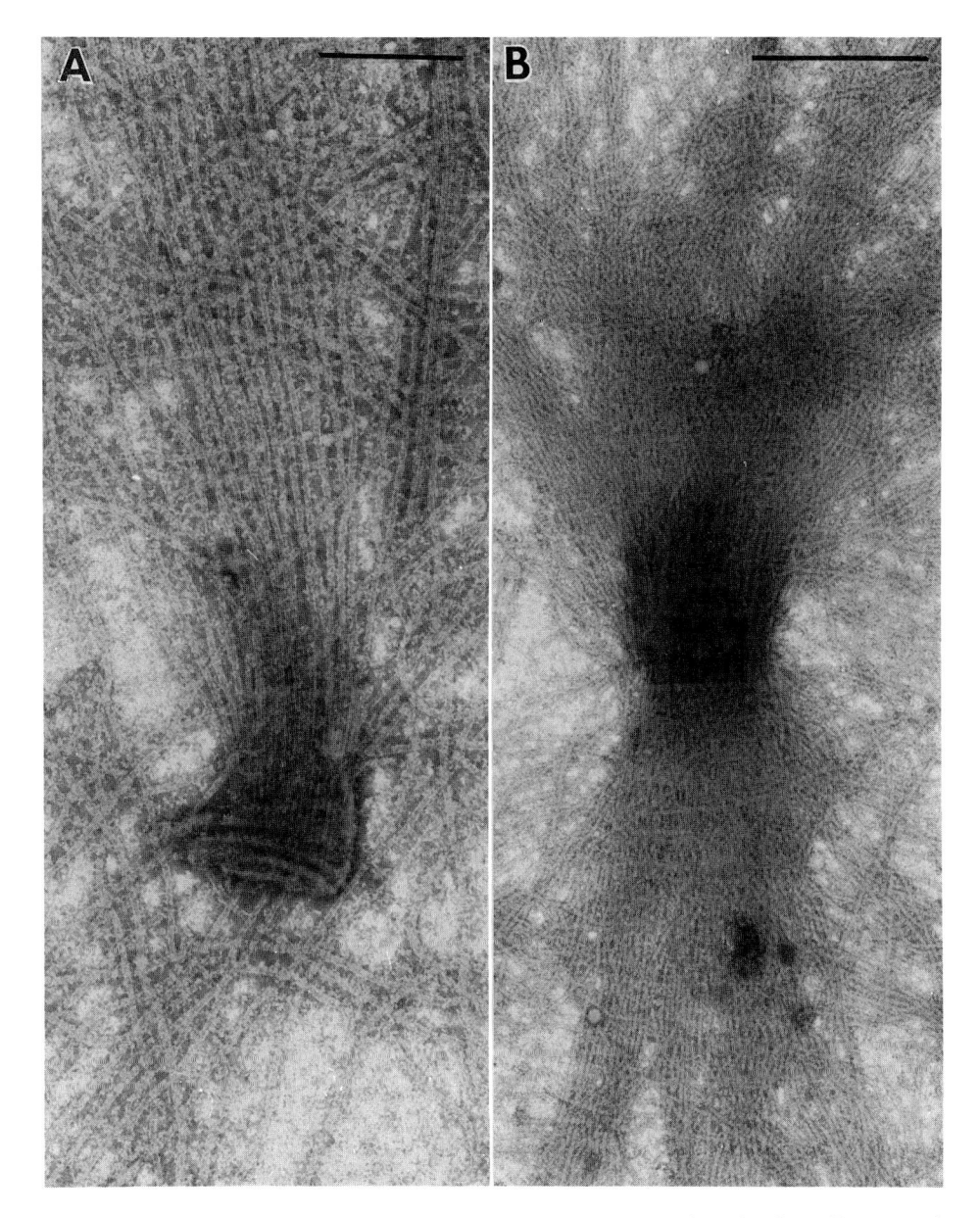

Fig. 11. Nucleation of microtubule assembly *in vitro* by components isolated from *Giardia* sp. Fragments of sheared cytoskeletons were collected on poly-L-lysine films and incubated with 2-3 mg/ml soluble rat brain tubulin for up to 90 min at 37°C. Extensive nets of microtubules formed around the 2 types of structure illustrated here. A. An isolated banded collar. Most microtubules spring from the convex (cytoskeleton) face, although some form also at the lateral edges and the concave (basal body) face. Bar equals 500 nm. B. A median body with a large number of microtubules assembled at the 2 free ends. Bar equals 1 μm.

3.3. Flagella

A feature of the mastigont in *Giardia* is that the basal bodies occupy a central position but the flagella emerge at remote points on the surface of the trophozoite. This unusual arrangement requires that the eight axonemes travel substantial distances (4-10 μm) in the cytoplasm before they enter the flagella. The caudal axonemes are retained in the body for at least two-thirds of their total length.

The arrangement of the basal bodies is shown in Fig. 10. They are clustered between the nuclei in two groups of four (tetrads). Brugerolle (1975a) first recognized that the symmetry about the midline is not truly bilateral. In terms of the flagella types they give rise to the positions of equivalent basal bodies and are inverted dorsoventrally in the two halves of the body. Six of the basal bodies are pointed towards the tail. The four at the center are attached directly to the disc cytoskeleton in two pairs superimposed vertically. The outer two (left ventral and right posterior-lateral) are joined obliquely end-to-end to the basal bodies of the two anterior flagella which face forward. The latter are slightly tilted and partly located in shallow pits on the surface of the two nuclei.

The different intracellular axonemes are accompanied by various other structures (Feely et al., 1984). Irregular dense fibrous masses or dense rods (Friend, 1966) run alongside the intracellular portions of the anterior and posterior-lateral axonemes (Fig. 4). Each anterior rod follows the inner radius of the axoneme for about three-quarters of the distance between the basal body and the beginning of the free flagellum. The posterior-lateral rods are shorter and lie above the axonemes where they pass over the ventral disc cytoskeleton. These rods may be dissimilar in composition. Immunostaining for the muscle proteins actin and α-actinin is present in the region of the posterior-lateral rods, but there is no reaction from the anterior rods (Feely et al., 1982). The effect on flagellar activity of these additional structures, and of the funis microtubules, is not clear. They may add to the stiffness of the axonemes within the body to dampen and possibly regulate contortions when the flagella are bending.

The cross-section of each flagellum shows the usual eukaryotic pattern of nine doublet and two central single microtubules. In addition, the two free ventral flagella develop paraflagellar structures that run alongside the axoneme. These appear in section as dense rods without a discernible substructure (Fig. 12B). They are linked to three doublets of the axoneme by a series of fine filaments (Holberton, 1973). The flagellar membrane is distended around the paraflagellar rod, to which it appears fused, forming a fin along one side. Opposite the rod, across the axoneme, a second less well-developed paraflagellar density is present beneath the membrane.

A preliminary biochemical characterization of *Giardia* flagella has been attempted recently (Clark, 1985). These studies used flagella sheared from trophozoites and purified from cell body material by centrifugation in Percoll density gradients. Electron microscopy showed that the isolated flagella were still enclosed by plasma membrane, and that about one quarter of the profiles contained paraflagellar rods. After treatment with Triton X-100, the membranes, rods and matrix material normally surrounding the

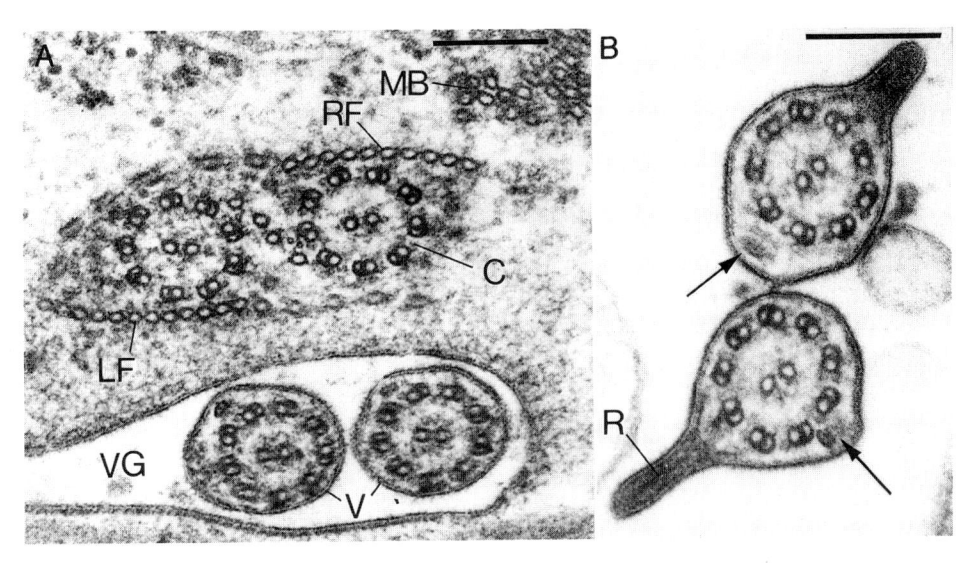

Fig. 12. TEM of *G. muris* showing structures associated with axonemes. A. A transverse section behind the disc in the region where the ventral flagella (V) emerge in the ventral groove (VG). In the cytoplasm, the caudal axonemes (C) are surrounded by microtubules of the funis. The microtubules are connected in 2 sheets by short bridges. Those in the right funis (RF) run above the axonemes and peel away on the left. The ventrally-placed left funis (LF) splays out towards the right. Some microtubules in the median body (MB) are linked by similar bridges. Bar equals 200 nm. B. Ventral flagella. A dense paraflagellar rod (R) extends the flagellar membrane on one side. The rod appears to be linked by fine connectives to the 3 nearest microtubule doublets. Also visible is a dense fiber between the axoneme and the membrane (arrows). Bar equals 200 nm.

axonemes disappeared. The intact purified flagella contained axonemal proteins and an additional set of $\sim$ 30 kDa polypeptides. The later resolved on SDS-PAGE gels as five bands not comigrating with cytoskeleton giardins. They also charged differently to the giardins. When compared on two-dimensional gels employing IEF in the first dimension, the flagellar polypeptides mapped to new positions separated from the giardins (Fig. 9). Furthermore, polyclonal antigiardins did not bind to the flagellar bands in immunoblots, confirming that the flagellar proteins are different chemical species (Crossley et al., 1986).

The 30 kDa flagellar proteins are removed by Triton, therefore they are not integral to the axoneme. Two other prominent flagellar proteins that disappeared after Triton extraction had mobilities on gels corresponding to molecular weights of 67 000 and 76 000. All of these Triton-labile polypeptides are candidates for components of the paraflagellar structures or flagellar membranes (see below). An antiserum from rabbits immunized with the flagellar 30 kDa bands has been used to localize these proteins (Crossley et al., 1986). In immunofluorescence tests there was no reaction from the disc. Instead, only the two free ventral flagella where the rods are located were brightly immunostained. This result suggests that the flagellar 30 kDa antigens are rod-associated proteins.

3.4. The plasma membrane

The plasma membrane of *Giardia* has few morphological features. Scanning electron microscope (SEM) studies, and freeze-fracture replicas, show the dorsal surface to be uneven with a large number of shallow pits (Erlandsen and Feely, 1984). These probably mark the sites of infolding of vacuoles that are visible in sections and freeze-fracture preparations in the cortex beneath the membrane (Friend, 1966; Feely et al., 1984). The ventral membrane covering the disc cytoskeleton is generally smooth, but often shows the imprint of the spiral of microtubules beneath. Intramembranous particles with no regular alignment are present in both dorsal and ventral membranes. They are typically more numerous in the dorsal membrane.

Details of the biochemical composition of the plasma membrane have emerged only recently. The impetus for these studies is the anticipated role of membrane proteins in inducing an immune reaction from the host during an infection. Several laboratories have used external radio-labelling of trophozoites to identify proteins exposed at the surface. Radio-iodine is transferred to tyrosine residues under the action of a catalyst such as lactoperoxidase or 1,3,4,6-tetrachloro-$3\alpha,6\alpha$-diphenylglycoluril (Iodogen). Labelled protein bands are subsequently detected on gels by autoradiography. The catalyst is too large to penetrate cells and label internal proteins.

Einfeld and Stibbs (1984) catalogued the accessible proteins labelled by this method on four cloned cultured strains (P-1, WB, LT, RS) of *Giardia* derived from human infections. The results were similar in each case. A major labelled band corresponded to a molecular weight of 82 000. Fainter bands were detected at 180 000, 105 000, 63 000, 55 000, 37 000, 30 000 and 24 000. The prominent antigen, as well as the 105, 30 and 24 kDa antigens, respectively, were Triton-extractable and could be precipitated by antibodies that agglutinated live and fixed trophozoites. The mobility of the main band was affected by periodate oxidation, suggesting that the protein might be glycosylated. Earlier it has been shown by Erlich et al. (1983) that antibodies from resistant BALB/c mice also recognized an 82 kDa antigen and a series of proteins from 32 to 25 kDa. A complex of four 32 kDa proteins could be extracted from *Giardia* lysates by binding to a column of the lectin wheat germ agglutinin (WGA), and eluting with *N*-acetyl-glucosamine. Nash et al. (1983) also used sera from rabbits or goats immunized with *Giardia* to precipitate surface-labelled components gradually released into the medium by P-1 and WB strain trophozoites. However, cross-immunoprecipitations by the heterologous antisera did not occur, indicating that different surface components were involved on each strain. The precipitated antigenic material did not in this case migrate on gels as a discrete band, but occurred as a smear of protein from 225 000 to 94 000 molecular weight.

A direct analysis of membrane proteins has been undertaken by Clark and Holberton (1986) following successful isolation of a pure membrane fraction. The plasma membrane was initially detached from the cytoplasm either by osmotic shock or by inducing external vesiculation in a low concentration of detergent. The isolated membranes were then collected and washed on density gradients. They were found to have a fuzzy filamentous coat on one side. Examined by SDS-PAGE, these fractions contained proteins broadly corresponding to some of the iodinated bands in the study of Einfeld and Stibbs (1984). These were a major broad band at molecular weight 75 000, a double band at 58 000 and 54 000 (comigrating with tubulin), five bands between 30 000 and 38 000, and diffuse bands in the region 15 000-20 000. Of these, only the 75, 58-54 and 22 kDa bands were iodinated in membranes prepared from surface-labelled cells, although other labelled bands appeared (at 190, 160, 120 and 28 kDa) that were not visible in the stained gels. The 75 kDa component of pure membrane and the 82 kDa iodinatible antigen described earlier may be the same protein, since they appear to be the major membrane species in each case. The difference in mobility may be due to anomalous behavior on gels run in two different buffer systems. Alternatively, the membrane protein may have suffered a limited chain cleavage during the purification stages. It is not yet clear to what extent the 30-38 kDa proteins in purified membranes correspond to the labile flagellar 30 kDa chains, nor whether the iodinatible 30 and 37 kDa polypeptides on *Giardia* sp. (Einfeld and Stibbs, 1984) and the group of four 32 kDa acidic glycoproteins from *Giardia muris* (Erlich et al., 1983) are the same or related proteins.

The iodinatible 58-54 kDa proteins are probably a membrane form of tubulin. There is increasing evidence for membrane tubulin in a variety of cells (Stephens, 1981; Rubin, 1984).

3.5. The vacuolar system

Endomembranes in *Giardia* trophozoites are few. Mitochondria are absent, and no profiles corresponding to a classic Golgi body have been found. Most noticeable are the cortical vacuoles, which are mainly confined to the ectoplasmic layer beneath the plasma membrane (Fig. 4). They are excluded from the ventral disc region where the membrane is attached to the disc cytoskeleton, but elsewhere they are found in large numbers adjacent to the ventral and dorsal surfaces. In the cytoplasm there are also scattered profiles of rough endoplasmic reticulum. For some reason, the endoplasmic reticular membranes do not always image clearly by conventional TEM fixation and staining so that the profiles appear as clefts in the cytoplasm (Fig. 4A). Although Friend (1966) considered these areas were not membrane-delimited, freeze-fracture preparations have demonstrated the presence of membranes (Feely et al., 1984).

The function of the sub-membrane vacuoles has been the subject of speculation. They have been thought to be either secretory (Friend, 1966), or endocytic (Bockman and Winborn, 1968). Less than 0.5 μm wide, the vacuoles are fairly uniform in size and mostly appear empty of inclusions. Friend (1966) noticed that a small proportion of the vacuoles contained clusters of particles embedded in a matrix. An experimental study of *Giardia* in the mouse has shown that dorsal and ventral vacuoles take up ferritin from the gut (Bockman and Winborn, 1968). Cytochemical evidence favors a digestive, lysosome-like function, whether or not hydrolytic enzymes are released to the outside. Kosjuk (1973) reported that the dorsal vacuoles stain vitally with acridine orange. More

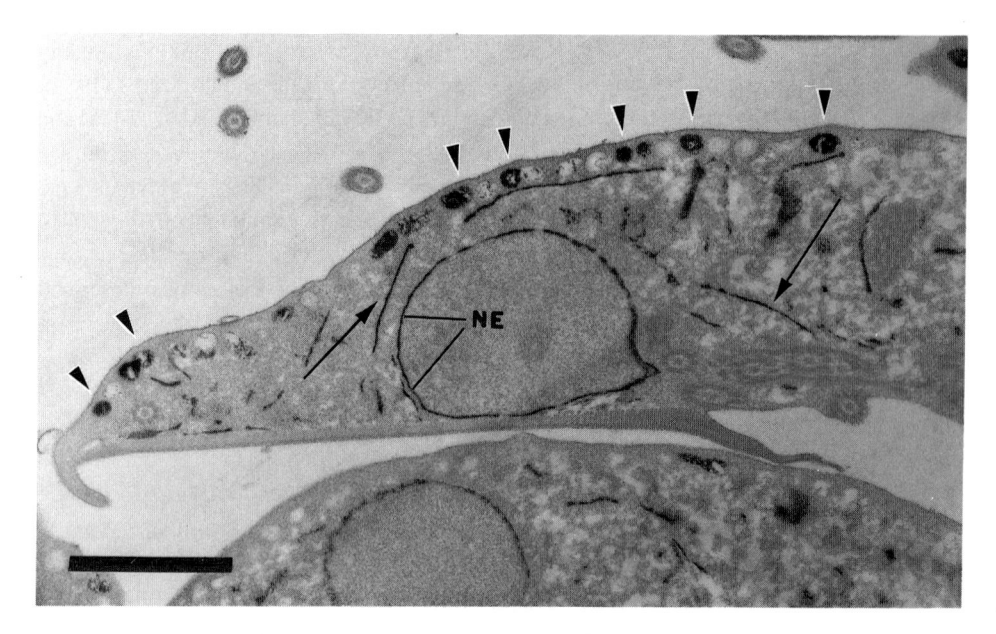

Fig. 13. This TEM shows the distribution of reaction product for acid phosphatase in a human source *Giardia* trophozoite. Note the presence of staining in the peripheral vacuoles (arrowheads), in the endoplasmic reticulum (arrows) and within the cisternae of the nuclear envelope (NE). Bar = 1 μm.

recently, acid phosphatase activity has been demonstrated in vacuoles in TEM sections of both mouse *Giardia* and a cultured *Giardia* sp., the WB strain (Feely and Dyer, 1987). The cytochemical reaction was widespread throughout the vacuolar system of the human *Giardia*, including the cisternae of the endoplasmic reticulum and the nuclear envelope (Fig. 13). In *Giardia* from the mouse the reaction was sensitive to the fixation process. Reaction product deposited in only some of the peripheral vacuoles. The two *Giardia* isolates were found to have different isoenzymes of acid phosphatase when acrylamide gels of extracts were visualized by the histochemical reaction.

These results identify the vacuoles provisionally as lysosomes derived from endocytotic vacuoles, but the detection of other hydrolases will be required for confirmation. The endoplasmic reticulum is also implicated as a site of formation and transport of acid phosphatase. In the absence of a Golgi body it seems probable that the vacuoles receive the processed enzyme directly from the tubules of the endoplasmic reticulum, although the existence of this pathway has not been shown. Also obscure is the location within the endomembrane system of sites where transit forms of enzymes, and the lectin-binding membrane proteins and cyst wall components, might be glycosylated.

3.6. Cyst

The cysts of human source *Giardia*, ovoid or elliptical in appearance, are approximately 7 to 10 μm long. They are somewhat refractile to light when viewed with brightfield

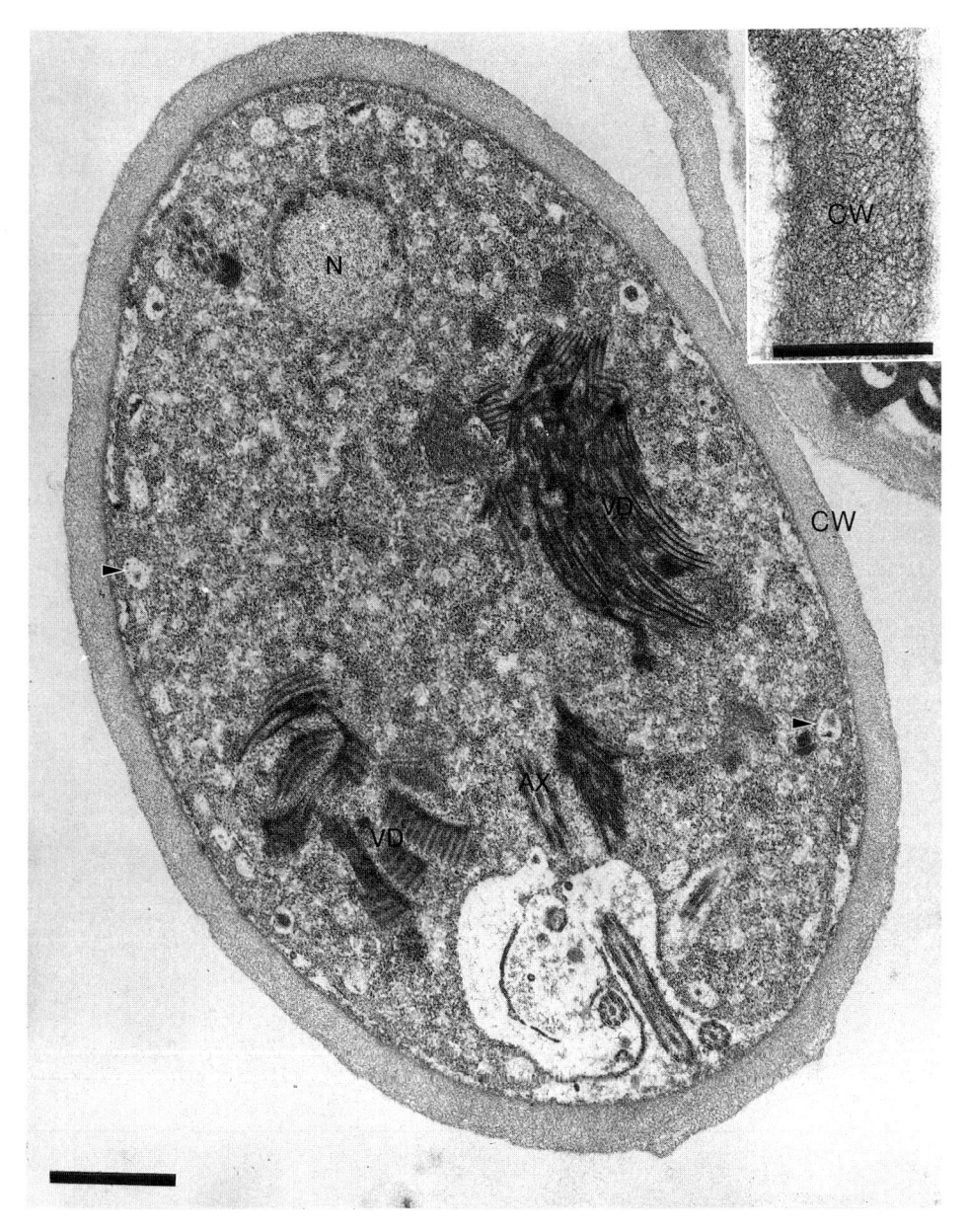

Fig. 14. This TEM shows the internal structure of a *G. muris* cyst. Note the fragments of the ventral disc, axonemes, the peripheral vacuoles, (arrowheads) and the nucleus (N). The cyst wall (CW) is composed of a felt-like web of fine fibrils. Bar = 1 μm. The inset shows a higher magnification of a cyst wall. Bar = 0.5 μm.

microscopy and can be quickly and easily found in wet preparations with a little practice. The cyst wall is approximately 0.3-0.5 μm thick and, upon examination by TEM, is seen to be composed of a layer of fibrils (7-30 nm in width) arranged in a felt-like web (Fig.

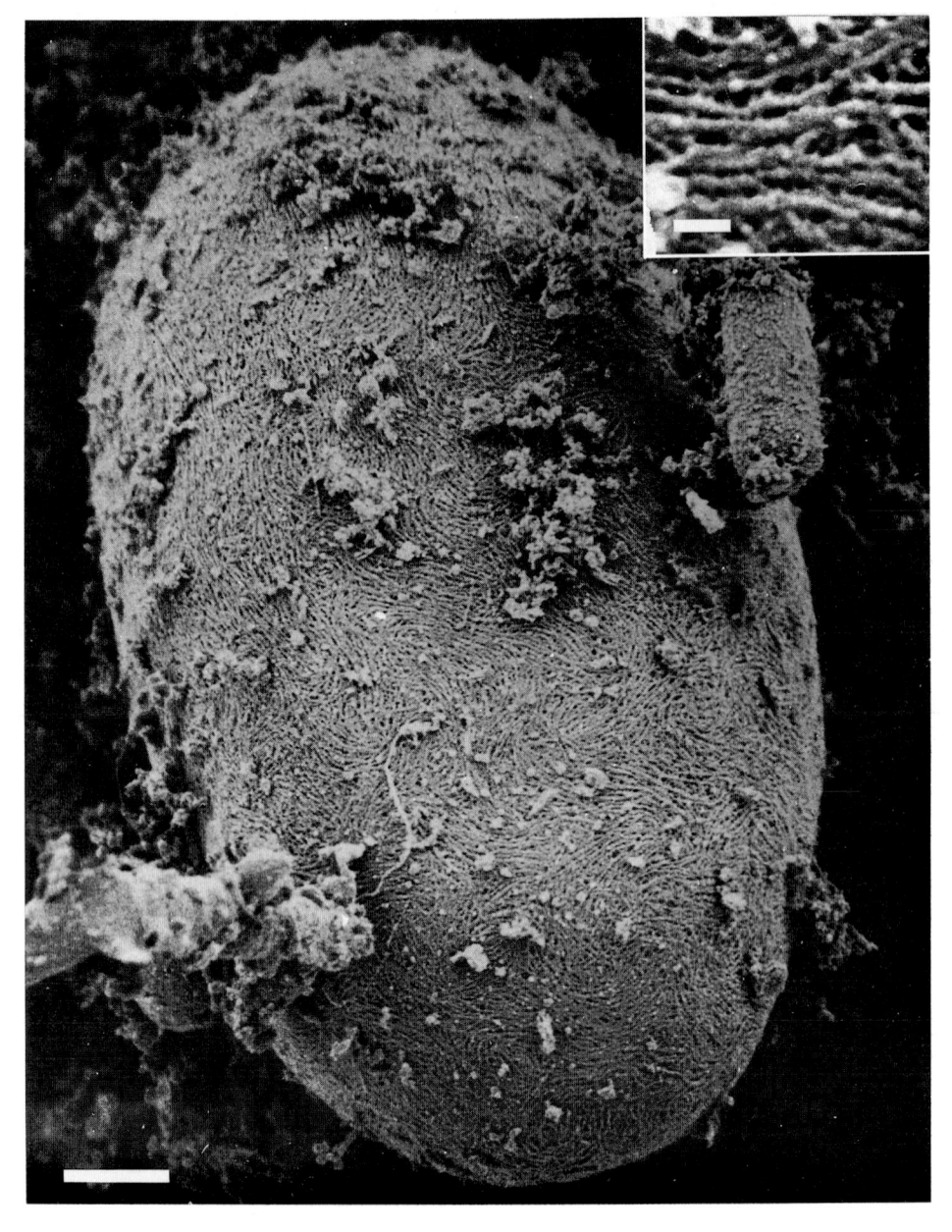

Fig. 15. A high resolution, low voltage SEM of a *G. muris* cyst showing the fine surface detail of the cyst wall. Note the arrangement of the fibrils of the cyst wall. Bar = 1 μm. A higher magnification of the fibrils is seen in the inset. Bar = 0.1 μm.

14). Examination of the cysts prepared for conventional SEM show few details and the surface of the cyst appears smooth in appearance (Fig. 1B). However, examination of

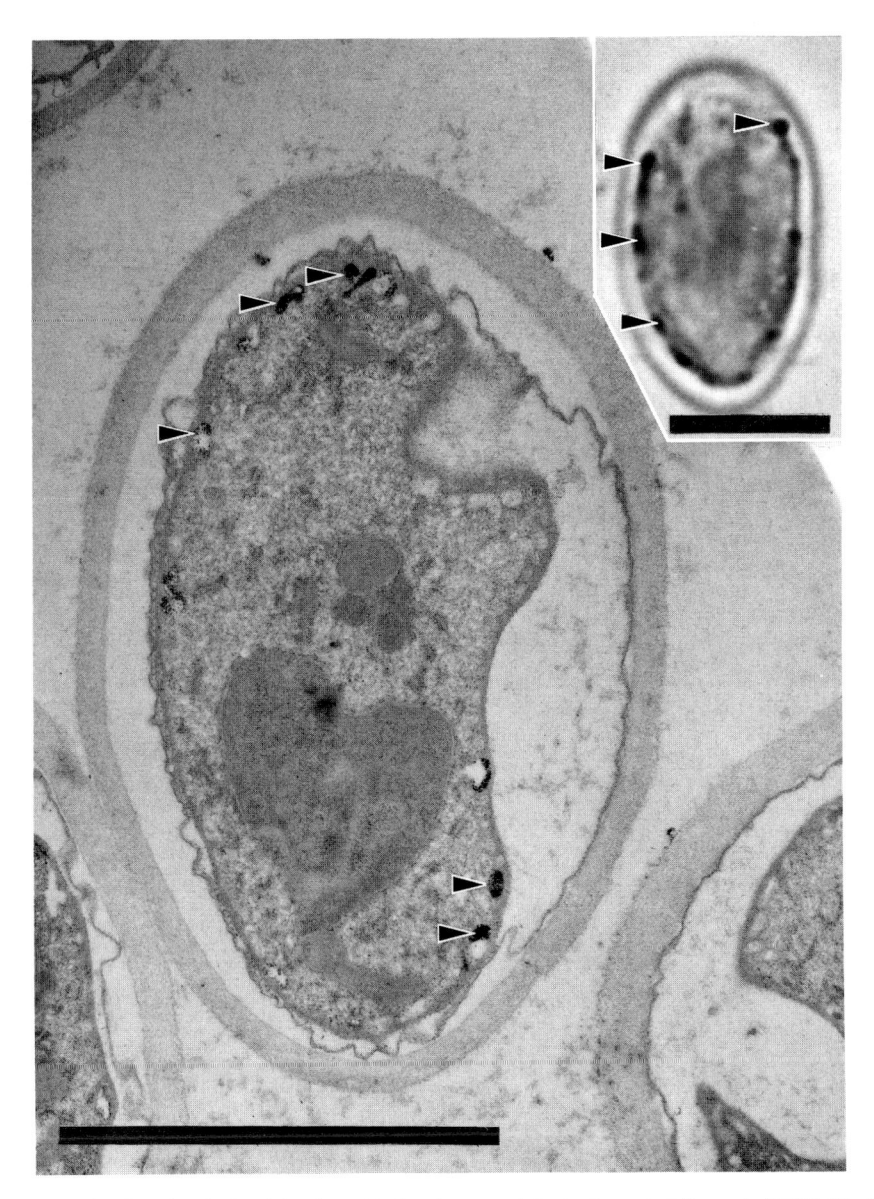

Fig. 16. Cytochemical staining for acid phosphatase activity in the cyst of *G. muris* (TEM). The inset shows the localization of reaction product (arrowheads) by light microscopy in the periphery of the cyst. Bar = 5 µm. The TEM shows the reaction product in the peripheral vacuoles (arrowheads). Bar = 5 µm.

isolated cysts prepared for high resolution, low voltage SEM shows fine detail of the cyst surface (Fig. 15). The fine fibrils of the cyst wall are arranged in curved arrays. These fibrils are approximately 7-30 nm wide and are of undetermined length (Fig. 15, inset). The chemical nature of the cyst wall is not completely understood. It has been reported that the cyst wall of organisms of the *G. duodenalis* and *G. muris* types contain chitin based on lectin binding studies (Ward et al., 1985). However, Jarroll et al. (1989) have questioned the presence of chitin in the cyst wall. Their studies, using gas chromatography and mass spectrometry on *G. muris* and two human source *Giardia* cyst isolates, demonstrated that *n*-acetylgalactosamine is the primary amino sugar of the cyst wall. They were unable to detect *n*-acetylglucosamine, the primary amino sugar of chitin.

Beneath the fibrous cyst wall, the organelles and structures found in the trophozoite can be found in the encysted organism. However, some of them are modified in shape. Two or four nuclei (depending on the maturity of the cyst) are found at one pole of the cyst (Fig. 2B and 14). Axonemes of the flagella are seen as linear structures by light microscopy (Fig. 2B) and in section by TEM showing the familiar '9+2' arrangement of microtubules (Fig. 14). The cytoplasm also contains profiles of the median body, segments of rough endoplasmic reticulum, and basal bodies. The cytoskeleton of the ventral disc is found in fragments (Sheffield and Bjorvatn, 1977) which may appear in stacks or crescents (Fig. 14). This arrangement of the ventral disc components in the cyst raises questions on the reassembly of the disc after excystation. Sheffield and Bjorvatn (1977) suggested that the fragments may serve as templates for disc formation or may be reassembled after excystation is completed. The periphery is marked by an array or layer of vacuoles or tubules. These are approximately 400 nm in diameter and resemble the peripheral vacuoles of the trophozoite. They stain positively for acid phosphatase activity (Fig. 16) and have been suggested to participate in the mechanism of excystation. It has also been suggested that these vacuoles may be responsible for the secretion of the components of the cyst wall (Friend, 1966).

4. Microbial symbionts of Giardia

Bacterial symbionts are commonly found in many protozoans, including those which are parasitic (Ball, 1969). The first report of bacteria in *Giardia* was made by Boeck (1917). His iron-hematoxylin preparations of *G. microti* had several dark staining inclusions in the trophozoites which he interpreted as endosymbiotic bacteria. Similar structures were observed in the cysts but were interpreted as nuclei produced by multiple fission rather than endosymbiotic microorganisms. Subsequent studies on *G. microti* cysts have demonstrated these inclusions to be bacteria (Feely et al., 1988). Endosymbionts were reported by Wenrich (1940) and Brug (1942) in human source *Giardia* and *G. muris*, respectively. In recent studies, endosymbiotic bacteria have been demonstrated in *G. muris* trophozoites and cysts by Nemanic et al. (1978). The bacteria were suggested to be Gram-negative based on their ultrastructure. Nemanic et al. (1978) speculated that endosymbionts might influence the infectivity of *G. muris* in mammalian hosts and possibly insert plasmids into the genome of the protozoan. Radulescu et al. (1986) reported the presence of a bacterial symbiont in the cysts of *Giardia* isolated from children

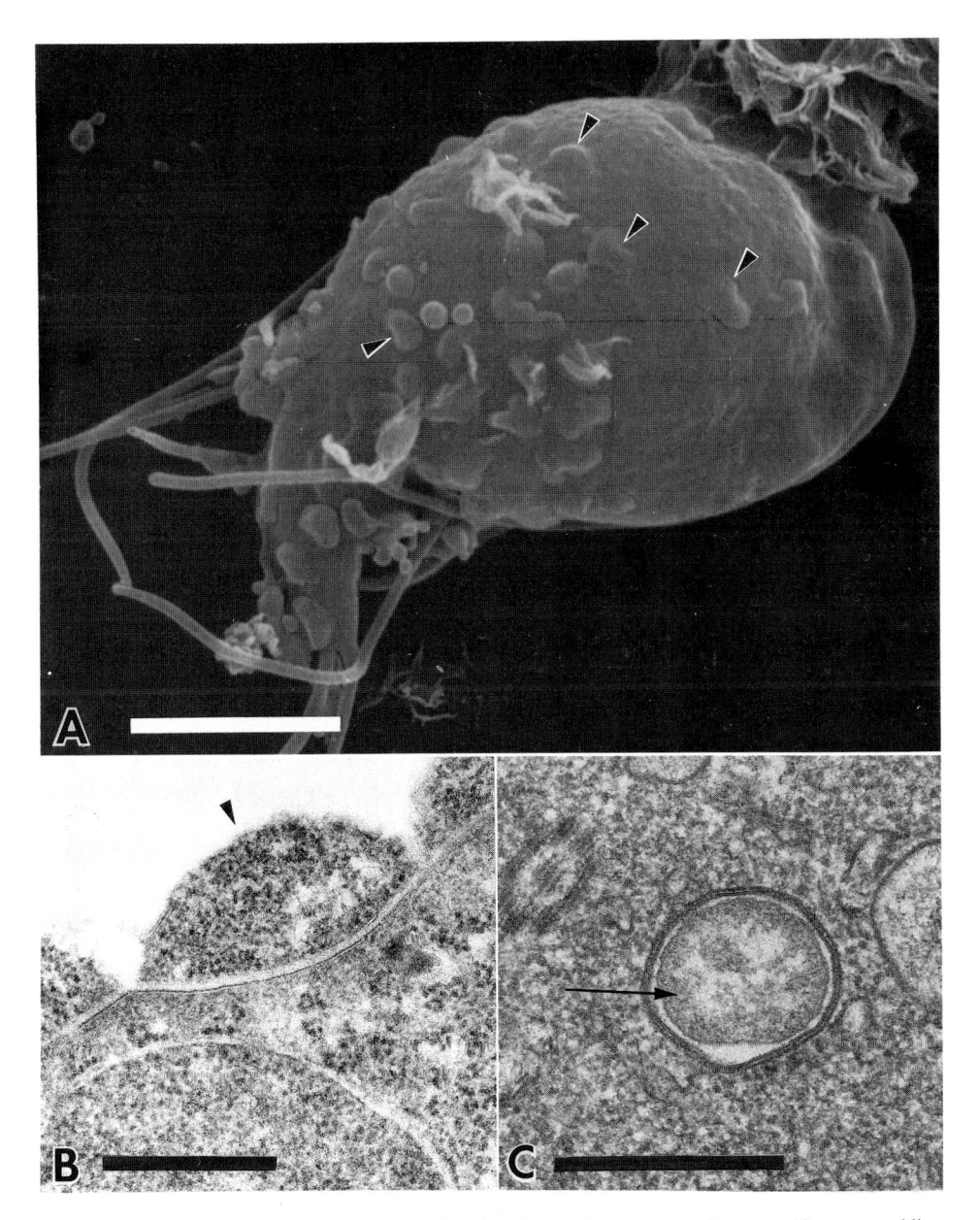

Fig. 17. A. This SEM of a *G. microti* trophozoite shows the presence of ectosymbionts resembling mycoplasma-like organisms (MLO, arrowheads) adherent to the dorsal surface. Bar = 1 μm. B. Examination by TEM shows that the MLOs (arrowhead) are found in shallow depressions of the surface of the trophozoite. Bar = 0.5 μm. C. Intracellular bacteria are found in both the cyst and trophozoite. This TEM shows an intracellular bacterium (arrow) within the cytoplasm of a cyst of *G. microti*. Bar = 0.5 μm.

who had received a live vaccine for *Shigella flexneri* and in cysts of *G. muris* from mice inoculated with the same bacteria. We have recently examined trophozoites and cysts from a number of hosts and found bacterial symbionts in several *Giardia* species (Feely et al., 1988). Initial observations of *G. microti* trophozoites and cysts by electron microscopy have shown the presence of many bacterial symbionts. This is the same species in which Boeck (1917, 1919) first described microbial symbionts in *Giardia*. Our studies have shown that trophozoites of this species are host to both ectosymbionts resembling

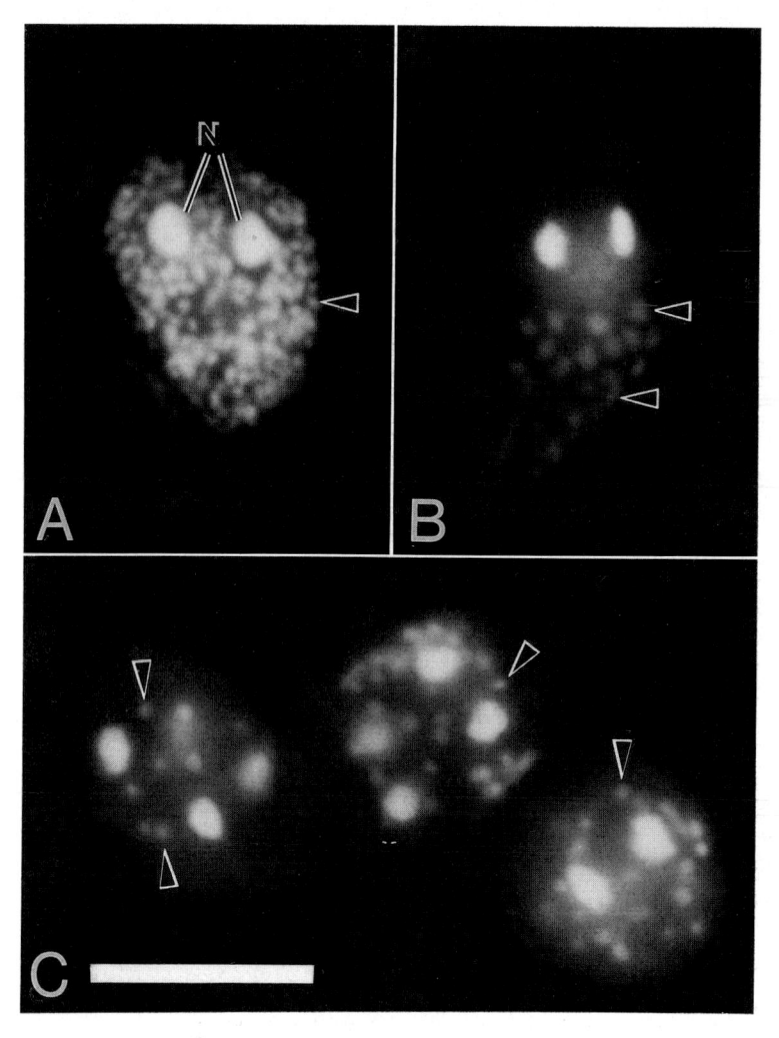

Fig. 18. Fluorescent staining for bacterial symbionts with Hoechst 33258. A. A *G. microti* trophozoite showing numerous fluorescent foci representing intracellular bacteria (arrowhead; N=nuclei). B. MLOs (arrowheads) are clearly seen on the surface of this *G. microti* trophozoite and can be differentiated from the intracellular bacteria by their greater size. C. Intracellular bacteria can be detected in *G. microti* cysts by the same method. Numerous bacteria (arrowheads) are visible in these cysts isolated from vole feces. Bar = 10 μm.

mycoplasma-like organisms (MLOs) and bacterial endosymbionts (Fig. 17A-C). MLOs were observed on the surfaces of *G. microti* (Fig. 17A) and *G. ondatrae* trophozoites. By transmission electron microscopy, these were seen to be attached in shallow depressions of the plasmalemma (Fig. 17B). Endosymbiotic bacteria were observed by TEM in the trophozoites and cysts of *G. microti* (Fig. 17C) and were found to be similar in appearance to those reported in other species. We have recently developed a method (Feely et al., 1988) to screen *Giardia* trophozoites and cysts for bacterial symbionts by application of a DNA-specific fluorochrome, Hoechst 33258, based on the technique published by Chen (1977) for staining of cultured mammalian cells. The technique adapted for use on *Giardia* is as follows: (1) Attach trophozoites and cysts to poly-*l*-lysine coated cover glass or slides (Mazia et al., 1975). (2) Fix the cells for 10 min in methanol:acetic acid (3:1). (3) Postfix in 4% neutral buffered formalin for 2 min followed by a 2 min rinse in absolute methanol and allow to air dry. (4) Stain for 10 min in Hoechst 33258 (0.5

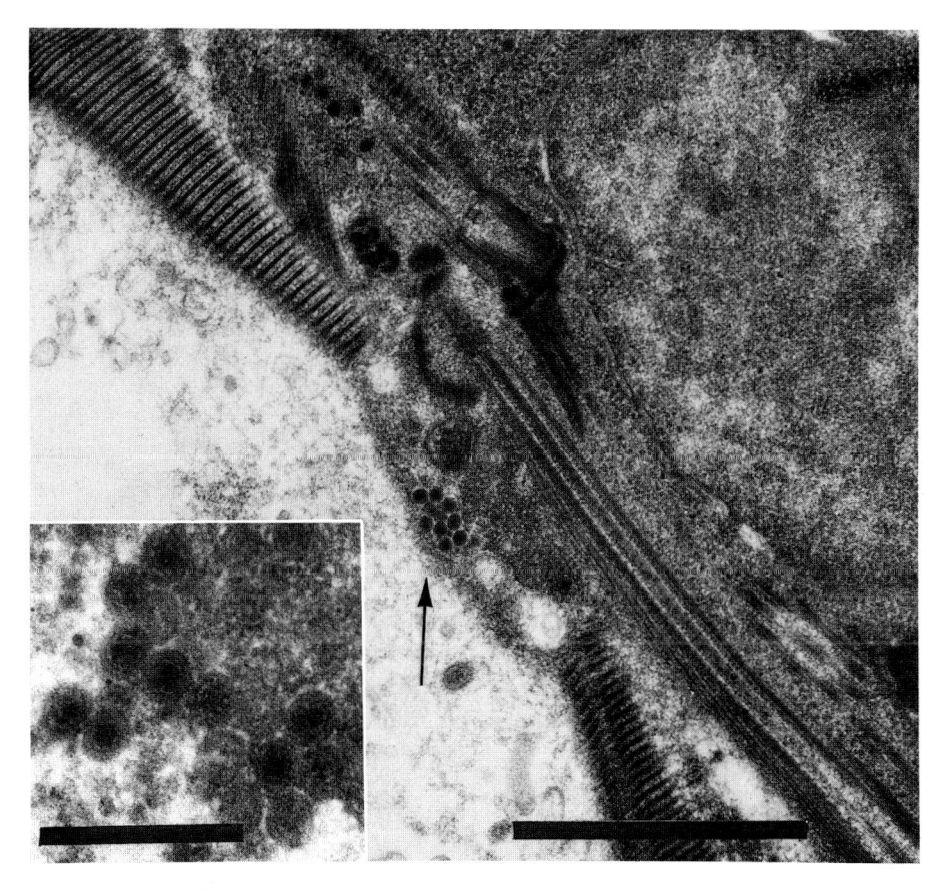

Fig. 19. TEM of a *G. muris* trophozoite showing viral-like particles (arrow). Bar = 1 μm. Higher magnification (inset) shows the polyhedral appearing particles. Bar = 0.1 μm.

µg/ml PBS). (5) Rinse in distilled water and mount in glycerol:phosphate buffered saline (9:1). (6) Examine by UV epifluorescence with fluorite objectives.

Endosymbiotic bacteria appeared as small, brightly fluorescent foci in the cytoplasm of the protozoan (Fig. 18A-C). The nuclei of the protozoan also stained but were easily recognized by their larger size and morphology. The majority of the trophozoites and cysts of *G. microti* were observed to have bacterial endosymbionts. Some individual trophozoites had surprisingly large numbers of bacteria (100 or more; Feely et al., 1988; see Fig. 18A) while others had few or none. MLOs were easily detected as well but were differentiated from the endosymbionts by (a) their greater size (Fig. 18B) and (b) by differential focusing which showed them to be found on the surface of the organism rather than intracellular. Cysts generally had fewer symbionts than the trophozoites (Fig. 18C). Trophozoites and cysts of other *Giardia* species from a variety of hosts (great-blue heron, green heron, beaver and muskrat) were found to have bacterial symbionts based on this method.

Viruses have been demonstrated unequivocally in *Giardia* only in recent years. Brug (1942) reported the presence of cytoplasmic granules in the cytoplasm of *G. muris* and suggested that they were viral particles. However, Ball (1969) considered this interpretation to be questionable based on the nature of Brug's material and published illustrations, and suggested that they were possibly inclusions of fungi. The presence of double-stranded RNA (dsRNA) has been documented in several strains of *Giardia*. Wang and Wang (1986) reported the presence of dsRNA in the Portland-1 strain which is commonly cultured in the laboratory for experimental use. This virus was transmittable to the WB strain and was characterized ultrastructurally as a 33 nm viral sphere in the nucleoplasm of both nuclei. In addition, Dejonckheere and Gordts (1987) demonstrated the presence of a dsRNA virus in 18 strains of human derived *Giardia* strains and in two of *G. cati* and *G. caviae*. Viral-like particles have been demonstrated in *G. muris* trophozoites from rat small intestine (Feely et al., 1988). These 60 nm particles (Fig. 19) were observed in the cytoplasm rather than the nucleoplasm and were not associated with any obvious deleterious effects on the protozoan or vertebrate hosts.

It is reasonable to assume that the symbionts which have been demonstrated in the laboratory in *Giardia* find their way into the vertebrate host. It is not known if any of the documented symbionts are potential pathogens. Wang and Wang (1986) noted no homology in the DNA of the host trophozoite and the dsRNA, suggesting no insertion of the viral genome into that of the *Giardia*. However, it appears that the presence of microbial symbionts in *Giardia* trophozoites and cysts is more frequent than has been previously recognized. The transmission of a pathogenic microorganism using the cysts as a vehicle and the insertion of bacterial or viral plasmids into the human genome are possibilities which deserve further research.

5. Attachment to substrates

The ability of the *Giardia* trophozoite to attach to the host epithelium has been of considerable interest since its discovery. This phenomenon has been observed in the host intestine and can be demonstrated easily in the laboratory by the experimental attachment of the organism to artificial substrates (Holberton, 1975; Feely and Erlandsen, 1982; Erlandsen and Feely, 1984). Trophozoites may attach in large numbers to the host intestinal epithelium (Fig. 20A). Attachment is secure and intimate and may produce the unique lesion (Fig. 20B, C) on the microvillous border of the enterocytes which has been demonstrated to be the mirror-image of the ventral disc (Erlandsen, 1974). Trophozoite attachment was recognized and described by early investigators of this organism. Muller (1890) and Zabel (1901) suggested the ventral disc was the responsible organelle for attachment to the host epithelium. Simon (1921) reported a rhythmic contraction and expansion of the periphery of the ventral disc which suggested a mechanism for attachment. The concept of the ventral disc as the primary organelle of attachment has persisted and several theories on the mechanism of attachment have been proposed. These suggested theories are based largely on morphological evidence and include mediation by microtubules, a hydrodynamic model, activity of contractile proteins and adherence by the interaction of lectins with surface bound sugars.

As previously described, the ventral disc is a complex structure of several cytoskeletal elements which may act as a supporting pontoon or to attach actively to the substrate. Mueller et al. (1974) suggested that the microtubules of the ventral disc underwent a coiling and uncoiling to change its diameter and thereby effect attachment. Although initially an appealing hypothesis, further morphological studies (Holberton, 1973, 1974) demonstrated that the microtubules of the disc are physically linked to one another and to the ventral plasmalemma. It would seem unlikely that such physical linkages would allow movement of the microtubules.

Ultrastructural observations by Holberton (1975) led to the suggestion of a hydrodynamic model for attachment. It was noted that the ventral flagella are continuously active in trophozoites attached to glass substrates. It was suggested that this activity caused a low pressure area under the ventral disc due to the flow of fluids around the ventral groove and marginal grooves of the attached organisms. Although lacking direct experimental confirmation, this model has been supported by the mathematical analysis of Jones et al. (1983). Recently, it has been reported that in the trophozoites of *Giardia psittaci* (Erlandsen and Bemrick, 1987), the ventrolateral flange was incomplete and did not encircle the ventral disc. Since no marginal groove was present, and these trophozoites were observed to attach to both the host intestinal epithelium and to glass substrates in vitro, it seems unlikely that a hydrodynamic model in itself would explain the mechanism of attachment adequately.

Contractile proteins have been demonstrated immunocytochemically in the periphery of the ventral disc by Feely et al. (1982), and have been suggested to participate in the mechanism of attachment. Examination of the periphery of the ventral disc by electron

44

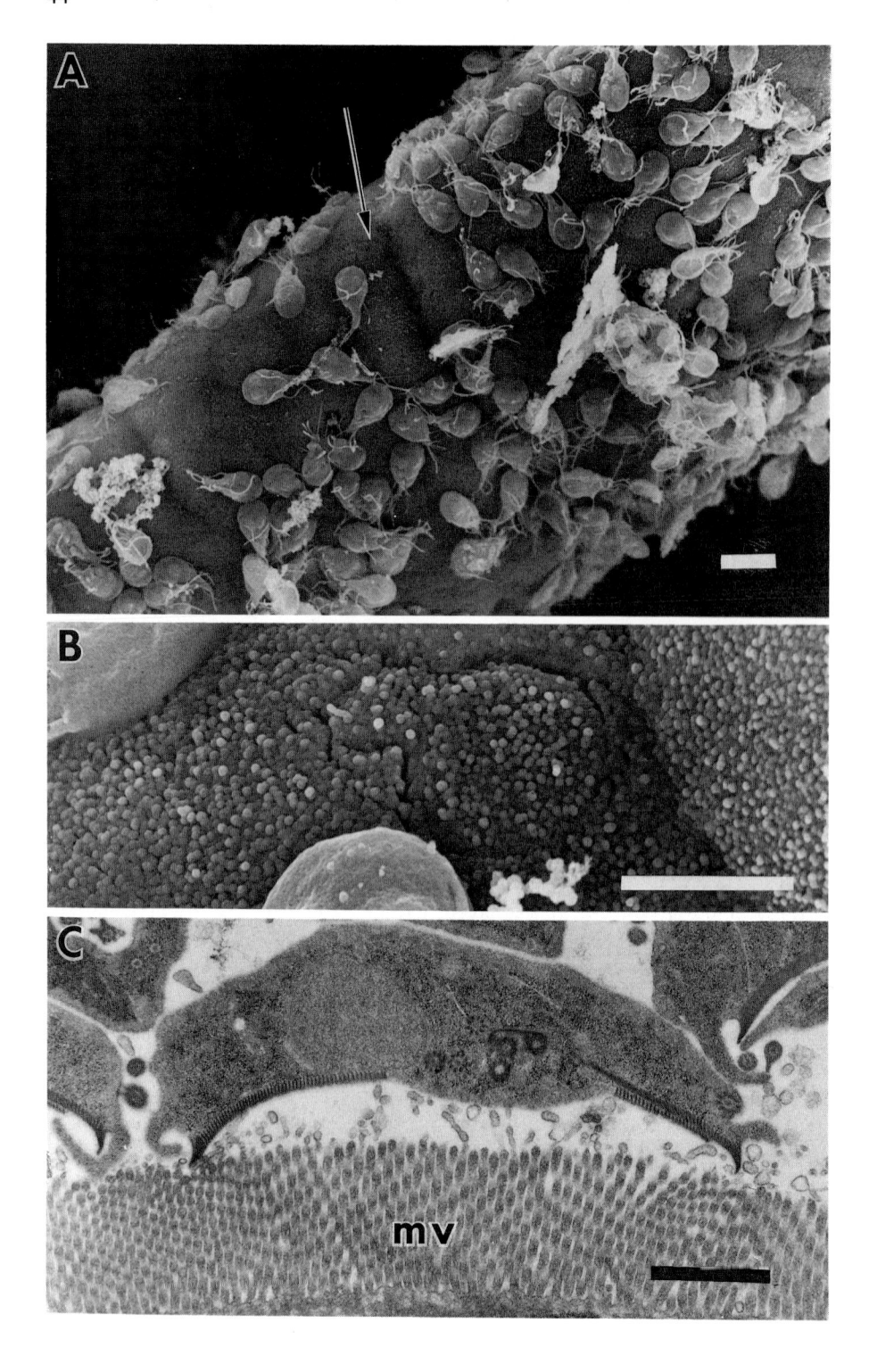

microscopy showed the presence of a fibrous dense material in the area called the lateral crest (Fig. 21A). This structure is responsible for the characteristic area of asymmetry discussed above and is evident by SEM (Fig. 21B). Immunostaining for actin is evident in the periphery of the ventral disc in an area corresponding to the lateral crest (Fig. 21C). Comparison of B and C shows this overlapping area clearly. In addition to actin, the contractile proteins α-actinin, tropomyosin and myosin were also localized in the ventral disc. The localization of these proteins suggested their participation in attachment. Further evidence for such a role exists in studies on the effect of cytochalasin-B and low Ca^{2+} concentration on trophozoite attachment (Feely and Erlandsen, 1982). Exposure to cytochalasin-B, which disassociates microfilaments, including actin, caused rapid detachment of trophozoites from artificial substrates. Similarly, incubation of trophozoites in a medium containing a concentration of calcium lower than that required for actin-myosin interaction also produced detachment. These reports have provided strong evidence that contractile proteins may be directly involved in the mechanism of attachment.

The physical attachment of human source *Giardia*, *G. muris* and *G. agilis* trophozoites to artificial substrates has been directly observed by Erlandsen and Feely (1984) by use of interference-reflexion microscopy. This technique demonstrates focal contact (10 nm or less) of a cell to underlying substrate as well as close contacts (up to 100 nm distance) of the cell and substrate. They reported the rapid formation and loss (1 s or less) of direct focal contacts between the lateral crest of the ventral disc and the substrate surface. In addition, focal contacts were observed between the substrate and the ventrolateral flange and close contacts between the central portions of the ventral disc and the lateral shield regions of the trophozoite. These studies support the possible active role of the ventral disc in the attachment mechanism.

Lectins have been suggested to participate in the attachment mechanism. Farthing et al. (1986) have described a surface lectin from human source *Giardia* specific for D-glucosyl and D-mannosyl residues. Since D-mannosyl residues have been reported on the microvillous border of enterocytes, it was suggested that this lectin may be responsible for the adherence of the trophozoite to the host cells. Although this lectin may play a role in adherence, there is no experimental confirmation on whether or not it is required for attachment. The contributions of lectin binding are difficult to evaluate since (a) this mechanism does not explain the orientation (ventral side toward the microvilli) of trophozoites attached to host tissue, or (b) the attachment of trophozoites in PBS or Hanks balanced salt solution to artificial substrates such as polystyrene and glass, which have no carbohydrate residues.

Fig. 20. Human source *Giardia* trophozoites attached to a mouse intestinal villus. A. Note numerous trophozoites attached to the microvillous border by their ventral surfaces. Bar = 10 μm. A lesion of the microvillous border is indicated by the arrow. B. The attachment lesion is shown at higher magnification and in greater detail. Bar = 5 μm. C. A similar preparation prepared for TEM. Note the trophozoite attached to the microvillous border (MV). Bar = 1 μm.

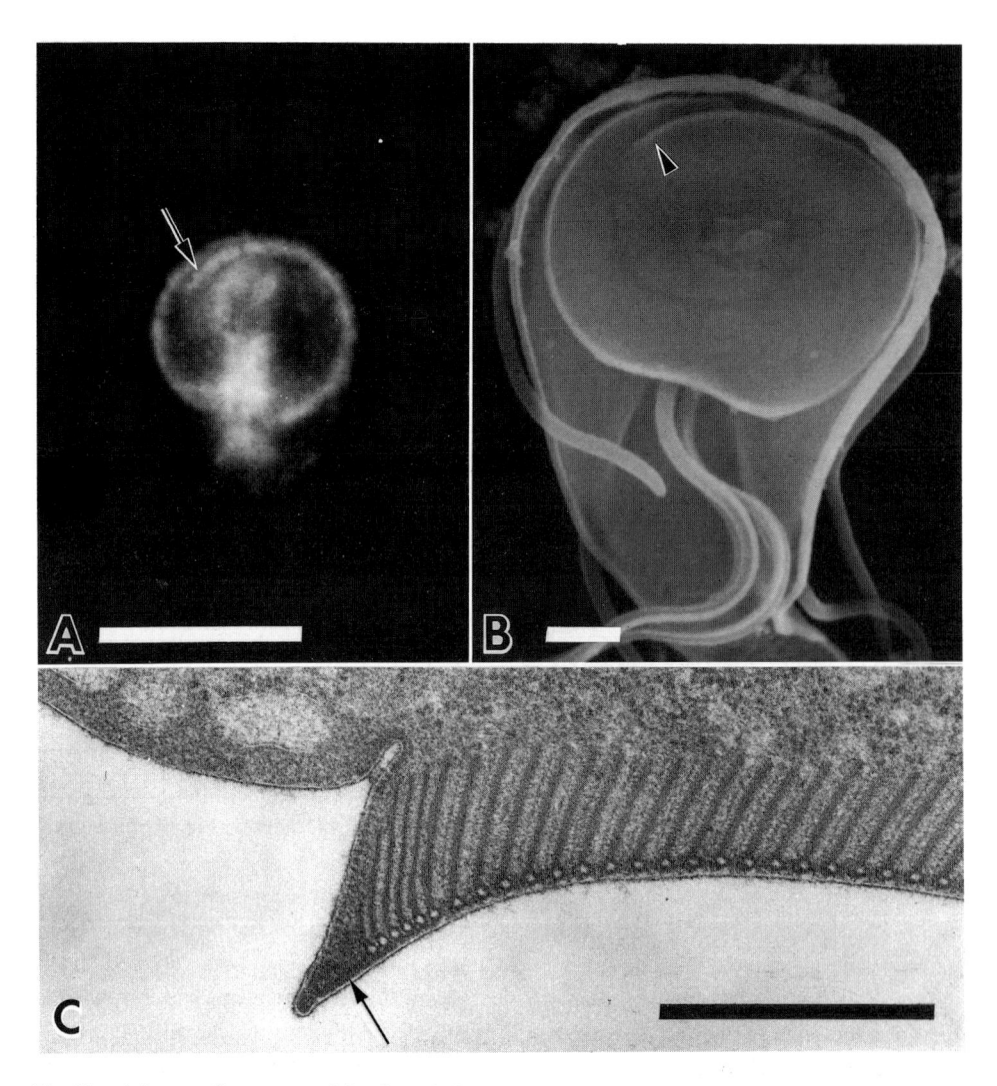

Fig. 21. A. Immunofluorescent staining for actin in a trophozoite. Note staining in the periphery of the ventral disc corresponding to the lateral crest and the presence of the overlapping area (arrowhead). Bar = 5 µm. B. This SEM of the ventral surface of a trophozoite shows the peripheral border of the ventral disc including the overlapping area (arrowhead) which closely resembles the pattern seen in the immunofluorescent staining for actin. Bar = 1 µm. C. This TEM of the ventral disc shows the presence of a fibrous-like material (arrowhead) in the lateral crest. Bar = 0.25 µm.

Acknowledgements

The authors would like to express their thanks to Ms. Marjorie Gardner and Mr. Chris Frethem for their technical assistance, and to Mrs. Edna Manning and Ms. Chris Cary for preparation of the manuscript. Financial support was provided, in part, by USPHS grant AI 20502 to DEF, cooperative agreement CR814622 from the Environmental Protection Agency to SLE, and the Minnesota Medical Foundation. The views expressed in this article do not necessarily reflect the views of the Environmental Protection Agency and official endorsements should not be inferred. Mention of trade names, materials or products does not constitute endorsement or recommendation for use.

References

Ansari, M.A.R. (1952) Contribution à l'étude du genre *Giardia*. Ann. Parasitol. 27, 477-490.
Ball, G.H. (1969) Organisms living in and on protozoa, In: T.T. Chen (Ed.), Research in Protozoology, Vol. 3, pp. 565-718. Pergamon Press, Oxford.
Bockman, A.K. and Winborn, W.B. (1968) Electron microscopic localization of exogenous ferritin within vacuoles of *Giardia muris*. J. Protozool. 15, 26-30.
Boeck, W.C. (1917) Mitosis in *Giardia microti*. Univ. Calif. Publ. Zool. 18, 1-26.
Boeck, W.C. (1919) Studies on *Giardia microti*. Univ. Calif. Publ. Zool. 19, 85-134.
Brug, S.L. (1942) Eigentümliche Einschlüsse in *Lamblia muris*. Zentralbl. Bakteriol. 148, 166-168.
Brugerolle, G. (1975a) Contribution à l'étude cytologique et phylétique des diplozoaires (Zoomastigophorea, Diplozoa, Dangeard 1910). V. Nouvelle interpretation de l'organisation cellulaire de *Giardia*. Protistologica 11, 99-109.
Brugerolle, G. (1975b) Contribution a l'étude cytologique et phylétique des diplozoaires (Zoomastigophorea, Diplozoa, Dangeard 1910). VI. Caractères généraux des Diplozoaires. Protistologica 11, 111-118.
Chavez, B., Knaippe, F., Gonzalez-Mariscal, L. and Martinez-Palomo, A. (1986) *Giardia lamblia*: electrophysiology and ultrastructure of cytopathology in cultured epithelial cells. Exp. Parasitol. 61, 379-389.
Cheissin, E.M. (1964) Ultrastructure of *Lamblia duodenalis*. 1. Body surface, sucking disc, and median bodies. J. Protozool. 11, 91-98.
Cheissin, E.M. (1965) Ultrastructure of *Lamblia duodenalis*. 2. The locomotory apparatus, axial rod and other organelles. Arch. Protistenkd. 108, 8-18.
Chen, T.R. (1977) In situ detection of mycoplasma contamination in cell cultures by fluorescent Hoechst 33258 stain. Exp. Cell Res. 104, 255-262.
Clark, J.T. (1985) Studies on the protein components from the plasma membrane and the extra-axonemal compartment of culture forms of the flagellate *Giardia intestinalis* (*lamblia*). Ph.D. Thesis, University of Hull.
Clark, J.T. and Holberton, D.V. (1986) Plasma membrane isolated from *Giardia lamblia*: identification of membrane proteins. Eur. J. Cell Biol. 42, 200-206.
Crossley, R. and Holberton, D.V. (1983a) Characterization of proteins from the cytoskeleton of *Giardia lamblia*. J. Cell Sci. 59, 81-103.
Crossley, R. and Holberton, D.V. (1983b) Selective extraction with Sarkosyl and repolymerization in vitro of cytoskeletal proteins from *Giardia*. J. Cell Sci. 62, 419-438.
Crossley, R. and Holberton, D.V. (1985) Assembly of 2.5 nm filaments from giardin, a protein associated with cytoskeleton microtubules in *Giardia*. J. Cell Sci. 78, 205-231.
Crossley, R., Marshall, J., Clark, J.T. and Holberton, D.V. (1986) Immunocytochemical differentiation of microtubules in the cytoskeleton of *Giardia lamblia* using monoclonal antibodies to α-tubulin and polyclonal antibodies to associated low molecular weight proteins. J. Cell Sci. 80, 233-252.
DeJonckheere, J.F. and Gordts, B. (1987) Occurrence and transfection of a *Giardia* virus. Mol. Biochem. Parasitol. 23, 85-89.

Einfeld, D.A. and Stibbs, H.H. (1984) Identification and characterization of a major surface antigen of *Giardia lamblia*. Infect. Immun. 46, 377-383.

Erlandsen, S.L. (1974) Scanning electron microscopy of intestinal giardiasis: lesions of the microvillous border of villus epithelial cells produced by trophozoites of *Giardia*. In: O. Johari (Ed.), Scanning Electron Microscopy, 1973, pp. 775-782. IIT Research Institute, Chicago.

Erlandsen, S.L. and Bemrick, W.J. (1987) SEM evidence for a new species, *Giardia psittaci*. J. Parasitol. 73, 623-629.

Erlandsen, S.L. and Chase, D.G. (1974) Morphological alterations in the microvillous border of villous epithelial cells produced by intestinal microorganisms. Am. J. Clin. Nutr. 27, 1277-1286.

Erlandsen, S.L. and Feely, D.E. (1984) Trophozoite motility and the mechanism of attachment. In: S.L. Erlandsen and E.A. Meyer (Eds), *Giardia* and Giardiasis. Biology, Pathogenesis, and Epidemiology, pp. 33-63. Plenum, New York.

Erlich, J.H., Anders, R.F., Roberts-Thomson, I.C., Schrader, J.W. and Mitchell, G.F. (1983) An examination of differences in serum antibody specificities and hypersensitivity reactions as contributing factors to chronic infection with the intestinal protozoan parasite, *Giardia muris*, in mice. Aust. J. Exp. Biol. Med. Sci. 61, 599-615.

Farthing, M.J.G., Pereira, M.E.A. and Keusch, G.T. (1986) Description and characterization of a surface lectin from *Giardia lamblia*. Infect. Immun. 51, 661-667.

Feely, D.E., Chase, D.G., Hardin, E.L. and Erlandsen, S.L. (1988) Ultrastructural evidence for the presence of bacteria, viral-like particles, and mycoplasma-like organisms associated with *Giardia* spp. J. Protozool. 35, 151-158.

Feely, D.E. and Dyer, J.K. (1987) Localization of acid phosphatase activity in *Giardia lamblia* and *Giardia muris* trophozoites. J. Protozool. 34, 80-83.

Feely, D.E. and Erlandsen, S.L. (1982) Effect of cytochalasin-B, low Ca^{2+} concentration, iodoacetic acid and quinacrine-HCl on the attachment of *Giardia* trophozoites in vitro. J. Parasitol. 68, 869-873.

Feely, D.E., Erlandsen, S.L. and Chase, D.G. (1984) Structure of the trophozoite and cyst. In: S.L. Erlandsen and E.A. Meyer (Eds), *Giardia* and Giardiasis. Biology, Pathogenesis, and Epidemiology, pp. 3-31. Plenum, New York.

Feely, D.E., Schollmeyer, J.V. and Erlandsen, S.L. (1982) *Giardia* sp.: distribution of contractile proteins in the attachment organelle. Exp. Parasitol. 53, 145-154.

Filice, F.P. (1952) Studies on the cytology and life history of *Giardia* from the laboratory rat. Univ. Calif. Publ. Zool. 57, 53-143.

Friend, D.S. (1966) The fine structure of *Giardia muris*. J. Cell Biol. 29, 317-332.

Garnier, J., Osguthorpe, D.J. and Robson, B. (1978) Analysis of the accuracy and implications of simple methods for predicting the secondary structure of globular proteins. J. Mol. Biol. 120, 97-120.

Holberton, D.V. (1973) Fine structure of the ventral disk apparatus and the mechanism of attachment in the flagellate *Giardia muris*. J. Cell Sci. 13, 11-41.

Holberton, D.V. (1981) Arrangement of subunits in microribbons from *Giardia*. J. Cell Sci. 47, 167-185.

Holberton, D.V., Crossley, R. and Marshall, J. (1981) Morphogenesis of the disc cytoskeleton in *Giardia*. Studies of microtubule assembly in vitro. 6th Int. Cong. Protozool. Warsaw.

Holberton, D.V. and Ward, A.P. (1981) Isolation of the cytoskeleton from *Giardia*. Tubulin and a low-molecular-weight protein associated with microribbon structures. J. Cell Sci. 47, 139-166.

Jarroll, E.L., Manning, P., Lindmark, D.G., Coggins, J.R. and Erlandsen, S.L. (1989) *Giardia* cyst wall-specific carbohydrate: evidence for the presence of galactosamine. Mol. Biochem. Parasitol. 32, 121–132.

Jones, R.D., Lemanski, C.L. and Jones, T.J. (1983) Theory of attachment in *Giardia*. Biophys. J. 44, 185-190.

Kilmartin, J.V., Wright, B. and Milstein, C. (1982) Rat monoclonal antitubulin antibodies derived by using a new nonsecreting rat cell line. J. Cell Biol. 93, 576-582.

Kosjuk, P.M. (1973) Functional morphology of *Lamblia duodenalis*. 4th Int. Cong. Protozool. Clermont-Ferrand.

Kulda, J. and Nohynkova, E. (1978) Flagellates of the human intestine and of intestines of other species. In:

J.P. Kreier (Ed.), Parasitic Protozoa, Vol. 2, pp. 69-104. Academic Press, New York.

Mazia, D., Schatten, G. and Sale, W. (1975) Adhesion of cells to surfaces coated with polylysine: applications to electronmicroscopy. J. Cell Biol. 66, 198-200.

McKeithan, T.W. and Rosenbaum, J.L. (1981) Multiple forms of tubulin in the cytoskeletal and flagellar microtubules of *Polytomella*. J. Cell Biol. 91, 352-360.

Mueller, J.C., Jones, A.L. and Brandborg, L.L. (1974) Scanning electron microscope observations in human giardiasis. In: O. Johari (Ed.), Scanning Electron Microscopy, 1973, pp. 557-564. IIT Research Institute, Chicago.

Muller, E. (1890) Ein Fund von *Cercomonas intestinalis* im Jejenum des Menschen. Biol. Forsch. Forh. Stockholm 2, 42-54.

Nash, T.E., Gillin, F.D. and Smith, P.D. (1983) Excretory-secretory products of *Giardia lamblia*. J. Immunol. 131, 2004-2010.

Nemanic, P.C., Owen, R.L., Stevens, D.P. and Mueller, J.C. (1978) Ultrastructural observations on giardiasis in a mouse model. II. Endosymbiosis and organelle distribution in *Giardia muris* and *Giardia lamblia*. J. Infect. Dis. 140, 222-228.

Owen, R.L., Nemanic, P.C. and Stevens, D.P. (1979) Ultrastructural observations on giardiasis in a murine model. I. Intestinal distribution, attachment, and relation to the immune system of *Giardia muris*. Gastroenterology 76, 757-769.

Radulescu, S., Burghelea, B., Meitert, T., Petrovici, A. and Meyer, E. (1986) Ultrastructural studies on the bacterial symbiont in *Giardia lamblia*. Arch. Roum. Pathol. Exp. Microbiol. 45, 285-292.

Rubin, R.W. (1984) Membrane tubulin: fact or fiction? BioEssays 1, 157-160.

Russell, D.G., Miller, D. and Gull, K. (1984) Tubulin heterogeneity in the trypanosome *Crithidia fasciculata*. Mol. Cell Biol. 4, 779-790.

Sheffield, H.G. and Bjorvatn, B. (1977) Ultrastructure of the cyst of *Giardia lamblia*. Am. J. Trop. Med. Hyg. 26, 23-30.

Simon, C.E. (1921) *Giardia enterica*: a parasitic flagellate of man. Am. J. Trop. Med. Hyg. 1, 440-491.

Stephens, R.E. (1981) Chemical differences distinguish ciliary membrane and axonemal tubulins. Biochemistry 20, 4716-4723.

Taylor, D.G. and Wenman, W.M. (1987) Human immune response to *Giardia lamblia* infection. J. Infect. Dis. 155, 137-140.

Wang, A.L. and Wang, C.C. (1986) Discovery of a specific double-stranded RNA virus in *Giardia lamblia*. Mol. Biochem. Parasitol. 21, 269-276.

Ward, H.D., Alroy, J., Lev, B.I., Keusch, G.T. and Pereira, M.E. (1985) Identification of chitin as a structural component of *Giardia* cysts. Infect. Immun. 49, 629-634.

Wehland, J., Schroder, H.C. and Weber, K. (1984) Amino acid sequence requirements in the epitope recognized by the α-tubulin-specific rat monoclonal antibody YL 1/2. Eur. Mol. Biol. Organ. J. 3, 1295-1300.

Wenrich, D.H. (1940) Observations on parasites and inclusion bodies in certain intestinal protozoa. Science 92, 416-417.

Zabel, E. (1901) *Megastoma intestinale* und andere Parasiten in der Zotten eines Magenkrebes. Arch. Verdau. Kr. 7, 509-554.

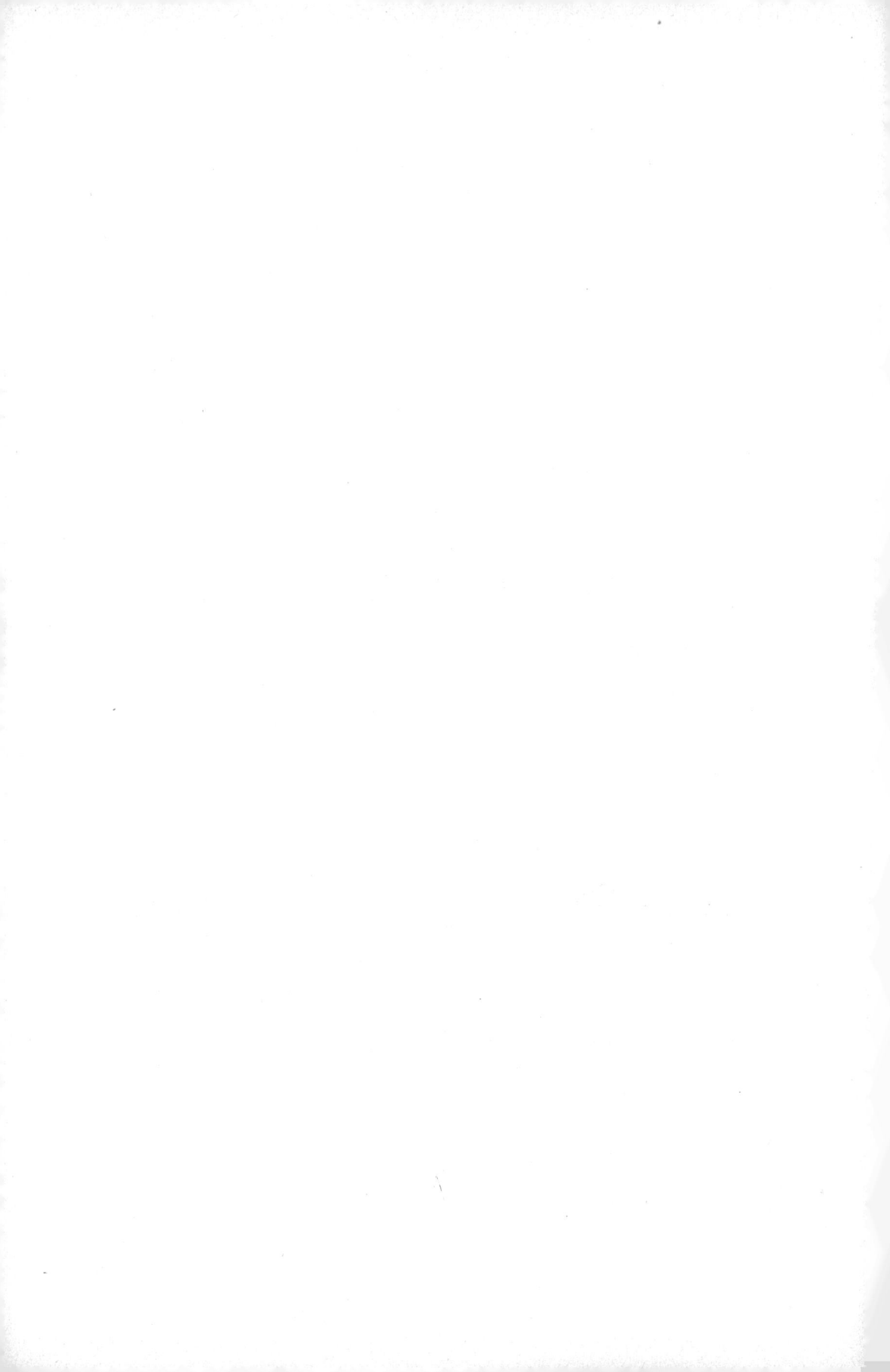

Giardiasis (E.A. Meyer, ed.)
© 1990 Elsevier Science Publishers B.V. (Biomedical Division)

2

Taxonomy and nomenclature

ERNEST A. MEYER

Department of Microbiology and Immunology, Oregon Health Sciences University, Portland, OR 97201, U.S.A.

1. *Giardia* classification: Phylum to Family	51
2. *Giardia* classification: Genus, species and race	52
2.1. Traditional criteria for naming *Giardia* species	52
2.2. The recommendations of Filice	53
2.3. Chemotaxonomy	54
2.3.1. Antigenic comparisons	54
2.3.2. Restriction endonuclease analysis	56
2.3.3. Isozyme determinations	56
2.4. Host specificity as a criterion for defining *Giardia* species	57
2.5. The demonstration of morphologically different *Giardia*	57
References	58

1. Giardia *classification: Phylum to Family*

In 1964, a committee of the Society of Protozoologists, recognizing the need for a thorough revision of the schemes then used for classifying the groups of organisms comprising the Phylum Protozoa, published its 'modern' classification of the Phylum (Honigberg et al., 1964). Subsequently, changes in that classification were proposed by two major figures in the systematics of parasitic protozoa. Levine's (1973) recommended changes principally involved the Sporozoa; in the subphylum Sarcomastigophora, in which the *Giardia* belong, he changed the ending of the names of some taxa. Baker's (1977) proposal was a compromise between that offered by the Society of Protozoologist's committee and Levine; Baker's classification of *Giardia* adhered to the scheme put forth by the Society of Protozoologist's committee. According to that committee's classification, organisms in the genus *Giardia* (Kunstler, 1983) belong to the

Subphylum: SARCOMASTIGOPHORA (Honigberg and Balamuth, 1963), with a single type of nucleus, vesicular; sexuality, if present, syngamy; with flagella, pseudopodia, or both types of locomotory organelles; typically no spore formation.

Superclass: MASTIGOPHORA (Diesing, 1866), one or more flagella typically present in trophozoites; asexual reproduction, basically by longitudinal binary fission; sexual reproduction unknown in many groups.

Class: ZOOMASTIGOPHOREA (Calkins, 1909), chromatophores absent; one to many flagella; ameboid forms, with or without flagella in some groups; sexuality absent in most groups; predominantly parasitic.

Order: DIPLOMONADIDA (Wenyon, 1926), with two karyomastigonts, each with four flagella; at least one of these flagella is recurrent; with two nuclei; without mitochondria or Golgi apparatus; with cysts; free-living or parasitic.

Further, the *Giardia* belong to the

Family: HEXAMITIDAE (Kent, 1980), six or eight flagella, two nuclei and sometimes axostyles and median or parabasal bodies; bilaterally symmetrical.

This family contains six genera, three of which (including *Giardia*) are exclusively parasitic. Discussions of the evolutionary relationships and taxonomy of this group are to be found in the papers of Brugerolle (1975), and Kulda and Nohynkova (1978).

2. Giardia *classification: Genus, species and race*

The evolution of genus and species names in this group has been alluded to in the introduction (Section 1.3). Organisms in the genus *Giardia* differ from other members of the family Hexamitidae in possessing an adhesive disk, which serves as an attachment organelle, on the flattened ventral surface of the trophozoite. While all of the members of this genus are parasites of vertebrates, members of only one of the several recognized morphological types have been shown to be capable of infecting humans. Parenthetically, some workers refer to organisms in this genus as belonging to the genus *Lamblia*.

2.1. Traditional criteria for naming Giardia species

Until the middle of this century, it was common practice to assign *Giardia* species names on the basis of host specificity, and on differences in various trophozoite dimensions. Many workers believed that these were valid species criteria, although little evidence was available to support it.

It was also recognized that all of the described 'species' in the genus could be divided into three morphological groups. Basis for this division was the shape and position of median bodies (intracellular organelles composed of microtubules) in the trophozoite and, in some cases, the shape of the trophozoite.

By 1978, Kulda and Nohýnková were able, in their review, to list references to more than 40 *Giardia* 'species'. Indeed, representatives of this genus appear to exist intestinally in virtually every mammalian species in which they have been systematically sought.

2.2. The recommendations of Filice

In 1952, Francis Filice published a monograph describing the results of his *Giardia* studies. Although most of the work involved describing the cytology and life history of organisms from a laboratory rat, Filice also addressed the problem of *Giardia* taxonomy. He concluded that the use of host specificity and body dimensions were untrustworthy species criteria in this genus. He further suggested assigning species status to each of the

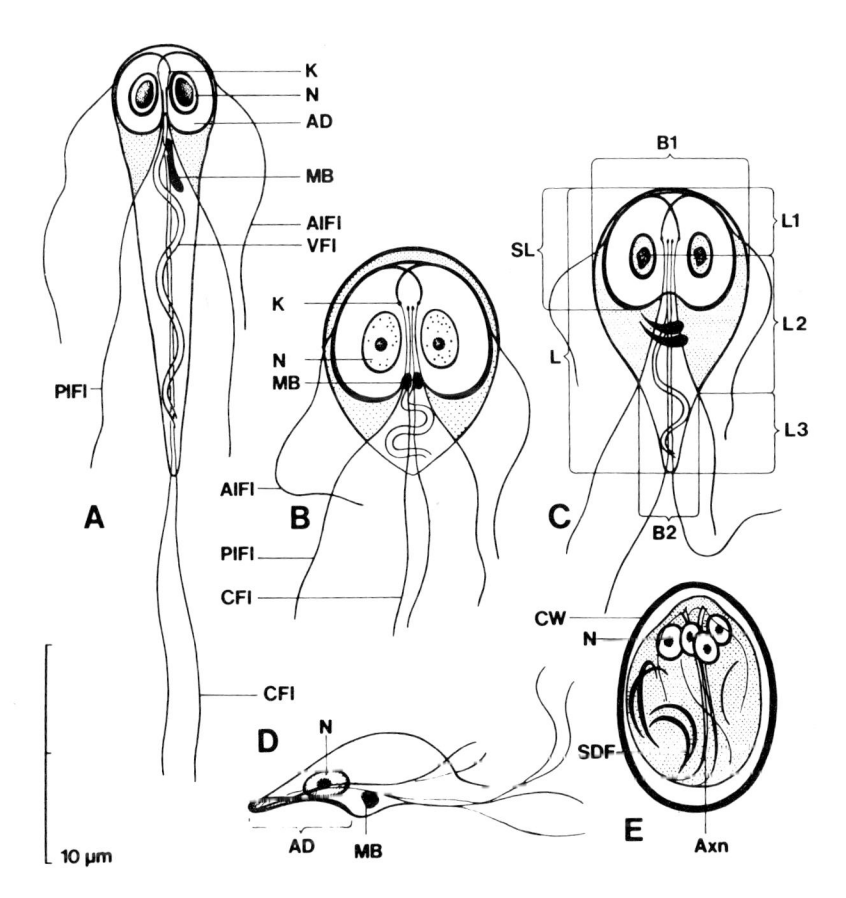

Fig. 1. Semidiagrammatic representation of three morphological types of *Giardia* viewed in the light microscope. (A-C) Ventral view of trophozoites of *G. agilis* from amphibians (A), *G. muris* from mice (B), and *G. duodenalis* from man (C). (D and E) *G. duodenalis*, lateral view of a trophozoites (D) and cyst (E). Trophozoites of the *G. agilis* group (A) have a long and narrow body, a relatively short adhesive disc and long club-shaped median bodies (MB) situated parallel to the longitudinal axis of the cell. Trophozoites of the *G. muris* group (B) have a broad, short body with a large adhesive disk overlapping in length one-half of the body length. Median bodies (MB) are small and round, situated parallel to the longitudinal axis of the cell. Trophozoites of the *G. duodenalis* group (C) have a pyriform body with an adhesive disk shorter than one-half of the body length. From Kulda and Nohýnková (1978).

three median body types which were clearly differentiable. He also proposed ascribing 'race' or other nontaxonomic but pragmatic status to all those *Giardia* of a given species to indicate their host origin or size. Finally, he recommended assigning new *Giardia* species names to organisms that differ from existing species on the basis of demonstrably constant biological differences. Presumably these differences might be morphologic or physiologic in nature.

Those *Giardia* of the median body type that parasitize humans (and a variety of other vertebrates) have been called *Giardia duodenalis* by Filice (1952); that terminology will be used in this volume. *G. duodenalis* median bodies are more often double than single. They resemble the claw of a claw hammer and lie transversely across the trophozoite body. The median bodies of other *Giardia* species are either teardrop-shaped (*G. agilis*), or small and rounded (*G. muris*) (see Fig. 1).

The *Giardia* species *duodenalis* thus includes all of the 23 'species' listed by Kulda and Nohýnková in their 1978 review, that have the 'duodenalis' type median body. Since that review, other *Giardia* of the same morphologic type have been described from other animal hosts [e.g., the llama (Kiorpes et al., 1987)].

It should be pointed out that there are proponents of the use of trophozoite measurements, along with host specificity, biochemical and immunologic studies, in defining *Giardia* species. The arguments in favor of the use of morphometrics are put forth in a paper by Woo (1984); the arguments against morphometrics have been presented by Bertram et al. (1984).

2.3. Chemotaxonomy

Increasingly, chemotaxonomy is being used to address the problem of classifying a variety of parasites, including the *Giardia*. For chemotaxonomic studies of parasitic protozoa, axenic cultures are greatly to be desired, both for the purpose of avoiding confusing results presented by contaminants, and to permit replication and comparison. In the case of *Giardia*, the number of axenic cultures available is still somewhat limited; cultures have only been available in relatively recent years. Not all *Giardia* of the *duodenalis* type can be cultured by existing methods.

Most *Giardia* chemotaxonomic studies have focused on three aspects of these organisms: (1) antigenic comparisons, determined by a variety of methods, (2) isozyme determinations, and (3) DNA analysis. A summary of references to much of this recent work is contained in Table 1.

2.3.1. Antigenic comparisons
In the studies cited above, common as well as different antigens have repeatedly been demonstrated between different axenic *Giardia* cultures. While it is to be hoped that advantage can be taken of antigenic analyses in identifying and classifying *Giardia*, several problems remain before this can be routine. First, the method of antigenic determination ideally should lend itself to quantitation; many such methods do not.

TABLE 1

The chemotaxonomic study of *Giardia*: references

Reference	Aspect of *Giardia* chemotaxonomy studied		
	Antigenic comparisons	Isozyme determinations	DNA analysis
Visvesvara et al., 1977	X		
Bertram, 1982	X	X	
Smith et al., 1982	X		
Bertram et al., 1983		X	
Nash et al., 1983	X		
Einfeld and Stibbs, 1984	X		
Nash et al., 1985			X
Nash and Keister, 1985	X		X
Baveja et al., 1986		X	
Korman et al., 1986	X	X	
Nash and Aggarwal, 1986	X		
Wenman et al., 1986	X		
Ungar and Nash, 1987	X		
Aggarwal and Nash, 1987	X		
Isaac-Renton et al., 1988	X		
Meloni et al., 1988		X	
Thompson et al., 1988		X	X

One quantitative approach to identifying these differences is to prepare monoclonal antibodies against a specific group of *Giardia*, and determine whether the antigen(s) in question are present on other trophozoites. Nash and Aggarwal (1986) describe such an approach. Alternatively, reaction of antibody to *Giardia* isolates with other *Giardia* can be quantitated using single antibody ELISA tests; by this means Ungar and Nash (1987) have quantitated differences between a number of *Giardia* isolates. Their data confirm earlier indications that these organisms have both different and common antigens.

A second problem: several recent papers include observations regarding antigenic variation in *Giardia*; these should be taken into account in studies aimed at antigenic characterization. Boreham et al (1987) suggest that the axenic *Giardia* stock cultures that they have studied were not homogeneous, but rather were composed of different populations of organisms. These workers made 11 and 15 clones of trophozoites from each of two stock cultures, then determined and compared the resistance to four anti-*Giardia* agents of the 26 clones and the two parent cultures. They concluded, because of the variation they observed in drug sensitivity of the clones studied, that each parent culture was composed of a mixture of different organisms. Presumably other supposed axenic *Giardia* cultures may consist of mixtures as well.

In a study of antigenic variation, Aggarwal and Nash (1988) report that a single *Giardia* trophozoite can give rise, in vivo as well as in vitro, to trophozoites with varying surface antigens. They believe that, in vitro, antibody may be a mechanism for selecting *Giardia* with varying surface antigens. On the other hand, the rapidity with which antigenic changes take place after infection suggested to them that factors other than immune pressure may confer a biological advantage on some organisms and result in the predominance of one antigenic variant.

The antigenic profile of a *Giardia* culture may also vary if the trophozoites harbor endosymbionts. The recent observations of Wang and Wang (1986) that some *Giardia* contain RNA viruses, and that of Feely (1988) and Radulescu et al. (1986) of endosymbiotic bacteria inside *Giardia* raise the possibility that such agents may affect antigenic, as well as other chemotaxonomic, determinations.

2.3.2. Restriction endonuclease analysis

A single comparison of *Giardia* DNA by restriction endonuclease analysis has been reported. Nash et al. (1985) employed this procedure to study 15 *Giardia* isolates; nine different patterns could be distinguished. While some animal and human isolates were indistinguishable in this analysis, the banding patterns of three isolates were quite dissimilar from any other. This method offers promise as an important means of distinguishing and characterizing *Giardia* isolates.

2.3.3. Isozyme determinations

Studies of isozymes (or isoenzymes), multiple molecular forms of a given enzyme produced by different representatives of the same species, have yielded much information useful in parasite characterization recently. Four such studies have involved *Giardia*. Bertram et al. (1983) studied six enzymes from five axenic *Giardia* isolates from cat, human and guinea pig hosts. They were able to divide their isolates into three zymodemes, groups with identical enzyme patterns. This study demonstrated that *Giardia* isozymes exist and can be used to characterize these organisms. Baveja et al. (1986) studied four enzymes of four *Giardia* isolates. They reported that their isolates could be grouped in three different zymodemes. Korman et al. (1986) studied five *Giardia* isolates by antiserum agglutination and by characterizing five enzymes. They demonstrated considerable heterogeneity both in surface antigens and in enzymes in their isolates.

The most extensive study to date of *Giardia* isozymes was that reported by Meloni et al. (1988). It involved the study of 25 cultures from humans, four from cats, and a single strain obtained from an infected rat and not cultured but maintained by passage in mice. In the latter instance, trophozoites for enzyme analysis were washed out of mouse small intestine. Ten different enzymes were studied; 13 zymodemes were identified. Analysis of the resultant data included determination of Euclidean distances, and construction of a phenogram based on these values. Of the three general approaches to *Giardia* chemotaxonomy (antigen comparison, DNA analysis, isozyme determination), isozyme characterization and analysis, as exemplified by the elegant studies of Meloni et al. (1988) would seem to offer a superior means of quantitating genetic relatedness among these organisms.

2.4. Host specificity as a criterion for defining Giardia *species*

Woo (1984), among others, has suggested that host specificity be used as one of the criteria for defining *Giardia* species. In meticulous cross-transmission studies, Woo has demonstrated that some *Giardia* are apparently highly host specific, and that others are capable of infecting several different animal species. The laboratory conditions that must be met to carry out these experiments appropriately are so detailed that such experiments can by no means be conducted routinely.

Further, because the initiation of *Giardia* infection depends on both parasite and host factors, it is difficult to interpret the failure of a challenge organism to infect an animal. How is one to interpret, for example, recent experiments by Nash et al. (1987) in which two groups of human volunteers were challenged with two *Giardia* isolates from humans? One of the isolates proved uniformly infectious; the other isolate failed to infect any of the challenged volunteers.

Recent cross-transmission experiments by Erlandsen et al. (1988) illustrate the difficulties involved in interpreting such studies. These workers challenged beavers and muskrats with graded doses of viable cysts from a variety of animals, including humans. They concluded that, at this time, it is not possible to assign a major role in waterborne transmission of human giardiasis, to beaver, muskrat, or, for that matter, any other nonhuman animal.

The Mongolian gerbil (*Meriones unguiculatus*) is probably the most used animal model (Belosevic et al., 1983) for studying infections caused by *G. duodenalis* organisms. Nevertheless, the variable success obtained in transmission experiments involving challenging the gerbil with *Giardia* from humans makes interpretation difficult. Visvesvara et al. (1988), for example, studying *Giardia* cysts from 10 human donors, found only one donor whose cysts consistently were infectious for, and resulted in cyst excretion in, the gerbil. Cysts from four patients were not infectious; cysts from the other five patients infected some but not all animals in the test groups. Swabby et al. (1988) had similar variable results; they reported successfully infecting gerbils with *Giardia* from 58% (14/24) of human donors. Results such as these underline the difficulties involved in interpreting cross-transmission studies. To complicate the picture, some strains of *Giardia* trophozoites from humans are apparently capable of colonizing the gerbil small intestine, yet are not excreted as cysts. Visvesvara et al. (1988) identified such infections at necropsy. In contrast, Belosevic et al. (1983) reported infections in all of the gerbils he inoculated with cysts from five human patients, and with trophozoites from culture; cysts were intermittently produced by all animals.

2.5. The demonstration of morphologically different Giardia

The differentiation of *G. duodenalis* from *G. muris* and *G. agilis* as proposed by Filice (1952) is based principally on median body descriptions; it was made at a time when examination of stained specimens by light microscopy was the principal means of describing these organisms. In the intervening years, advances in microscopy, both in electron and light microscopy, have made possible the examination of *Giardia* structure in greater detail, and the identification of morphological differences between organisms in the genus. Recently, two such morphologic differences have been reported among *Giardia duodenalis* organisms which might merit creating separate species.

Erlandsen and Bemrick (1987) studied by scanning electron microscopy (SEM) trophozoites of the budgerigar; the organisms have not been cultured. The organisms earlier had been described, by light microscopy, by Box (1981); she described its median bodies and, in keeping with Filice's proposal, had suggested the name *Giardia duodenalis* race psittaci. Erlandsen and Bemrick (1987) noted that, by SEM, the budgerigar organism differs from all other *G. duodenalis* in lacking a ventrolateral flange, and therefore lacked a marginal groove bordering the adhesive disk. The absence of such an organelle would seem to meet Filice's criterion for elevation to species status.

Feely studied another *Giardia* of the *duodenalis* type, a parasite of the prairie vole (*Microtus ochrogaster*). Kofoid and Christiansen had named an organism of this description from the meadow mouse *G. microti* in 1915; at this time species names were based on morphologic descriptions and assumed host specificity. The ultrastructure of *G. duodenalis* cysts and the process of excystation have only been described in detail in the last decade or so (Sheffield and Bjorvatn, 1977; Bingham et al., 1979). In studying these cysts by light and electron microscopy, Feely noted that they differed morphologically from other *G. duodenalis* cysts; cysts from the prairie vole contained two differentiated trophozoites, each having a mature ventral disk. Apparently one other *Giardia*, a parasite of voles and muskrats, has been described as exhibiting two ventral disks in the encysted organism (Waters et al., 1940). It will be of interest to determine the animal host distribution of parasites of this type. If this morphologic difference can be shown to be a constant one, organisms of this type would seem to qualify for consideration as a separate species.

References

Aggarwal, A. and Nash, T.E. (1987) *Giardia lamblia*: RNA translation products. Exp. Parasitol. 64, 336-341.

Aggarwal, A. and Nash, T.E. (1988) Antigenic variation of *Giardia lamblia* in vivo. Infect. Immun. 56, 1420-1423.

Baker, J.R. (1977) Systematics of parasitic protozoa. In: J.P. Kreier (Ed.), Parasitic Protozoa, Vol. 1, pp. 35-56. Academic Press, New York.

Baveja, U.K., Jyoti, A.S., Kaur, M., Agarwal, D.S., Anand, B.S. and Nanda, R. (1986) Isoenzyme studies of *Giardia lamblia* isolated from symptomatic cases. Aust. J. Exp. Biol. Med. Sci. 64, 119-126.

Belosevic, M., Faubert, G.M., MacLean, J.D., Law, C. and Croll, N.A. (1983) *Giardia lamblia* infections in Mongolian gerbils: an animal model. J. Infect. Dis. 147, 222-226.

Bertram, M.A. (1982) A comparison of axenic cultures of *Giardia* trophozoites from different mammalian hosts. Ph.D. Dissertation, Oregon Health Sciences University, Portland.

Bertram, M.A., Meyer, E.A., Lile, J.D. and Morse, S.A. (1983) A comparison of isoenzymes of five axenic

Giardia isolates. J. Parasit. 69, 793-801.
Bertram, M.A., Meyer, E.A., Anderson, D.L. and Jones, C.T. (1984) A morphometric comparison of five axenic *Giardia* isolates. J. Parasit. 70, 530-535.
Boreham, P.F.L., Phillips, R.E. and Sheperd, R.W. (1987) Heterogeneity in the responses of clones of *Giardia intestinalis* to anti-giardia drugs. Trans. R. Soc. Trop. Med. Hyg. 81, 406-407.
Box, E.D. (1981) Observations on *Giardia* of budgerigars. J. Protozool. 28, 491-494.
Brugerolle, G. (1975) Contribution à l'étude cytologique et phylétique des Diplozoaires (Zoomastigophorea, Diplozoa Dangeard, 1910). VI. Caractères généraux des Diplozoaires. Protistologica 11, 111-118.
Einfeld, D.A. and Stibbs, H.H. (1984) Identification and characterization of a major surface antigen of *Giardia lamblia*. Infect. Immun. 46, 377-383.
Erlandsen, S.L. and Bemrick, W.J. (1987) SEM evidence for a new species, *Giardia psittaci*. J. Parasit. 73, 623-629.
Erlandsen, S.L., Sherlock, L.A., Januschka, M., Schupp, D.G., Schaefer, F.W., Jakubowski, W. and Bemrick, W.J. (1988) Cross-species transmission of *Giardia* spp.: Inoculation of beavers and muskrats with cysts of human, beaver, mouse and muskrat origin. Appl. Environ. Microbiol. 54, 2777-2785.
Feely, D.E. (1988) Morphology of the cyst of *Giardia microti* by light and electron microscopy. J. Protozool. 35, 52-54.
Filice, F.P. (1952) Studies on the cytology and life history of a *Giardia* from the laboratory rat. Univ. Calif. Publ. Zool. 57, 53-145.
Honigberg, B.M., Balamuth, W., Bovee, E.C., Corliss, J.O., Gojdics, M., Hall, R.P., Kudo, R.R., Levine, N.D., Loeblich, A.R., Weiser, J. and Wenrich, D.H. (1964) A revised classification of the Phylum Protozoa. J. Protozool. 11, 7-20.
Isaac-Renton, J.L., Byrne, S.K. and Prameya, R. (1988) Isoelectric focusing of ten strains of *Giardia duodenalis*. J. Parasit. 74, 1054-1056.
Kiorpes, A.L., Kirkpatrick, C.E. and Bowman, D.D. (1987) Isolation of *Giardia* from a llama and from sheep. Can. J. Vet. Res. 51, 277-280.
Korman, S.H., Le Blancq, S.M., Spira, D.T., El On, J., Reifer, R.M. and Deckelbaum, R.J. (1986) *Giardia lamblia*: Identification of different strains from man. Z. Parasitenkund. 173-180.
Kulda, J. and Nohynkova, E. (1978) Flagellates of the human intestine and of intestine of other species. In: J.P. Kreier (Ed.), Parasitic Protozoa, Vol. II, pp. 2-139. Academic Press, New York.
Levine, N.D. (1973) Protozoan Parasites of Domestic Animals and of Man. Burgess Publishing Company, Minneapolis.
Meloni, B.P., Lymbery, A.J. and Thompson, R.C.A. (1988) Isoenzyme electrophoresis of 30 isolates of *Giardia* from humans and felines. Amer. J. Trop. Med. Hyg. 38, 65-73.
Nash, T.E. and Aggarwal, A. (1986) Cytotoxicity of monoclonal antibodies to a subset of *Giardia* isolates. J. Immunol. 136, 2628-2632.
Nash, T.E. and Keister, D.B. (1985) Differences in excretory-secretory products and surface antigens among 19 isolates of *Giardia*. J. Infect. Dis. 152, 1166-1171.
Nash, T.E., Gillin, F.D. and Smith, P.D. (1983) Excretory-secretory products of *Giardia lamblia*. J. Immunol. 131, 2004-2010.
Nash, T.E., McCutchan, T., Keister, D., Dame, J.B., Conrad, J.D. and Gillin, F.D. (1985) Restriction-endonuclease analysis of DNA from 15 *Giardia* isolates obtained from humans and animals. J. Infect. Dis. 152, 64-73.
Nash, T.E., Herrington, D.A., Losonsky, G.A. and Levine, M.M. (1987) Experimental human infections with *Giardia lamblia*. J. Infect. Dis. 156, 974-984.
Radulescu, S., Burghelea, B., Beitert, T., Petrovici, A. and Meyer, E. (1986) Ultrastructural study on the bacterial symbiont in *Giardia lamblia*. Arch. Roum. Path. Exp. Microbiol. 45, 285-292.
Smith, P.D., Gillin, F.D., Kaushal, N.A. and Nash, T.E. (1982) Antigenic analysis of *Giardia lamblia* from Afghanistan, Puerto Rico, Ecuador, and Oregon. Infect. Imm. 36, 714-719.
Swabby, K.D., Hibler, C.P. and Wegrzyn, J.G. (1988) In: P.M. Wallis and B.R. Hammond (Eds.), Advances in

Giardia Research, 1988, pp. 75–77. University of Calgary Press, Calgary. Infection of Mongolian gerbils (*Meriones unguiculatus*) with *Giardia* from human and animal sources.

Thompson, R.C.A., Meloni, B.P. and Lymebery, A.J. (1988) Humans and cats have genetically identical forms of *Giardia*: evidence of a zoonotic relationship. Med. J. Australia 143, 207-209.

Ungar, B.L.P. and Nash, T.E. (1987) Cross-reactivity among different *Giardia lamblia* isolates using immunofluorescent antibody and enzyme immunoassay techniques. Amer. J. Trop. Med. Hyg. 37, 283-289.

Visvesvara, G.S., Healy, G.R. and Meyer, E.A. (1977) Comparative antigenic analysis of *Giardia lamblia* trophozoites grown axenically in medium supplemented with either human, bovine, or rabbit serum. Fifth Intern. Cong. Protozool. New York, June 26-July 2. P. 175.

Visvesvara, G.S., Dickerson, J.W. and Healy, G.R. (1988) Variable infectivity of human-derived *Giardia lamblia* cysts for Mongolian gerbils (*Meriones unguiculatus*). J. Clin. Microbiol. 26, 837-841.

Wang, A.L. and Wang, C.C. (1986) Discovery of a specific double-stranded RNA virus in *Giardia lamblia*. Molec. Biochem. Parasitol. 21, 269-276.

Waters, P.C., Fiene, A.R. and Becker, E.R. (1940) Strains of *Giardia ondatrae* Travis. 1939. Trans. Am. Microsc. Soc. 59, 160-162.

Wenman, W.M., Meuser, R.U. and Wallis, P.M. (1986) Antigenic analysis of *Giardia duodenalis* strains isolated in Alberta. Can. J. Microbiol. 32, 926-929.

Woo, P.K. (1984) Evidence for animal reservoirs and transmission of *Giardia* infection between animal species. In: S.L. Erlandsen and E.A. Meyer (Eds.), *Giardia* and Giardiasis, pp. 341-364. Plenum Press, New York.

Giardiasis (E.A. Meyer, ed.)
© 1990 Elsevier Science Publishers B.V. (Biomedical Division)

3

Giardia metabolism

EDWARD L. JARROLL and DONALD G. LINDMARK

Department of Biology, Cleveland State University, 1983 E. 24th Street, Cleveland, Ohio 44115, U.S.A.

1. Introduction	61
2. Energy and carbohydrate mechanism	62
3. Lipid metabolism and composition	65
4. Nucleic acid metabolism	67
4.1. Pyrimidine metabolism	67
4.2. Purine metabolism	70
5. Hydrolases and synthetases	72
6. Summary	74
References	75

1. Introduction

Members of the genus *Giardia* have been characterized as being aerotolerant anaerobes which rely on substrate level phosphorylation, iron-sulfur protein and flavoprotein mediated electron transport for the production of energy (Lindmark, 1980; Weinbach et al., 1980; Lindmark and Jarroll, 1984). *Giardia* lacks mitochondria and microbodies, but these protozoans contain lysosome-like organelles that not only accumulate ferritin but also stain positively in histochemical reactions for acid phosphatase and aryl sulphatase (Feely, 1985; Feely and Dyer, 1987).

As recently as ten years ago, the paucity of knowledge on the biochemistry and metabolism of *Giardia* would have made an attempt to write this chapter futile, but this situation has changed markedly since 1980. Perhaps the single major advancement that has permitted this change was the successful axenic cultivation of human source *Giardia* trophozoites in vitro (Meyer, 1976). As a result of this breakthrough, several papers dealing with the biochemical and metabolic nature of this parasite have begun to appear.

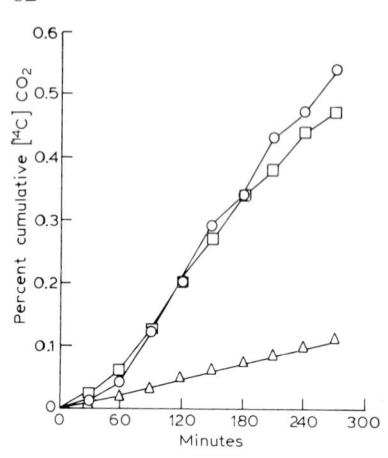

Fig. 1. Radiorespirometric patterns for the evolution of $^{14}CO_2$ from specifically labeled [^{14}C]glucose during the growth of *Giardia lamblia* trophozoites. ○, [3,4-^{14}C]glucose; □ [1-^{14}C]glucose; △ [6, ^{14}C]glucose. From Jarroll et al. (1981). With permission.

2. Energy and carbohydrate metabolism

Giardia trophozoites exhibit oxygen-independent endogenous respiration over the range 10-210 μM O_2 at a linear rate of approximately 93 nmoles of O_2/min/mg protein at 37°C (Lindmark, 1980).

Glucose (Lindmark, 1980), and ethanol (Weinbach et al., 1980) reportedly stimulated respiration in intact cells while NADH and NADPH increased respiration ten-fold only after the cells were lysed (Weinbach et al., 1980). Respiration was not stimulated by other carbohydrates (e.g., D-fructose, D-ribose, maltose, D-mannose, mannitol), Krebs cycle intermediates (e.g., succinate, fumarate, a-ketoglutarate, citrate), or organic acids (e.g. pyruvate, acetate, L-lactate) (Lindmark, 1980). Weinbach et al. (1980) stated that malate stimulated respiration, but Lindmark (1980) was unable to demonstrate similar results. Respiration was inhibited by iodoacetamide and quinacrine, but not by cyanide, 2,4-dinitrophenol, rotenone, malonate, sodium arsenate, or sodium arsenite (Lindmark, 1980; Weinbach et al., 1980).

Intact *Giardia* trophozoites in the presence of exogenous glucose produce ethanol and acetate as organic end product as demonstrated by silicic acid column chromatography and enzymatic analysis (Jarroll et al., 1981; Lindmark, 1980). Aerobically, approximately six times more acetate than ethanol is produced; anaerobically, at least two times more ethanol than acetate is produced. Under either atmospheric condition, CO_2 is the only gaseous end product that has been detected (Lindmark, 1980). Based on the pattern of CO_2 evolution (Fig. 1) when specifically radiolabeled glucose was used as a substrate under anaerobic conditions, *Giardia* trophozoites metabolize glucose at approximately equivalent rates via the Embden-Meyerhof-Parnas (EMP) [3,4-^{14}C glucose and the hexose monophosphate (HM) pathways [1-^{14}C glucose] (Jarroll et al., 1981).

Besides radiorespirometric data suggesting the presence of the EMP pathways, two enzymes, hexokinase and fructose-biphosphate aldolase, have been demonstrated (Lindmark, 1980). The specific activity of these and some of the other enzymes of carbohydrate and energy metabolism are presented in Table 1. Citrate synthetase, isocitrate dehydrogenase, succinate dehydrogenase, fumarate hydratase, lactate dehydrogenase, acetate kinase, phosphate acetyltransferase, hydrogenase and catalase activities were below the limits of detection. All of the energy metabolism enzymes detected were nonsedimentable at 109 000 × g for 30 min (Lindmark, 1980).

TABLE 1
Specific activities of enzymes in *G. duodenalis (lamblia)*

Enzyme	Activity mU/mg protein ± SD (No. of determinations)
Hexokinase	24 ± 8 (2)
Fructose-biphosphate aldolase	61 + 21 (2)
Pyruvate kinase	122 ± 15 (6)
Phosphoenolpyruvate carboxykinase	21 ± 5 (3)
Malate dehydrogenase	921 ± 52 (10)
Malate dehydrogenase (decarboxylating)	120 ± 31 (6)
Pyruvate synthase	301 ± 63 (5)
Acetyl-CoA synthetase	20 ± 5 (3)
Alcohol dehydrogenase	461 ± 36 (3)
NADPH oxidoreductase	412 ± 25 (3)
NADPH dehydrogenase	310 ± 32 (8)
NADH dehydrogenase	201 ± 23 (7)
Superoxide dismutase	2400 ± 500 (2)
Acid phosphatase	77 ± 15 (8)

Homogenates were prepared as described in Materials and Methods. All assays were run at 30°C except alcohol dehydrogenase (19°C). From Lindmark (1980). With permission.

Until recently, studies on *Giardia* carbohydrate and energy metabolism were confined to trophozoites even though work by Bingham et al. (1979) suggested that *Giardia* cysts were metabolically active since their ability to excyst decreased as storage temperature and time increased. Recently, Lindmark and Miller (1988) using *G. duodenalis* trophozoites, cysts of *G. duodenalis* and *G. muris* purified (Sauch, 1984) from the feces of gerbils and mice, respectively, and *G. muris* trophozoites obtained by excystation of purified *G. muris* cysts investigated the activity of key enzymes of glucose metabolism in all of these forms. Lysates prepared by exposure of intact cells to 0.1% Triton X-100 produced the following results: hexokinase, pyruvate kinase, phosphoenolpyruvate carboxykinase, pyruvate:ferredoxin oxidoreductase (pyruvate synthase), alcohol dehydrogenase, NADPH oxidoreductase, malate dehydrogenase, and malate dehydrogenase (decarboxylating) activities were detected in the trophozoites and cysts of both *Giardia* species. All of these enzymes exhibited similar specific activities in both species regardless of the life cycle stage (Tables 1 and 2). Evidence for respiration in *G. muris* cysts

TABLE 2

Specific activities of enzymes in *Giardia**

Enzyme	Activity mU/mg protein ± SD (No. of determinations)		
	G. lamblia	*G. muris*	
	Cyst	Trophozoite	Cyst
Hexokinase	20 ± 6 (5)	15 ± 3 (4)	10 ± 4 (4)
Pyruvate kinase	101 ± 20 (3)	190 ± 39 (3)	110 ± 5 (2)
Phosphoenolpyruvate carboxykinase	18 ± 14 (6)	22 ± 4 (3)	10 ± 2 (3)
Malate dehydrogenase	701 ± 15 (5)	600 ± 40 (5)	510 ± 18 (5)
Malate dehydrogenase (decarboxylating)	85 ± 10 (3)	100 ± 30 (3)	60 ± 10 (2)
Pyruvate:ferredoxin oxidoreductase (Pyruvate synthase)	210 ± 54 (11)	200 ± 41 (2)	240 ± 33 (3)
Alcohol dehydrogenase	200 ± 35 (4)	390 ± 26 (2)	210 ± 40 (4)
NADPH oxidoreductase	300 ± 20 (3)	300 ± 38 (2)	200 ± 51 (3)
Acid phosphatase	60 ± 10 (12)	85 ± 10 (3)	42 ± 10 (4)

* The specific activity of *G. duodenalis* trophozoite enzymes are in Table I. All assays were conducted at 30°C except alcohol dehydrogenase (19°C). Modified from Lindmark and Miller (1987).

has now come to light as well. Paget et al. (1989) showed that *G. muris* cysts respire oxygen at a rate approximately 10 to 20% of that observed in trophozoites. Respiration is not stimulated by exogenous glucose, but it is stimulated by exogenous ethanol. Oxygen thresholds exist above which respiration decreases, and these thresholds are much higher in cysts than in trophozoites. This suggests that respiration in cysts is resistant to higher oxygen concentrations than in trophozoites. Additionally, respiration in cysts decreases as water temperature decreases; below 7°C, respiration is negligible. This observation might well explain the increased cyst viability with decreased storage temperature reported by Bingham et al. (1979).

One of the most unexpected results of the work of Paget et al. (1989) was the observation that metronidazole, which completely inhibited respiration and motility in *G. muris* trophozoites, failed to inhibit cyst viability or respiration. This suggests that patients treated with metronidazole may excrete viable cysts until the infection is resolved.

Fig. 2 depicts the proposed pathway of energy metabolism in *Giardia*. From the evidence presented, it seems clear that *Giardia* is an aerotolerant anaerobe that oxidizes endogenous and exogenous glucose incompletely to ethanol, acetate and CO_2. Energy

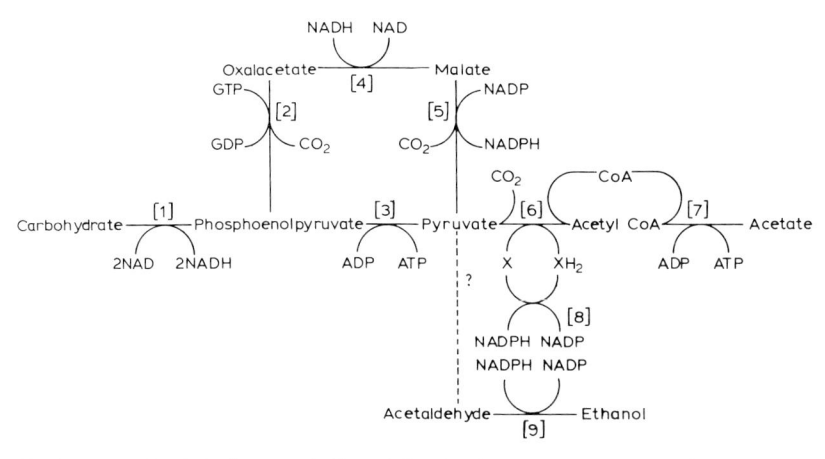

Fig. 2. Map of carbohydrate metabolism of *Giardia*. Glycolytic enzymes [1]; phosphoenolpyruvate carboxykinase (GDP) [2]; pyruvate kinase (ADP) [3]; malate dehydrogenase (NAD) [4]; malate dehydrogenase (decarboxylating) (NADP) [5]; pyruvate synthase [6]; acetyl-CoA synthetase (ADP) [7]; alcohol dehydrogenase (NADP) [8]; NADPH oxidoreductase [9]. From Lindmark (1980). With permission.

is apparently generated by substrate-level phosphorylation, and iron-sulfur proteins and flavins are probably involved in electron transport. No supporting evidence exists for the presence of a cytochrome-mediated electron transport system or oxidative phosphorylation.

2. Lipid metabolism and composition

G. lamblia trophozoites appear to rely on the salvage rather than the de novo synthesis of lipids (Jarroll et al., 1981), but appear to be able to incorporate arachidonic and palmitic acids into cellular phospho- and neutral lipids (Blair and Weller, 1987). The phospholipid, fatty acid and neutral lipid composition of *G. lamblia* trophozoites was similar to that of the medium in which they were grown. The total cellular lipid composition of *G. lamblia* trophozoites from in vitro culture (Jarroll et al., 1981; Jarroll et al., 1989), as well as the lipid composition of *G. lamblia* and *G. muris* cysts (Jarroll et al., 1989) have been studied. The cysts of *G. lamblia* and *G. muris* were purified from the feces of gerbils and mice, respectively, using sucrose gradient and Percoll velocity sedimentation methods (Sauch, 1984). Fecal preparations from uninfected gerbils and mice, processed in the same manner as those containing cysts, were extracted as described previously (Jarroll et al., 1981) and used as controls. Polar and neutral lipids from these controls were below the level of thin layer chromatographic (TLC) detection. All lipid analyses were performed as previously described (Jarroll et al., 1981) except that lipids were purified and fractionated by sephadex and florisil column chromatography prior to TLC analysis. The tentatively identified phospholipids (Fig. 3) and neutral lipids (see Jarroll et al., 1981) of both

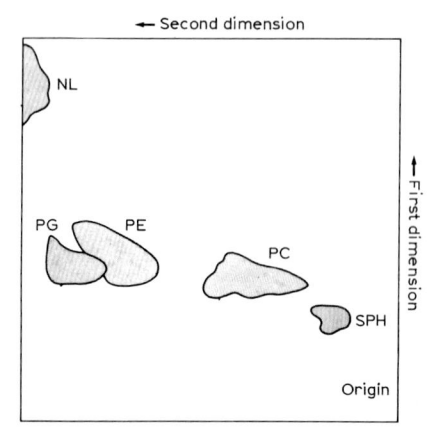

Fig. 3. Representative two-dimensional thin layer chromatogram of phospholipids extracted from *Giardia* trophozoites grown in vitro, human-source *Giardia* cysts isolated from gerbils, and *G. muris* cysts isolated from mice. Phospholipids were visualized by charring plates after spraying with $K_2Cr_2O_7$ dissolved in H_2SO_4. Abbreviations: NL, neutral lipids; PG, phosphatidylglycerol; PE, phosphatidylethanolamine; PC, phosphatidylcholine; SPH, sphingomyelin. (Jarroll et al., 1989.)

stages (cyst and trophozoite) of both *Giardia* species were identical. The phospholipids include phosphatidylcholine (PC), phosphatidylethanolamine, sphingomyelin (SPH), and phosphatidylglycerol (PG). The latter was not detected in *Giardia* trophozoites in an earlier study (Jarroll et al., 1981). Additionally, Blair and Weller (1987) reported the presence of phosphatidylserine and phosphatidylinositol, but these were not reported in a subsequent study by Kaneda and Goutsu (1988). The neutral lipids included mono-, di-, triacylglycerides, sterols (the most abundant), and sterol esters (Jarroll et al., 1981; Kaneda and Goutsu, 1988).

The inability to synthesize cellular lipids de novo was demonstrated previously (Jarroll et al., 1981) by showing that radiolabeled lipid precursors (i.e., glucose, threonine, acetate and glycerol) were not incorporated into cellular lipids. Radiolabeled cholesterol, however, was readily incorporated into cellular sterols directly from the growth medium. In in vitro culture, the lipids required for trophozoite growth appear to be supplied primarily by the serum. Recent reports suggest that in the small intestine, lipid requirements may be met, at least in part, by the incorporation of bile lipids (i.e., PC and cholesterol) (Farthing et al., 1985; Farthing et al., 1983; Gillin et al., 1986). Gillin and her coworkers (1986) have reported the growth of *Giardia* (WB strain) on serum-free medium supplemented with PC, cholesterol and six bile salts including glycocholate, glycochenodeoxycholate, glycodeoxycholate, taurocholate, taurochenodeoxycholate, and taurodeoxycholate.

4. Nucleic acid metabolism

4.1. Pyrimidine metabolism

Pyrimidine metabolism in *G. lamblia* trophozoites has been examined extensively (Aldritt et al., 1985; Lindmark and Jarroll, 1982; Vitti et al., 1987). Orotate, bicarbonate and aspartate are not incorporated into pyrimidine nucleotides even when the trophozoites were incubated in phosphate-buffered saline containing glucose rather than growth medium (Aldritt et al., 1985; Lindmark and Jarroll, 1982). Pyrimidine requirements are apparently met by salvage of preformed pyrimidines. The activity of enzymes associated with pyrimidine salvage have been detected in cell homogenates (Aldritt et al., 1985; Lindmark and Jarroll, 1982; Vitti et al., 1987), but the activity of enzymes of de novo pyrimidine synthesis (i.e., carbamoylphosphate synthetase, aspartate transcarbamoylase, dihydrooratase, and dihydroorotate dehydrogenase) were below the level of detection (Lindmark and Jarroll, 1982; Vitti et al., 1987). Fig. 4 represents a schematic of the proposed pyrimidine salvage pathways of *Giardia*. The specific activity of the pyrimidine salvage enzymes are presented in Table 3. Uridine and cytidine appear to be converted first to uracil by uridine hydrolase and cytidine deaminase, respectively, and cytosine is directly salvaged to a limited extent by cytosine phosphoribosyltransferase. Thymine incorporation into cellular nucleotide pools is below the level of detection, but thymidine is incorporated into nucleotide pools by the action of thymidine phosphotransferase. Dihydrofolate reductase and thymidylate synthetase activities were not detected in *Giardia* (Aldritt et al., 1985; Vitti et al., 1987).

Trophozoites of *Giardia* appear to transport uridine, cytidine and thymidine by a carrier mediated mechanism (Jarroll et al., 1987). This conclusion is supported by several lines of experimental evidence. Saturation kinetics are evident for all three of the nucleosides when their concentrations exceeded 1.6 nmoles/ml. The K_m values for uridine, cytidine and thymidine were 0.77, 6.67 and 0.57 μM, respectively (Fig. 5). At least 100 times more uridine and cytidine are accumulated than thymidine at the substrate concentrations used. A 15 min preincubation of trophozoites with either 5 mM iodoacetate or 2.5 mM *N*-ethylmaleimide almost completely inhibits the uptake of uridine (98.8%), cytidine (95%), and thymidine (99%) compared to controls which were preincubated in phosphate buffered saline. Furthermore, the uptake of each of the labeled nucleosides is inhibited by at least 95% by the addition of homologous unlabeled nucleosides at a ratio (unlabeled:labeled) of 10:1 for thymidine and at a ratio of 30:1 for uridine and cytidine. Inhibition of each nucleoside by analog pyrimidines and pyrimidine nucleosides is shown in Fig. 6–9. Unlabeled uridine competitively inhibits the uptake of labeled cytidine (Fig. 6, $K_i = 20$ μM), and unlabeled cytidine competitively inhibits the uptake of labeled uridine (Fig. 7, $K_i = 8$ μM). The uptake of thymidine is not inhibited by either cytidine or uridine (data not shown), but at ratios above 100:1 (Fig. 8, thymidine:uridine or cytidine), thymidine partially inhibits cytidine uptake, but has little or no effect

TABLE 3

Pyrimidine salvage enzymes in *Giardia* trophozoites

	Specific activity [nmol/(min · mg) protein]	
	Pellet	Supernatant
Thymidine kinase	0.0142 ± 0.007	0.0123 ± 0.001
Uridine kinase	<0.001	<0.001
Cytidine kinase	<0.001	<0.001
Thymidine phosphotransferase	0.090 ± 0.003	0.01505 ± 0.0045
Uridine phosphotransferase	0.058 ± 0.019	<0.001
Cytidine phosphotransferase	<0.001	<0.001
Uracil phosphoribosyltransferase	0.025 ± 0.004	1.87 ± 0.62
Cytosine phosphoribosyltransferase	<0.001	0.1325 ± 0.04
Thymidine hydrolase	<0.001	155 ± 18
Uridine hydrolase	<0.001	168 ± 14
Cytidine hydrolase	<0.001	7.6 ± 0.4
Cytidine deaminase	<0.001	183 ± 33
Cytosine deaminase	<0.001	<0.001

Each data value was from four independent experiments. From Aldritt et al. Reproduced from *The Journal of Experimental Medicine*, 1985, 161, 437-445, by copyright permission of the Rockefeller University Press.

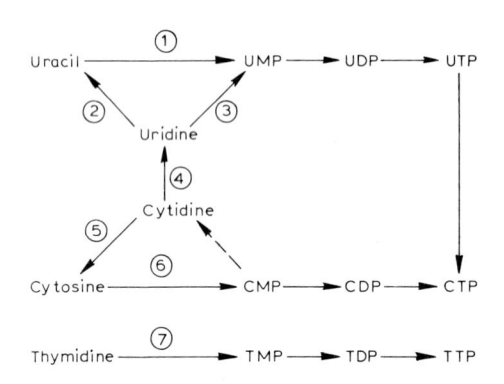

Fig. 4. The pyrimidine salvage pathway in *Giardia*: (1) uracil phosphoribosyltransferase, (2) uridine hydrolase, (3) uridine phosphotransferase, (4) cytidine deaminase, (5) cytidine hydrolase, (6) cytosine phosphoribosyltransferase, (7) thymidine phosphotransferase. From Aldritt et al. (1985). Reproduced from the Journal of Experimental Medicine, 1985, 161, 437-445, by copyright permission of the Rockefeller University Press.

on uridine uptake. Unlabeled uracil competitively inhibits uridine uptake (Fig. 9, K_i = 12 μM), but cytosine only partially inhibits cytidine uptake (Fig. 8, cytosine:cytidine = 100:1 gave a maximum of 36% inhibition). Even at a ratio of 100:1 (thymine:thymidine), thymine does not appear to inhibit thymidine uptake (data not shown).

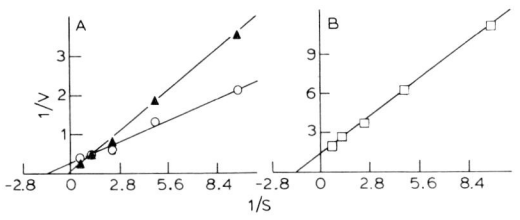

Fig. 5. (A) A comparison of the K_m and V_{max} values for uridine (○) and cytidine (▲), and (B) the K_m and V_{max} values for thymidine. 1/V is the reciprocal of the velocity (pmole/10^6 *Giardia duodenalis* trophozoites/min) and 1/S is the reciprocal of the substrate concentration (nmole/ml). Data points are reciprocals of the mean of at least three sets of replicates. From Jarroll et al. (1987). With permission.

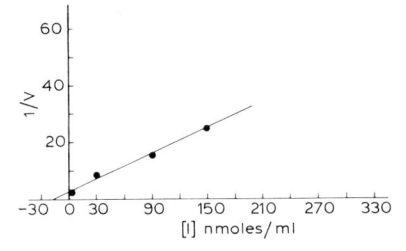

Fig. 6. Inhibition of [^{3}H]cytidine uptake (1/V represents the reciprocal of the uptake velocity in pmole/10^6 *Giardia duodenalis* trophozoites/min of cytidine) by unlabeled uridine (I equals inhibitor) as determined by the method of Dixon (1953). Data points represent the mean of at least three sets of replicates. $K_i = 20$ μM. From Jarroll et al. (1987). With permission.

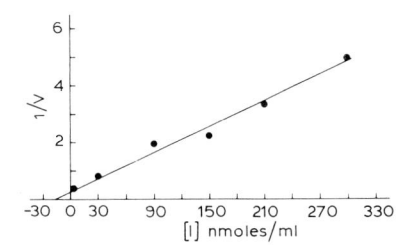

Fig. 7. Inhibition of [^{3}H]uridine uptake (1/V represents the reciprocal of the uptake velocity in pmole/10^6 *Giardia duodenalis* trophozoites/min of uridine) by unlabeled cytidine (I equals inhibitor) as determined by the method of Dixon (1953). Data points represent the mean of at least three sets of replicates. $K_i = 8$ μM. From Jarroll et al. (1987). With permission.

The results of the inhibition studies suggest that uridine and cytidine, perhaps uracil and cytosine as well, are transported at a common site which is different from the site for thymidine transport. The relatively low K_m for uridine suggests that the uridine/cytidine transport site has a higher affinity for uridine than cytidine. Similarly, the low K_m of the thymidine site for thymidine indicates a high affinity for that substrate.

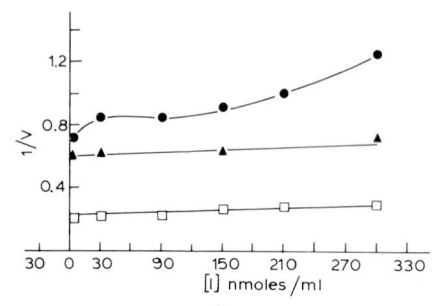

Fig. 8. Inhibition of [³H]cytidine (●) uptake and [³H]uridine uptake by unlabeled thymidine (I equals inhibitor), and the inhibition of [³H]cytidine (▲) uptake by unlabeled cytosine (I equals inhibitor). In all cases, 1/V represents the reciprocal of the uptake velocity in pmole/10⁶ *Giardia* trophozoites/min of the radiolabeled nucleoside, and the data points represent means of at least three sets of replicates. From Jarroll et al. (1987). With permission.

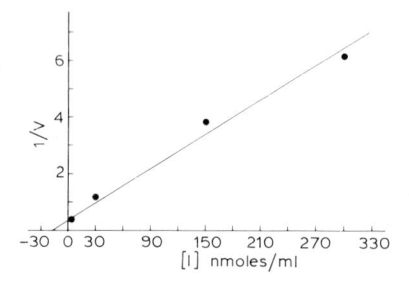

Fig. 9. Inhibition of [³H]uridine uptake (1/V represents the reciprocal of the uptake velocity in pmole/10⁶ *Giardia* trophozoites/min of uridine) by unlabeled uracil (I equals inhibitor) as determined by the method of Dixon (1953). Data points represent the mean of at least three sets of replicates. K_i = 12 μM. From Jarroll et al. (1987). With permission.

4.2. Purine metabolism

Purine metabolism has also been studied in trophozoites of *Giardia* by assaying the incorporation of radiolabeled precursors into purine nucleotides using high pressure liquid chromatography [HPLC], and by assaying for the presence of enzymes associated with purine salvage (Wang and Aldritt, 1983; Aldritt and Wang, 1986). Adenine, adenosine, guanine and guanosine were incorporated into purine nucleotides, but the incorporation of formate, glycine, hypoxanthine, xanthine and inosine were below the level of detection. Of further interest was the observation that adenosine is first converted to adenine, and guanosine is first converted to guanine before either is incorporated into their respective nucleotides. No interconversion between the two purines has been detected. Additionally, the activities of only four purine salvage enzymes (i.e., adenosine hydrolase, guanosine hydrolase, adenine phosphoribosyltransferase, and guanine phosphoribosyltransferase) were detected in supernatants of sonicated cells (Table 4). Purine nucleoside kinase, purine nucleoside phosphotransferase, hypoxanthine phosphoribosyltransferase (HPRT),

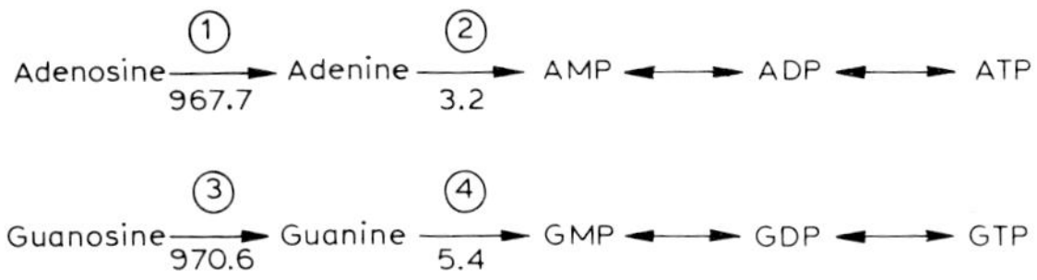

```
              ①              ②
Adenosine ─────► Adenine ─────► AMP ◄────► ADP ◄────► ATP
           967.7           3.2

              ③              ④
Guanosine ─────► Guanine ─────► GMP ◄────► GDP ◄────► GTP
           970.6           5.4
```

Fig. 10. The purine salvage pathways in *Giardia*. (1) Adenosine hydrolase, (2) adenine phosphoribosyltransferase, (3) guanosine hydrolase, (4) guanine phosphoribosyltransferase. Numbers beneath the arrows represent specific enzyme activities in nmol · min^{-1} · mg protein^{-1}. From Wang and Aldritt (1983). Reproduced from the Journal of Experimental Medicine, 1983, 158, 1703-1712, by copyright permission of the Rockefeller University Press.

and xanthine phosphoribosyltransferase (XPRT) were below the level of detection. Based on these results, Fig. 10 has been proposed as the purine salvage pathway in *G. lamblia*. This work has been verified in another laboratory in which the conversion of inosine to hypoxanthine was noted (Berens and Marr, 1986).

TABLE 4
Profile of purine salvage enzymes in *Giardia* trophozoites

Enzymes	Specific activities * (nmol · min^{-1} · mg protein^{-1})
HPRT	<0.001
GPRT	5.40 ± 1.61
XPRT	<0.001
APRT	3.16 ± 0.52
Adenosine hydrolase	967.7 ± 32.4
Guanosine hydrolase	970.6 ± 23.5

* The activities were detected in the 10^3 g supernatant fraction of the crude extract of *Giardia* trophozoites. Results are means from three independent experiments. From Wang and Aldritt. Reproduced from *The Journal of Experimental Medicine*, 1983, 158, 1703-1712, by copyright permission of the Rockefeller University Press.

Thus, *G. lamblia* trophozoites appear to depend solely on salvage pathways for their pyrimidines and purines. Furthermore, at pyrimidine concentrations similar to what one might expect under physiological conditions, *G. lamblia* trophozoites appear to assimilate pyrimidine nucleosides, and perhaps the pyrimidines as well, via carrier mediated transport with a common site for the transport of uridine and cytidine, but a different site for the transport of thymidine.

TABLE 5
Specific activities of hydrolases of G. lamblia

Enzyme	Activity mU/mg protein ± SD (No. of determinations)
Acid phosphatase	80 ± 4 (10)
Deoxyribonuclease	58 ± 15 (8)
Ribonuclease	42 ± 12 (10)
Proteinase (hemoglobin)	150 ± 18 (12)
Proteinase (BANA)	240 ± 25 (10)
β-N-acetylglucosaminidase	ND* (25)
β-galactosidase	ND (10)
β-D-glucosidase	ND (12)
α-D-glucosidase	ND (14)
β-glucuronidase	ND (14)
β-D-xylosidase	ND (7)

* Not detectable at 30°C or 37°C, at pH from 3-8. From Lindmark (1988). With permission.

5. Hydrolases and synthetases

The hydrolases of G. duodenalis have been the subject of two recent studies (Lindmark, 1988; Jarroll et al., unpublished data). G. duodenalis trophozoite homogenates exhibit enzyme activity for acid phosphatase, deoxyribonuclease, ribonuclease, and proteinase with urea denatured hemoglobin and N-benzoyl-DL-arginine-2-naphthylamide (BANA) as substrates (Table 5). Differential and isopycnic centrifugation of homogenates showed that these hydrolases of Giardia are localized in a single particle population (Figs. 11 and 12) that sediments at 10 000 rpm for 10 min, has an equilibrium density in sucrose of 1.15, and exhibits latency. Freezing and thawing (15 cycles) as well as Triton X-100 completely and simultaneously destroyed latency for all of the hydrolases, but even though latency was destroyed as described, the hydrolase activities were still sedimentable at 10 000 rpm. The latter suggests that these hydrolases are tightly bound to the particles. Further support for the particle bound nature of hydrolases, at least for acid phosphatase and aryl sulphatase, comes from light and electron microscopic cytochemical localization of these enzymes in Giardia of the duodenalis, muris, and agilis types (Feely, 1985; Feely

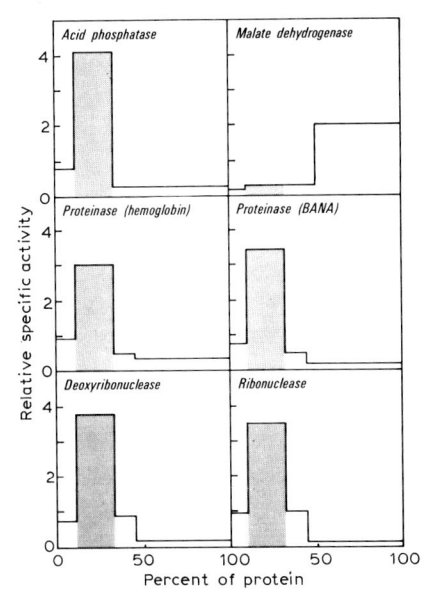

Fig. 11. Distribution of enzymes after differential centrifugation of a *G. duodenalis* homogenate. Relative specific activity of enzymes was plotted against cumulative percentage of protein recovered in each fraction. In the graph the direction from left to right corresponds to increasing centrifugal force. The far right hand block represents the final supernatant. Shaded area designates fraction subjected to isopycnic centrifugation. Percentage recoveries were 93 for acid phosphatase, 86 for deoxyribonuclease, 103 for ribonuclease, 95 for proteinase (hemoglobin), 85 for proteinase (BANA), 92 for malate dehydrogenase and 101 for protein. The figure represents the data of a typical experiment. From Lindmark (1988). With permission.

and Dyer, 1987). In the case of both of these enzymes, positive reactions were detected in numerous membrane-bounded vacuoles lying adjacent to the plasma membrane of the trophozoites. Similar enzyme activities (Lindmark and Miller, 1988) and cytochemical localizations have been observed in *Giardia* cysts (Feely, 1985). No conclusive evidence as yet exists to suggest that the particles referred to by Lindmark (1988) are the same particles that were visualized cytochemically by Feely (1985).

In light of a recent report suggesting that chitin is a major constituent of the *Giardia* cyst wall (Ward et al., 1985), it is quite interesting to note that none of the carbohydrate splitting hydrolases assayed for i.e., β-galactosidase, β-D-glucuronidase, β-N-acetylglucosaminidase (Lindmark, 1988) or chitinase (Jarroll et al., unpublished data) were detected in either trophozoite homogenates, cyst lysates, or cysts that had been induced to excyst.

Brief mention was made by Gillin et al. (1987) that they had detected an increase in chitin synthetase activity in encysting *G. lamblia* trophozoites above the level detected in control trophozoite cultures. Chitin synthetase activity was measured by the incorporation of ^{3}H-*N*-acetylglucosamine into trichloroacetic acid (TCA)-precipitable material. This incorporation was inhibited by Nikkomycin and Polyoxin D which inhibit chitin synthetase, and furthermore, the TCA-precipitable product was digested by the action

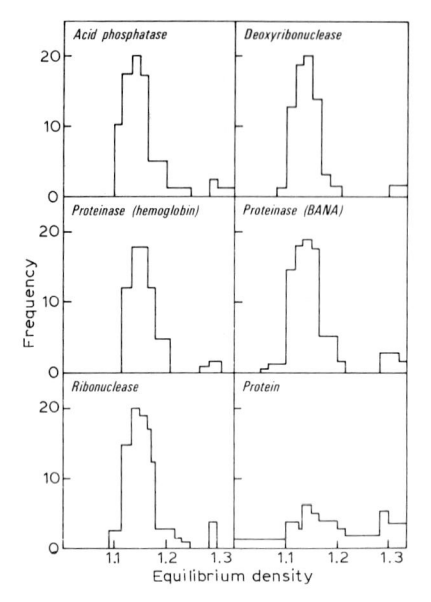

Fig. 12. Distribution of hydrolases after isopycnic centrifugation of the particle fraction represented by the shaded areas in Figure 11. Density-frequency plots are shown. Percentage recoveries were 92 for acid phosphatase, 77 for deoxyribonuclease, 105 for ribonuclease, 79 for proteinase (hemoglobin), 94 for proteinase (BANA) and 93 for protein. From Lindmark (1988). With permission.

of a purified chitinase. However, (1) that exact nature of the TCA precipitate was not determined [purified chitinase has been shown to have proteolytic as well as other glycolytic activities associated with it (Roberts and Cabib, 1982)]; (2) the specificity of this enzyme activity for N-acetylglucosamine was not shown, and (3) the fact that two inhibitors of chitin synthetase in yeast systems prevented labeled N-acetylglucosamine incorporation into an undefined TCA precipitate does not confirm that those inhibitors are not disrupting different processes in *Giardia*. The occurrence of chitin synthetase activity needs to be clarified further.

Thus, the hydrolases of *Giardia* appear to be localized in a single particle population of lysosome-like organelles, and this parasite, unlike other anaerobic protozoan parasites, appears to be virtually devoid of carbohydrate splitting enzymes. The possibility exists that *Giardia* produces chitin synthetase.

6. Summary

Giardia duodenalis can be classified as an aerotolerant anaerobe that respires in the presence of oxygen by a flavin, iron-sulfur protein-mediated electron transport system. Glucose is catabolized by the Embden-Meyerhof-Parnas and hexose monophosphate pathways, and energy is produced by substrate level phosphorylation. Substrates are incompletely oxidized to CO_2, ethanol and acetate by nonsedimentable enzymes.

Giardia trophozoites appear to rely on preformed lipids rather than synthesizing them de novo. The lipid composition of the cysts of *G. lamblia* isolated from gerbils and *G. muris* isolated from mice are similar to those obtained from the trophozoites of *G. duodenalis* grown in vitro. Phospholipids include phosphatidylcholine, phosphatidylethanolamine, phosphatidylglycerol, phosphatidylinositol, phosphatidylserine and sphingomyelin. Neutral lipids include sterols, mono-, di-, and triacylglycerides. Fatty acids can be incorporated into phospho- and neutral lipids.

G. duodenalis trophozoites appear to rely solely on the salvage of pyrimidines, purines and their nucleosides for their nucleic acid requirements. Trophozoites appear to transport pyrimidine nucleosides and perhaps their pyrimidine homologs as well by a carrier mediated mechanism. A two site system has been proposed in which uridine and cytidine are transported at a common site which is distinct from the site for thymidine transport.

The activities of several hydrolases of *Giardia* have been shown to be confined to a single lysosome-like particle population with an equilibrium density of approximately 1.15 in sucrose. In contrast to the trophozoites of *Entamoeba* and the trichomonads, trophozoites of *Giardia* appear to lack most carbohydrate splitting hydrolases. Additionally, these trophozoites may exhibit chitin synthetase activity while they are undergoing encystment.

References

Aldritt, S.M., Tien, P. and Wang, C.C. (1985) Pyrimidine salvage in *Giardia lamblia*. J. Exp. Med. 161, 437-445.
Aldritt, S.M. and Wang, C.C. (1986) Purification and characterization of guanine phosphoribosyltransferase from *Giardia lamblia*. J. Biol. Chem. 261, 8528-8533.
Blair, R.J. and Weller, P.F. (1987) Uptake and esterification of arachidonic acid by trophozoites of *Giardia lamblia*. Mol. Biochem. Parasitol. 25, 11-18.
Berens, R.L. and Marr, J.J. (1986) Adenosine analog metabolism in *Giardia lamblia*: implications for chemotherapy. Biochem. Pharmacol. 35, 4191-4197.
Farthing, M.J.G., Keusch, G.T. and Carey, M.C. (1985) Effect of bile and bile salts on growth and membrane lipid uptake by *Giardia lamblia*: possible implications for pathogenesis of intestinal disease. J. Clin. Invest. 76, 1727-1732.
Farthing, M.J.G., Varon, S.R. and Keusch, G.T. (1983) Mammalian bile promotes the growth of *Giardia lamblia* in axenic culture. Trans. R. Soc. Trop. Med. Hyg. 77, 467-469.
Feely, D.E. (1985) Acid hydrolase cytochemistry of *Giardia*. Microecol. Ther. 15, 149-156.
Feely, D.E. and Dyer, J.K. (1987) Localization of acid phosphatase activity in *Giardia lamblia* and *Giardia muris* trophozoites. J. Protozool. 34, 80-83.
Gillin, F.D., Gault, M.J., Hofmann, A.F., Gurantz, D. and Sauch, J.F. (1986) Biliary lipids support serum-free growth of *Giardia lamblia*. Infect. Immun. 53, 641-645.
Gillin, F.D., Reiner, D.S., Gault, M.J., Douglas, H., Das, S., Wunderlich, A. and Sauch, J.F. (1987) Encystation and expression of cyst antigens by *Giardia lamblia* in vitro. Science 235, 1040-1043.
Jarroll, E.L., Muller, P.J., Meyer, E.A. and Morse, S.A. (1981) Lipid and carbohydrate metabolism of *Giardia*

lamblia. Mol. Biochem. Parasitol. 2, 187-196.

Jarroll, E.L., Hammond, M. and Lindmark, D.G. (1987) *Giardia lamblia*: uptake of pyrimidine nucleosides. Exp. Parasitol. 63, 152-156.

Jarroll, E., Manning, P., Berrada, A., Hare, D. and Lindmark, D. (1989) Biochemistry and metabolism of *Giardia.* J. Protozool., 36, 190–197.

Kaneda, Y. and Goutsu, T. (1988) Lipid analysis of *Giardia lamblia* and its culture medium. Ann. Trop. Med. Parasitol. 82, 83-90.

Lindmark, D.G. (1980) Energy metabolism of the anaerobic protozoan, *Giardia lamblia.* Mol. Biochem. Parasitol. 1, 1-12.

Lindmark, D.G. (1988) *Giardia lamblia*: localization of hydrolase activities in lysosome-like organelles in trophozoites. Exp. Parasitol. 65, 141-147.

Lindmark, D.G. and Jarroll, E.L. (1982) Pyrimidine metabolism in *Giardia lamblia* trophozoites. Mol. Biochem. Parasitol. 5, 291-296.

Lindmark, D.G. and Jarroll, E.L. (1984) The metabolism of trophozoites. In: S.L. Erlandsen and E.A. Meyer (Eds.), *Giardia* and Giardiasis, Plenum, New York, 65-80.

Lindmark, D.G. and Miller, J.J. (1988) Enzyme activities of *Giardia lamblia* and *Giardia muris* trophozoites and cysts. In: P. Wallis and B. Hammond (Eds.), Advances in *Giardia* Research, University of Calgary Press, Calgary, Alberta, Canada, pp. 187–189.

Meyer, E.A. (1976) *Giardia lamblia*: isolation and axenic cultivation. Exp. Parasitol. 39, 101-105.

Paget, T.A., Jarroll, E.L., Manning, P., Lindmark, D.G. and Lloyd, D. (1989) Respiration in the cyst and trophozoite forms of *Giardia muris.* J. Gen. Microbiol. 135, 145–154.

Roberts, R. and Cabib, E. (1982) *Serratia marcescens* chitinase: one step purification and use for the determination of chitin. Anal. Biochem. 127, 402-412.

Sauch, J.F. (1984) Purification of *Giardia muris* cysts by velocity sedimentation. App. Environ. Microbiol. 48, 454-455.

Vitti, G.F., O'Sullivan, W. and Gero, A. (1987) The biosynthesis of uridine $5'$-monophosphate in *Giardia lamblia.* Int. J. Parasitol. 17, 805-812.

Ward, H., Alroy, J., Lev, B., Keusch, G. and Pereira, M. (1985) Identification of chitin as a structural component of *Giardia* cysts. Infect. Immun. 49, 629-634.

Wang, C.C. and Aldritt, S. (1983) Purine salvage networks in *Giardia lamblia.* J. Exp. Med. 158, 1703-1712.

Weinbach, E.C., Claggett, C.E., Keister, D.B., Diamond, L. and Kon, H. (1980) Respiratory metabolism of *Giardia lamblia.* J. Parasitol. 66, 347-350.

Giardiasis (E.A. Meyer, ed.)
© 1990 Elsevier Science Publishers B.V. (Biomedical Division)

4

Animal models for *Giardia duodenalis* type organisms

GAETAN M. FAUBERT and MIODRAG BELOSEVIC

Institute of Parasitology of McGill University, Macdonald College, Ste-Anne de Bellevue, Québec, Canada and Department of Zoology, Biological Sciences Building, University of Alberta Edmonton, Alberta Canada T6G 2E1

1. Introduction	78
1.1. Animal models	78
2. Pre-requisites for an animal model of human giardiasis	78
3. In search of an animal model for *G. duodenalis*	79
3.1. Rat	79
3.2. Mice	80
3.3. Dogs, cats, rabbits	81
3.4. Gerbils	81
4. The use of the gerbil-*Giardia* model in the laboratory	83
4.1. Epidemiology	83
4.2. Host immunity	85
4.3. Pathology	85
4.4. Genetic variability of *Giardia* isolates	87
4.5. Other uses	87
5. Conclusions	87
6. Preparation of the gerbils for inoculation with *G. duodenalis*-type organisms	88
6.1. Animals	88
6.2. The parasite	88
References	89

1. Introduction

1.1. Animal models

From the earliest days of modern biology and medicine, animals have been widely used to gain insights into human biology as well as general biology. The similarities in structure and function among mammals makes them obvious candidates for research. As experimental parasitology matured over the last 25 years, rats, mice, guinea pigs, gerbils, hamsters and rabbits came into favor because they were usually the only means available to keep the parasite alive in the laboratory. However, the selection of an animal to study the biology of the parasite and the disease is often based on our innate biases and we limit our potential as experimenters. One common bias is the use of animals with which we have worked during our early professional days. This bias results in an unwillingness to consider the entire animal kingdom as a source of potential models to study the biology of parasites.

The ultimate objective of modelling in experimental parasitology is generally to understand the disease in humans. Therefore, the animal chosen to study a particular parasitic disease should reflect, as much as possible, the sensitivity to the infection as it occurs in nature and the pathology that will develop later without any prior manipulation of the animal before the experimental infection. Within this context, it is important to realize that host susceptibility, which can depend upon many non-immunological factors, is different from host mechanisms of acquired resistance, which usually relies on specific immune mechanisms that vary from species to species (Capron and Capron, 1986). If this principle is respected, great dividends in understanding and controlling disease states should result. Unfortunately, animal models are often chosen in parasitology not through a planned search, but rather as a consequence of availability of a particular animal or because of our innate biases.

2. Pre-requisites for an animal model of human giardiasis

In the past decades, researchers have sought to develop an experimental laboratory model to study human giardiasis. The selection of a laboratory model should be based on the following considerations: (1) sensitivity of the animal to the *G. duodenalis*-type organisms; (2) successful infection including colonization and multiplication of trophozoites in the small intestine; (3) the formation and release of cysts in the feces; (4) infection must be transferable from humans or other hosts by oral inoculation; (5) the course of the infection and associated pathology in the animal host should mimic the changes observed in human giardiasis; (6) the animal should be inexpensive, breed under laboratory conditions and be easy to maintain in the laboratory; (7) background knowledge of the biological properties of the animal; (8) ethical implications.

3. In search of an animal model for G. duodenalis

Unlike *G. muris*, *G. duodenalis*-type organisms can be cultured in vitro; this suggests that major physiological and biochemical differences exist between these organisms. Due to these differences, an animal model employing *G. duodenalis*-type organisms would be invaluable in studies dealing with the mechanisms of pathogenicity of human giardiasis. Several laboratory animals have been tested for their suitability to serve as hosts for *Giardia* isolated from humans. The highlights from these studies are outlined below.

3.1. Rat

The possibility that rats might be susceptible to infection with *Giardia* isolated from humans was explored first by Hegner (1927) and subsequently by Armaghan (1937). These authors found that the inoculation of *Giardia* cysts isolated from humans to rats resulted in an infection. Armaghan (1937) reported that only 4 of 45 rats inoculated with cysts became infected, and that infections were short (15 days) and without cyst formation. Goritskaya and Vrublevskaya (1966) reported that suckling rats were susceptible to infection with cysts of *Giardia* isolated from humans. In their study, 58 of 85 suckling rats became infected following oral inoculation with cysts. They also showed that the size of the inoculum influences the infection rate in young rats. Sehgal et al. (1976) also reported that adult and weanling rats become infected when inoculated with cysts of *Giardia* isolated from human feces. In their study, 5 of 31 adult and 7 of 19 weanling animals became infected following oral inoculation with 1.9 to 3.3 × 10^3 cysts/rat. A significantly higher infection rate was observed once the parasite had been passaged through rats. This may be an indication that an adaptation to the new host species had occurred. Craft (1982) reported that specific pathogen-free weanling Spraque-Dawley rats were highly susceptible to infection with *Giardia* isolated from humans. All the rats became infected after oral inoculation of 150 cysts. Using adult Wistar albino rats, Anand et al. (1980) studied the pathogenesis of malabsorption during giardiasis. They found a significant fall in the transport of glucose and glycine tested on segments of intestine in vitro from rats infected with human-derived giardial cysts. Histologically, the mucosa showed no morphological abnormalities; the villi remained tall and finger-like with a normal villus:crypt ratio. The lamina propria was normal with no increase in the number of chronic inflammatory cells (Anand et al., 1980). On the other hand, Woo and Paterson (1987) were unable to infect adult Wistar rats with *G. duodenalis*-type organisms. The above reports suggest that rats are not very suitable hosts to study human giardiasis for two reasons: poor susceptibility to infection and the absence of pathology at the gut level.

3.2. Mice

Mice have been used to study the biology of *G. duodenalis* by several investigators. Vinayak et al. (1979) reported an infection rate of 100% in weanling Swiss mice inoculated orally with 1.5×10^5 cysts. Hill et al. (1983) demonstrated that oral inoculation of suckling mice with cultured trophozoites of *Giardia* resulted in infection as shown by cyst release in the feces. Cysts were recovered from the feces of suckling mice for up to three weeks after infection, and were infective to other suckling mice. These authors concluded that the susceptibility of CF-1 mice to infection was age specific, and that the infection was apparently without adverse effects on the murine host. The activities of drugs against *G. duodenalis* have been studied in suckling mice (Boreham et al., 1986). Litters of Quackenbush mice less than 5 days of age were infected with 10^5 trophozoites obtained from in vitro cultures. The course of infection in these mice was similar to that in CF-1 mice. These workers concluded that the suckling mouse model for giardiasis may be a useful tool in chemotherapeutic studies (Boreham et al., 1986).

Swiss albino mice between 2 to 3 weeks old have been used to study cell mediated immunity (Kanwar et al., 1984, 1985, 1987; Upadhyay et al., 1986), humoral antibody response (Kanwar et al., 1986), and acquired immunity against *Giardia* (Kanwar et al., 1985). The animals were inoculated orally with 10 000 cysts from infected patients. In these young outbred mice, the peak cyst excretion and trophozoite counts were observed 10 days after infection. Cysts were released consistently during a period of 29 days and by day 30, cyst excretion ceased in all animals (Kanwar et al., 1986). Four week old Swiss mice were also used to demonstrate the importance of the T-cell mediated immune response in giardiasis by Vasudev et al. (1982). The mice were thymectomized and irradiated before infection with 1000 cysts of *Giardia* from an infected patient.

Dose response studies were conducted in Swiss mice to determine the influence of parasite load on the absorption of nutrients in brush border membrane vesicles. Samra et al. (1987) found low uptake of D-glucose, L-phenylalanine, L-lysine and L-aspartic acid in mice infected with 100 000 or 10 000 cysts of *Giardia* from humans. Mucosal cells and fluids removed from the small bowel of non-infected mice were used in vitro as a model to study the functional and structural derangements caused by human source *Giardia* (Anand et al., 1985). Similarly, using Swiss mice, Upadhyay et al. (1985) studied the combined effects of malnutrition and giardiasis on malabsorption. Aggarwal et al. (1983) studied the virulence of various human isolates in Swiss mice infected with *Giardia* cysts obtained from symptomatic and asymptomatic patients. They found a difference between the isolates as judged by high cyst excretion rate and high trophozoite counts.

In summary, mice have been used to study the biology, immunology and pathology of giardiasis. It should be noted, however, that successful infections with *G. duodenalis*-type organisms can only occur in weanling and young mice, that is, at a time they are immunologically immature. The lack of an adequate immune response to *Giardia* during the establishment of the parasite in the small intestine may influence the outcome since the immune response could contribute to the pathology of the infection. Under these conditions, the results obtained using immature hosts may be difficult to interpret. Numerous attempts in our laboratory to infect different strains of adult mice (more than 8 weeks old) with *G. duodenalis*-type organisms were unsuccessful. In our opinion, the demonstrated age-dependent susceptibility of mice to *G. duodenalis*-type organisms dramatically reduces the usefulness of these hosts for studies on immunology and pathology of human giardiasis.

3.3. Dogs, cats, rabbits

Kirkpatrick and Greene (1985) reported that of six laboratory-reared cats inoculated with cultured *Giardia* trophozoites from humans, only one excreted fecal cysts over 80 days of observation. However, only two of eight cats inoculated with cysts from patients were found to produce fecal cysts. They concluded that adult cats are not very susceptible to *Giardia* from human sources. This study, however, did not exclude the possibility that cats may have been previously exposed to *Giardia* and, therefore, were immune at the time of experimentation. Woo and Paterson (1986) were not successful in infecting kittens with trophozoites obtained from axenic culture. We believe that additional studies are needed before an accurate assessment of susceptibility of cats to *Giardia* from human sources can be made.

Mongrel dogs were used as a model to demonstrate the concept of inter-species transmission of *Giardia* and also to demonstrate that infection can be transmitted by both trophozoite and cyst stages of the parasite. Before including any dogs in the study, Hewlett et al. (1982) carefully examined each animal for *Giardia* cysts 6 times per week for a period of 3 weeks. Of 37 dogs they examined, 68% were found to be infected with *Giardia* sp. and were thus excluded. After oral challenge, three of eight dogs became infected with cysts and two of three became infected with trophozoites (Hewlett et al., 1982). Further studies are needed, however, before a thorough assessment of dogs as possible hosts to study human giardiasis could be made. We believe that dogs bred in the laboratory and kept free of *Giardia* spp. may be of value in studies on pathophysiology of giardiasis.

3.4. Gerbils

Our knowledge on the biology of *Giardia* and giardiasis has been greatly advanced by the description of the *G. muris*-mouse model, as well as the development of appropriate techniques required for the assessment of the infection, by Roberts-Thomson et al. (1976) (see chapter 5). These authors reported that the administration of graded doses of cysts to CF-1 mice resulted in a reproducible pattern of infection, as assessed by counting cysts in the feces and trophozoites in the small intestine. This well-defined host-parasite association is currently an animal model of choice when studying immunological responses of the host to *Giardia*. Due to the major physiological differences between *G.*

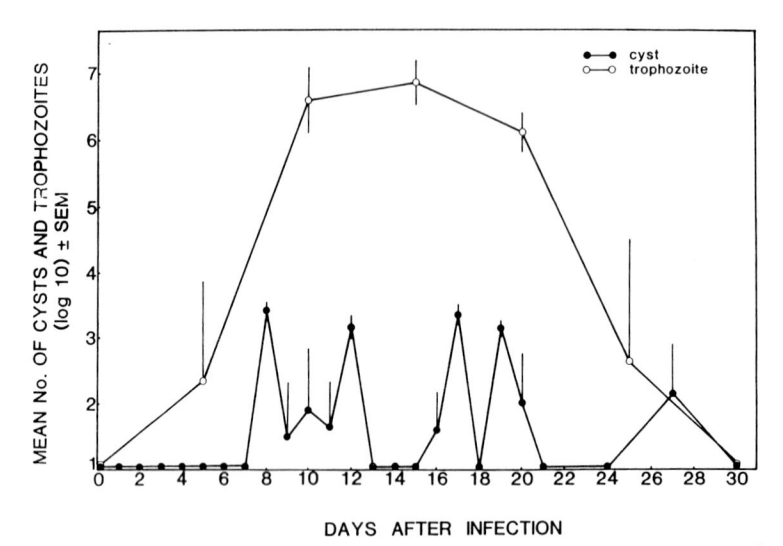

Fig. 1. The course of infection in Mongolian gerbils after administration of 5 × 10³ human source *Giardia* cysts/gerbil. For cyst release, each point represents the mean number of cysts released per 2 h collection period for four animals. For trophozoite colonization, each point represents the mean number of trophozoites per gerbil (*N* = 2).

muris and *G. duodenalis*-type organisms, it was desirable to develop an animal model using *G. duodenalis*-type organisms.

Belosevic et al. (1983) were first to propose the Mongolian gerbil (*Meriones unguiculatus*) animal model to study human giardiasis. These authors reported that gerbils were highly susceptible to infection with *Giardia* cysts obtained from stool specimens of infected humans and cultured trophozoites. Cysts were first detected in feces on day 8 after inoculation (Fig. 1) and the period of cyst release in individual animals varied from 13 to 39 days. Typically, cyst release was intermittent and most cysts were released during the second and third weeks of infection. Periods of positive fecal examinations were frequently followed by periods of negative fecal examinations. The pattern of infection observed after oral inoculation with trophozoites was similar to that obtained after inoculation with cysts. On day 5 after inoculation (Fig. 2), all trophozoites were found in the duodenum and proximal jejunum. As the number of trophozoites increased, they were seen in all sections of the small intestine. At day 20, which corresponded to the beginning of the self-cure, trophozoites were not observed in distal jejunum and ileum, and by day 30, small numbers of trophozoites were seen only in the duodenum. The location of trophozoites in the small intestine was similar when the inoculum was either trophozoites (orally or duodenally administered) or cysts obtained from humans (Belosevic and Faubert, unpublished observations).

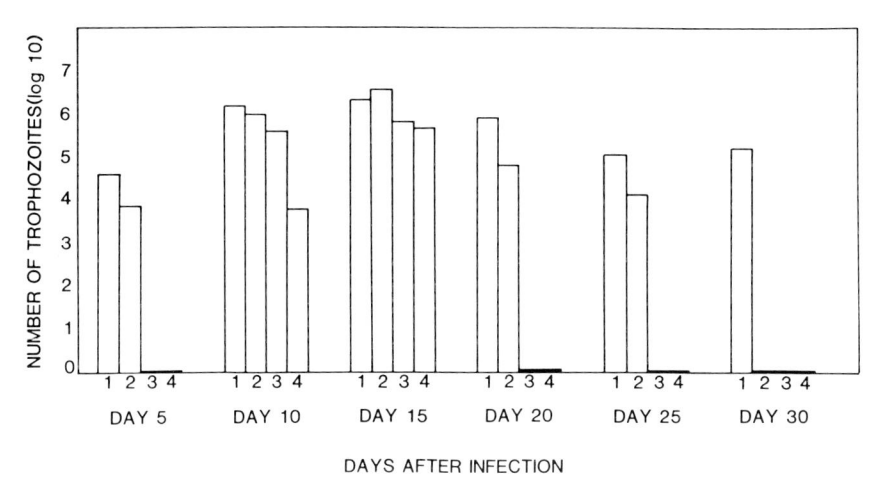

Fig. 2. The distribution of trophozoites in the small intestine of Mongolian gerbils infected with 2×10^5 G. duodenalis trophozoites (WB strain) grown in TYI-S-33 medium. 1 = duodenum; 2 = proximal jejunum; 3 = distal jejunum; 4 = ileum.

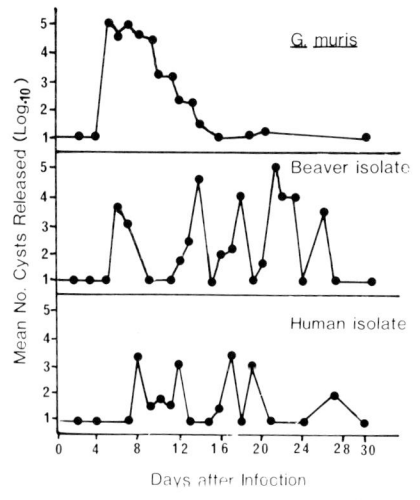

Fig. 3. Patterns of infection in Mongolian gerbils inoculated orally with cysts of Giardia spp. The infection dose for the beaver isolate and Giardia muris was 6×10^4 cysts/gerbil and for the human isolate 5×10^3 cysts/gerbil. Each point is the geometric mean number of cysts released by five gerbils for each isolate.

4. The use of the gerbil-Giardia model in the laboratory

4.1. Epidemiology

The susceptibility of gerbils to both G. muris and G. duodenalis-type organisms has been demonstrated by Faubert et al. (1983). The results of this study support the general concept of inter-species transmission of Giardia. Not only were gerbils susceptible to G.

muris but also to beaver and human isolates of *Giardia* (Fig. 3). Uniform susceptibility of gerbils to both *G. muris* and *G. duodenalis*-type organisms may be useful in attempts to identify and characterize *Giardia* of unknown origin, especially when combined with in vitro cultivation of trophozoites obtained from the small intestine of infected gerbils (Faubert et al., 1983). This approach was used to excyst *Giardia* spp. isolated from meadow voles, dogs, beavers and humans (Wallis et al., 1984). Thus far, trophozoites obtained from the gut of gerbils infected with dog, human and beaver cysts were successfully cultured in TYI-S-33 medium (Wallis and Wallis, 1986; Wallis et al., 1984). Belosevic et al. (1984) used the gerbil-*Giardia* model to examine the role of cats in possible zoonotic transmission of giardiasis. The trophozoites recovered from gerbils infected with cysts isolated from the feces of cats were found to be of *G. duodenalis*-type with a typical claw-hammer shaped median body. Thus, the gerbil-*Giardia* model is becoming invaluable in studies of the epidemiology of giardiasis, because it allows for biological assessment of different *Giardia* isolates.

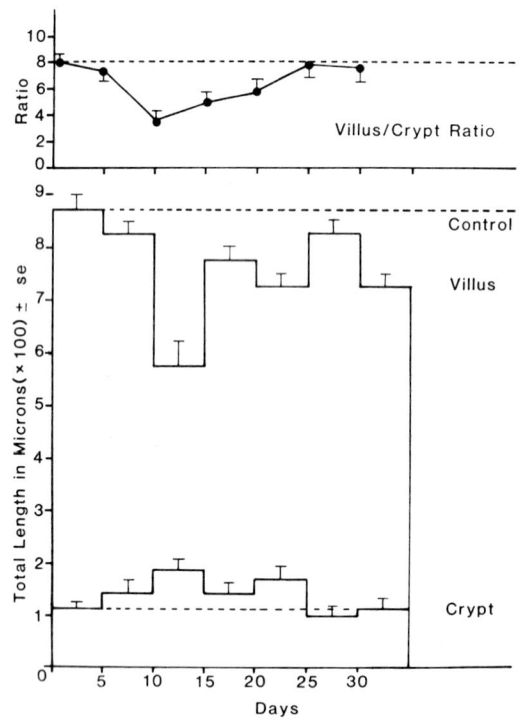

Fig. 4. Intestinal villus to crypt ratio of gerbils infected with 2×10^5 *G. duodenalis* trophozoites (WB strain) grown in TYI-S-33 medium. The bottom part of the diagram represents the total length of the villus and the crypt for different days after the infection. The data represent the mean value of six gerbils.

4.2. Host immunity

Both Belosevic et al. (1983) and Lewis et al. (1987) reported that gerbils develop long lasting immunity after primary *Giardia* infection. Animals were found to be resistant to reinfection as long as 5 to 8 months after elimination of the primary infection. Lewis et al. (1987) also showed that acquired immunity after a primary infection can be abrogated in some animals by administration of hydrocortisone acetate. Aggarwal and Nash (1987) used the gerbil-*Giardia* model to compare the antigenicity of two different human isolates. They studied the course of infection, host responses and ability of gerbils to resist reinfection to both homologous and heterologous challenge.

4.3. Pathology

During an epidemiological survey done in 3 provinces in China, Wang et al. (1986) studied the pathology in gerbils infected with cysts obtained from infected individuals. Diarrhea occurred in 14 of the 35 gerbils from day 3 to day 9 after infection. The gerbils started to lose weight 7 days after infection. The mucosal surface was covered with a mucoid exudate. The villi were broadened and intestinal tissue was edematous with a mild lymphocytic infiltration. The authors concluded that the gerbil-*Giardia* model

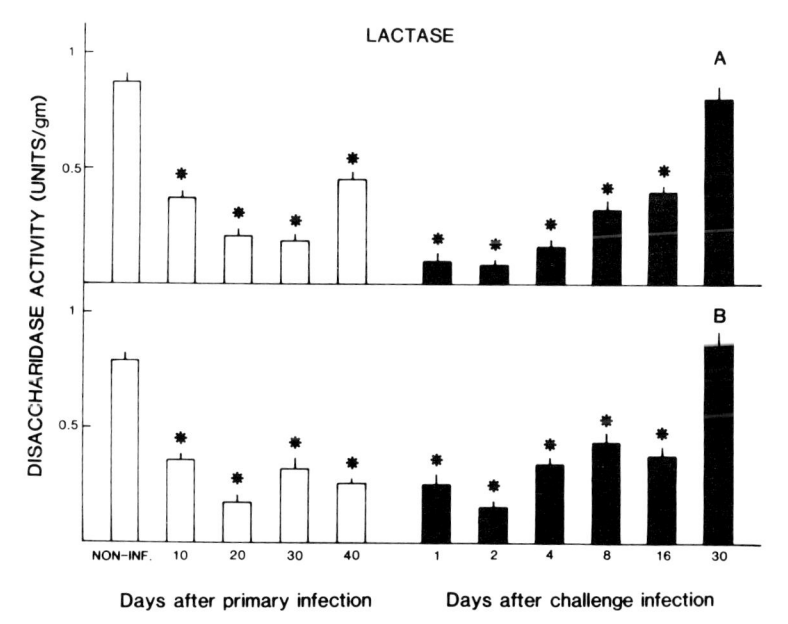

Fig. 5. Lactase activity in the anterior (A) and posterior (B) small intestine of gerbils during the primary infection and at various times after challenge infection with trophozoites of *Giardia duodenalis*. Each bar on the graph represents the mean lactase activity ± SEM of six gerbils. Infection dose for the primary infection was 2×10^5 trophozoites/gerbil. Gerbils were challenged orally with 2×10^5 trophozoites each on day 40 after the primary infection. (*) = significantly different ($P < 0.05$, ANOVA) when compared to the non-infected group.

paralleled some of the clinical manifestations seen in humans and that histopathological changes in the small intestine were comparable to those observed in human giardiasis. We also observed that gerbils inoculated with human origin *Giardia* cysts or trophozoites grown in vitro show a reduction in the villus to crypt ratio in the jejunal mucosa (Fig. 4) (Belosevic and Faubert, unpublished observations). These changes were transient and are similar to those observed in human giardiasis (Gillon and Ferguson, 1984). Studies on disaccharidase deficiency during giardiasis conducted in our laboratory showed that the reduction of lactase activity in the primary *Giardia* infection, was related to the period of highest trophozoite density in the small intestine (Fig. 5). Interestingly, secondary exposure of gerbils to the parasite caused a sharp decrease in lactase activity even in the absence of live trophozoites in the small intestine (Belosevic and Faubert, unpublished observations).

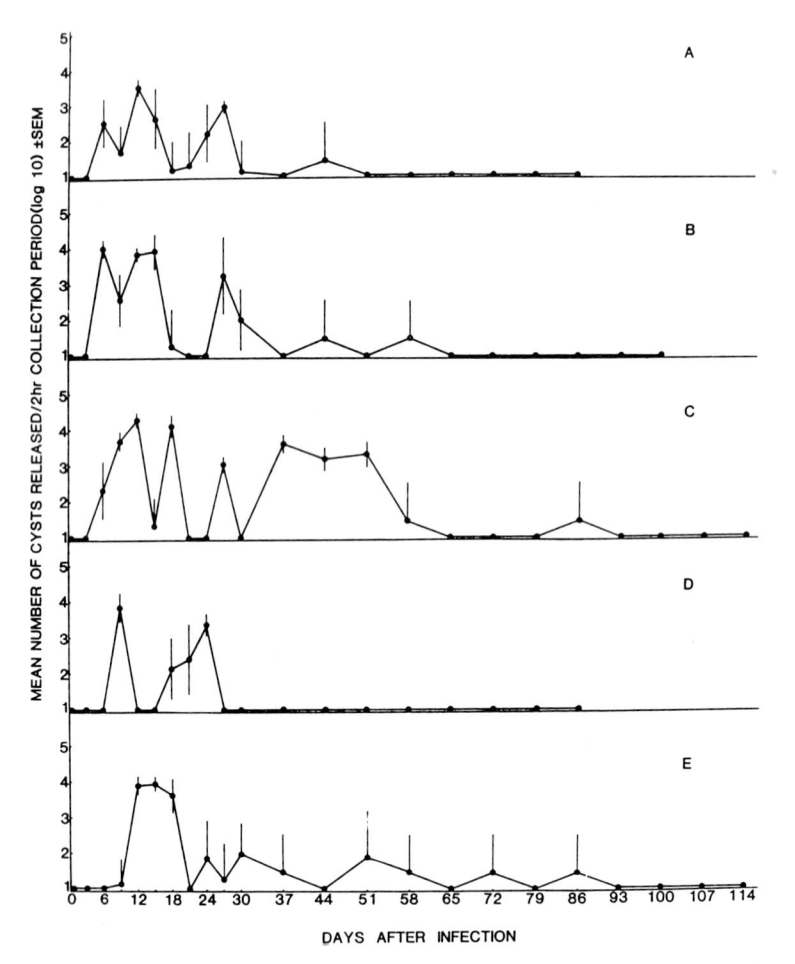

Fig. 6. The course of infection in Mongolian gerbils after administration to five animals 5×10^3 *Giardia* cysts from different human sources. See Table 1.

4.4. Genetic variability of Giardia isolates

Using the gerbil-*Giardia* model, we observed that the mode of cyst release varies between different human isolates (Table 1). Isolate A produced in gerbils a constant cyst release for a period of 33 days (Fig. 6). Isolate B also produced constant cyst release for 24 days followed by intermittent cyst release from day 32 to day 68. Isolate C produced a high number of cysts over several consecutive days, whereas gerbils inoculated with isolate D produced low number of cysts and for a short period of time. Finally, gerbils infected with isolate E exhibited constant cyst output for 6 days, followed by intermittent cyst release (Faubert and Belosevic, unpublished observations). It appears, therefore, that the pattern of cyst release in infected gerbils is a characteristic of the parasite and is independent of the host, suggesting the presence of behavioral heterogeneity among different *Giardia* isolates.

TABLE 1
Source of *Giardia duodenalis* isolates obtained from patients with symptomatic giardiasis

Isolate *	Source of infection	No. cysts $\times 10^5$/g feces counted in patients
A	Ethiopia	40
B	Canada	5
C	Spain	15
D	Haiti	0.1
E	Cuba	13

* All patients were cured with metronidazole treatment.

4.5. Other uses

Swabby et al. (1988) employed the gerbil as a 'live culture' for the *G. duodenalis*-type organisms. They were able to supply from 20 to 100×10^6 cysts for use in engineering studies designed to verify the efficacy of water treatment facilities, as well as for quality control of diagnostic procedures for waterborne pathogens.

5. Conclusions

In our opinion, the gerbil-*Giardia* model is very useful to study human giardiasis for the following reasons: (1) the animal is highly susceptible to infection with *G. duodenalis*-type organisms; (2) adult animals can be infected with either cysts or trophozoites cultured in vitro; (3) trophozoites recovered from gerbils can be used to initiate new in vitro cultures; and, (4) it is an ideal model to study the pathophysiologic changes caused by the infection.

6. Preparation of the gerbils for inoculation with G. duodenalis-*type organisms*

6.1. Animals

Six to ten week old male Mongolian gerbils (*Meriones unguiculatus*) bred under laboratory conditions should be used in order to exclude previous contacts with *Giardia* spp. The animals must be kept in separate animal quarters, preferably in filter-top cages. Prior to use gerbils should be acclimated for a minimum of 10 days. Ten days prior to experimental infection, animals are treated orally for 3 consecutive days with metronidazole (20 mg/gerbil/day per os). This treatment ensures that the gerbils are free from all previous intestinal infections (Belosevic et al., 1983; Swabby et al., 1988).

6.2. The parasite

Feces from gerbils are usually collected over a period of 2 hours, weighed and soaked in 0.85% saline for 1 hr prior to isolation of cysts. *Giardia* cysts collected for infection of gerbils must be separated from fecal debris as soon as possible, because prolonged storage in fecal matter may affect cyst infectivity (Faubert and Belosevic, unpublished observations). Cysts can readily be isolated from the feces using the sucrose flotation method of Roberts-Thomson et al. (1976) with the following modifications: centrifugation speeds and times should be decreased to $300 \times g$ for 7 min and $500 \times g$ for 5 min for first and second spin, respectively. Usually, 5×10^3 freshly isolated cysts administered in 0.2 ml of 0.85% saline by gastric intubation are sufficient to infect gerbils. However, for consistent infection, a higher dose (2×10^5 cysts/gerbil) is recommended.

For experimental inoculation of gerbils with trophozoites, actively growing organisms (log phase) in Diamond's TYI-S-33 culture medium are chilled on ice and sedimented by centrifugation at $200 \times g$ for 5 min. They are washed in phosphate buffered saline, pH 7.2, and resuspended in 0.2 ml PBS to contain 10^6 organisms and are administered to gerbils by gastric intubation.

References

Aggarwal, A., Bhatia, A., Naik, S.R. and Vinayak, V.K. (1983) Variable virulence of isolates of *Giardia lamblia* in mice. Ann. Trop. Med. Parasitol. 77, 163-167.

Aggarwal, A. and Nash, T.E. (1987) Comparison of two antigenically distinct *Giardia lamblia* isolates in gerbils. Am. J. Trop. Med. Hyg. 36, 325-332.

Anand, B.S., Chaudhari, R., Jyothi, A., Yadev, R.S. and Baveja, U.K. (1985) Experimental examination of the direct damaging effects of *G. lamblia* on intestinal mucosal scrapings of mice. Trans. R. Soc. Trop. Med. Hyg. 79, 613-617.

Anand, B.S., Kumar, M., Chakravarti, R.N., Sehgal, A.K. and Chhuttani, P.N. (1980) Pathogenesis of malabsorption in *Giardia* infection: an experimental study in rats. Trans. R. Soc. Trop. Med. Hyg. 74, 565-569.

Armaghan, V. (1937) Biological studies on the *Giardia* of rats. Am. J. Hyg. 26, 236-258.

Belosevic, M., Faubert, G.M., Croll, N.A. and MacLean, J.D. (1982) *Giardia lamblia*: axenic growth in autoclaved and filtered Diamond's TYI-S-33 medium. Can. J. Zool. 60, 1673-1675.

Belosevic, M., Faubert, G.M., Guy, R. and MacLean, J.D. (1984) Observations on natural and experimental infections with *Giardia* isolated from cats. Can. J. Comp. Med. 48, 241-244.

Belosevic, M., Faubert, G.M., MacLean, J.D., Law, C. and Croll, N.A. (1983) *Giardia lamblia* infections in Mongolian gerbils: an animal model. J. Infect. Dis. 147, 222-226.

Boreham, P.F.L., Phillips, R.E. and Shepherd, R.W. (1986) The activity of drugs against *Giardia intestinalis* in neonatal mice. J. Antimicrobiol. Chem. 18, 393-398.

Capron, M. and Capron, A. (1986) Rats, mice and men: models for immune effector mechanisms against schistosomiasis. Parasitol. Today 2, 69-75.

Craft, J.C. (1982) Experimental infection with *Giardia lamblia* in rats. J. Infect. Dis. 145, 495-498.

Faubert, G.M., Belosevic, M., Walker, T.S., MacLean, J.D. and Meerovitch, E. (1983) Comparative studies on the pattern of infection with *Giardia* spp. in Mongolian gerbils. J. Parasitol. 69, 802-805.

Gillon, J. and Ferguson, A. (1984) Changes in the small intestinal mucosa in giardiasis. In: S.L. Erlandsen and E.A. Meyer (Eds.), *Giardia* and Giardiasis. Plenum Press, New York, pp. 163-183.

Goritskaya, V.V. and Vrublevskaya, L.A. (1966) Experimental invasion of white rats with *Lamblia intestinalis*. Med. Parazitol. Parazit. Bol. 35, 206-208.

Hegner, R.W. (1927) Excystation and infection in the rat with *Giardia lamblia* from man. Am. J. Hyg. 7, 782-785.

Hewlett, E.L., Andrews Jr., J.S., Ruffier, J. and Schaefer III, F.W. (1982) Experimental infection of mongrel dogs with *Giardia lamblia* cysts and cultured trophozoites. J. Infect. Dis. 145, 89-93.

Hill, D.R., Guerrant, R.L., Pearson, R.D. and Hewlett, E.L. (1983) *Giardia lamblia* infection of suckling mice. J. Infect. Dis. 147, 217-221.

Kanwar, S.S., Ganguly, N.K., Mahajan, R.C. and Walia, B.N.S. (1985) Acquired resistance to *Giardia lamblia* infection in mice. Trop. Geog. Med. 37, 32-36.

Kanwar, S.S., Ganguly, N.K., Walia, B.N.S. and Mahajan, R.C. (1984) Enumeration of small intestinal lymphocyte population in *Giardia lamblia* infected mice. J. Diar. Dis. Res. 2, 243-248.

Kanwar, S.S., Ganduly, N.K., Walia, B.N. and Mahajan, R.C. (1985) Changes in mouse splenic lymphocyte sub-population during primary and secondary course of *Giardia lamblia* infection. Ind. J. Med. Res. 82, 393-397.

Kanwar, S.S., Ganguly, N.K., Walia, B.N.S. and Mahajan, R.C. (1986) Direct and antibody dependent cell mediated cytotoxicity against *Giardia lamblia* by splenic and intestinal lymphoid cells in mice. Gut 27, 73-77.

Kanwar, S.S., Walia, B.N.S., Ganguly, N.K. and Mahajan, R.C. (1987) The macrophages as an effector cell in *Giardia lamblia* infections. Med. Microbiol. Immunol. 176, 183-188.

Kirkpatrick, C.E. and Greene IV, G.A. (1985) Susceptibility of domestic cats to infections with *G. lamblia* cysts and trophozoites from human sources. J. Clin. Microbiol. 21, 678-680.

Lewis Jr., P.D., Belosevic, M., Faubert, G.M., Curthoys, L. and MacLean, J.D. (1987) Cortisone-induced recrudescence of *Giardia lamblia* infections in gerbils. Am. J. Trop. Med. Hyg. 36, 33-40.

Roberts-Thomson, I.C., Stevens, D.P., Mahmoud, A.A.F. and Warren, K.S. (1976) Giardiasis in the mouse: an animal model. Gastroenterology 71, 57-61.

Samra, H.K., Garg, U.R., Ganguly, N.K. and Mahajan, R.C. (1987) Effect of different *Giardia lamblia* inocula on glucose and amino acids transport in the intestinal brush border membrane vesicles of infected mice. Ann. Trop. Med. Parasitol. 81, 367-372.

Sehgal, A.K., Grewal, M.S., Chakravarti, R.N., Broor, S.L., Deka, N.C. and Chuttani, P.N. (1976) Experimental giardiasis in albino rats. Ind. J. Med. Res. 64, 1015-1018.

Swabby, K.D., Hibler, C.P. and Wegrzyn, J.G. (1988) Infection of Mongolian gerbils (*Meriones unguiculatus*) with *Giardia* from human and animal sources. In: P.M. Wallis and B.R. Hannon (Eds.), Advances in *Giardia* Research, pp. 75–77. University of Calgary.

Upadhyay, P., Ganguly, N.K., Mahajan, R.C. and Walia, B.N.S. (1985) Intestinal uptake of nutrients in normal and malnourished animals infected with *G. lamblia*. Digestion 32, 243-248.

Upadhyay, P., Ganguly, N.K., Walia, B.N. and Mahajan, R.C. (1986) Kinetics of lymphocyte subpopulation in intestinal mucosa of protein deficient *Giardia lamblia* infected mice. Gut 4, 386-391.

Vasudev, V., Ganguly, N.K., Anand, B.S., Krishna, V.R., Dilawari, J.B. and Mahajan, R.C. (1982) A study of *Giardia* infection in irradiated and thymectomized mice. J. Trop. Med. Hyg. 85, 119-122.

Vinayak, V.K., Sharma, G.L. and Naik, S.R. (1979) Experimental *Giardia lamblia* infection in Swiss mice, a preliminary report. Ind. J. Med. Res. 70, 195-198.

Wallis, P.M. and Wallis, H.M. (1986) Excystation and culturing of human and animal *Giardia* spp. by using gerbils and TYI-S-33 medium. App. Environ. Microbiol. 51, 647-651.

Wallis, P.M., Buchanan-Mappin, J.M., Faubert, G.M. and Belosevic, M. (1984) Reservoirs of *Giardia* spp. in southwestern Alberta. J. Wildl. Dis. 20, 279-283.

Wang, Z.Y., Lu, S.Q., Zhang, Y.Q., Song, J.L., Wen, Y. and Gui, S.H. (1986) Investigations on the prevalence, immunodiagnosis and experimental model of giardiasis. Chinese Med. J. 99, 961-968.

Woo, P.T.K. and Paterson, W.B. (1986) *Giardia lamblia* in children in daycare centres in southern Ontario, Canada, and susceptibility of animals to *G. lamblia*. Trans. R. Soc. Trop. Med. Hyg. 80, 56-59.

Giardiasis (E.A. Meyer, ed.)
© 1990 Elsevier Science Publishers B.V. (Biomedical Division)

5

Animal model of *Giardia muris* in the mouse

DAVID P. STEVENS

Department of Medicine, Case Western Reserve University School of Medicine, University Hospitals of Cleveland, Cleveland, OH 44106, U.S.A.

1. Introduction	91
2. Early development of a murine model	92
3. Murine infection as a model of human disease	92
4. Immunologic studies in murine giardiasis	93
5. Conclusion	96
References	96

1. Introduction

Unanswered questions pertaining to the natural history, protective immunity, and immunopathogenesis of human giardiasis suggested a role for an animal model of this infection. Selection of the mouse for such a model was based on several advantages. Considerable technology existed for the study of the immune response in mice. Moreover, many well-defined inbred strains were available. Finally, the size and life span of this host made it an economical choice.

The model has led to preliminary insights into the role of the host's immune system in both the pathogenesis and development of resistance to this small intestinal protozoan (Stevens and Roberts-Thomson, 1978). Moreover, while *Giardia* infection had been described in dozens of host species in the natural state, the model has provided the opportunity for controlled and prospective observations of the natural history of this infection (Roberts-Thomson et al., 1976a; Stevens, 1982; Belosevic and Faubert, 1983; Belosevic et al., 1986).

2. Early development of a murine model

A semi-quantitative flotation technique for isolation of fecal cysts was developed by Roberts-Thomson et al. (1976a). The *Giardia* strain which was employed in these studies was isolated from a golden hamster screened for *Giardia* in the Case Western Reserve University School of Medicine Animal Quarters in 1975. This same *Giardia* strain has been maintained by passage in CF-1 mice at six to eight week intervals in this and other laboratories. Multiple murine strains have subsequently been infected and details of their susceptibility are reviewed below. Morphologic aspects of this *Giardia* strain were described by Owen et al. (1979).

After oral inoculation with 10^3 cysts, the peak infection, as determined by the number of cysts excreted in stool, occurred in seven to 14 days. Subsequently, cyst excretion gradually diminished until six to ten weeks when cysts were generally undetectable.

Correlation was made between the number of trophozoites present in the small intestine and the quantity of cysts excreted in stool (Roberts-Thomson et al., 1976a). They found that the intensity of trophozoite infection in small intestine correlated directly with the number of cysts excreted in stool. This observation permitted the assumption that cyst excretion from live animals was a measure of the intensity of infection in the small bowel at any given point. The most heavily infected area of the small intestine in these experiments was the proximal jejunum. In contrast, Olveda, Andrews and Hewlett (1982) found trophozoites in proximal jejunum late in infection at a time when cysts were undetectable in stool. The absence of cysts in stool when trophozoites are detectable in jejunum remains unexplained. A similar observation was made by earlier investigators in a somewhat different murine model (Iwanczuk et al., 1965). Thus, cyst excretion in stool appears to be reliable as a measure of infection up to 8 weeks after inoculation when jejunal infection is moderate to heavy; however, low intensity infection in jejunum is inconsistently detectable by cyst excretion.

3. Murine infection as a model of human disease

Morphologic studies of the small intestinal mucosa by light microscopy demonstrated a reduction in villous height during peak infection (Roberts-Thomson et al., 1976b; Stevens and Roberts-Thomson, 1978; Brett, 1983). Severe mucosal atrophy, however, such as that seen in human infection was not observed.

The rate of weight gain in infected growing animals was retarded compared to uninfected controls. Weight loss was not observed in otherwise healthy, immune-competent, mature mice. Possible explanations for reduced weight gain in infected animals include mucosal abnormalities resulting in true malabsorption and competition for nutrients by infecting organisms. Diarrhea or change in stool weight were not observed in infected animals.

4. Immunologic studies in murine giardiasis

Initially studies were performed to establish that prior infection by oral inoculation was protective against subsequent infection with *Giardia* cysts (Roberts-Thomson, 1976b). CF-1 mice were infected and studied by quantification of cysts in stools over time to verify the disappearance of infection. Subsequent oral challenge with 10^3 *Giardia* cysts failed to result in recurrence of infection. Previously uninfected control animals of the same age were readily infected by oral challenge with *Giardia* cysts.

The role for humoral immunologic mechanisms in resistance to *Giardia* infection remains incompletely defined (Anders et al., 1983). Snider and Underdown (1986) demonstrated in BALB/c and C57BL/6 strains specific anti-*G. muris* IgA in intestinal secretions which were associated with clearance of *G. muris* by these animals. An additional group of experiments which implicated the role for circulating immunity were those of Snider et al. (1985) in which BALB/c mice were treated from birth with rabbit anti-IgM antiserum. This treatment resulted in marked IgA, IgG and IgM deficiency. These animals contained no demonstrable anti-*G. muris* antibody either in serum or gut washings. Moreover, they developed chronic *Giardia* infection. In contrast, untreated controls developed identifiable antibodies in the circulation and gut washings and cleared the infection. As these authors pointed out, these results did not distinguish between a direct primary role for anti-*Giardia* antibody or a secondary effect for B-cell function in resistance to this infection.

The role for cellular immunity was first suggested by the demonstration by scanning electron microscopy of a direct interaction between lymphocytes and *G. muris* in this model by Owen et al. (1979). Studies from the laboratories of Owen and co-workers have also demonstrated by EM a potential role for cells found in Peyer's patches (Owen et al., 1981) as well as those found within the intestinal lumen (Heyworth et al., 1985a,b). Later studies (Carlson et al., 1986) showed that total Peyer's patch cell populations more than doubled during *G. muris* infection in BALB/c mice. The relative populations of T-helper and T-suppressor cells as demonstrated by flow cytometry did not change during infection.

Thymus-mediated immunity was studied in congenitally thymus-deficient nude (Nu/Nu) mice (Stevens et al., 1978). Orally inoculated Nu/Nu animals proceeded to excrete cysts for twenty weeks. Heterozygous, thymus-competent controls developed the previously observed course of infection with gradual elimination of cyst excretion after ten weeks. Oral challenge of previously infected Nu/Nu animals with *Giardia* cysts resulted in resumption of high levels of cyst excretion. Cyst excretion, however, continued for a shorter time than that observed during primary infection. Heterozygous, previously infected controls were resistent when challenged. Reconstitution experiments, in which spleen cell suspensions from immune animals were injected into Nu/Nu animals, resulted in the development of resistance to infection by subsequent oral challenge with cysts (Roberts-Thomson and Mitchell, 1978). Carlson et al. (1987) have shown that the

T-cell deficit in the nude strain persistently infected by *G. muris* in their laboratory was associated with a specific reduction of L3T4$^+$ lymphocytes.

Initial studies of the genetic control of immunity to *Giardia* were pursued by several laboratories. Protective immunity has been observed in most strains, but at least three strains, W/W, C3H/He and A/J, as well as Nu/Nu mice, were found to remain infected for prolonged periods after oral infection by *Giardia* (Roberts-Thomson et al., 1980; Roberts-Thomson and Mitchell, 1979; Underdown et al., 1981).

When poorly resistant C3H/He mice and resistant BALB/c mice were mated, the F1 hybrid was resistant, suggesting that resistance was inherited in a dominant fashion. However, when back-cross experiments were performed using matings between resistant (BALB/c × C3H/He) F1 hybrids and poorly resistant C3H/He animals, intermediate resistance was found. The absence of clear-cut segregation of these latter off-spring into resistant and susceptible characteristics argued against single gene control of resistance.

Additional studies by Belosevic et al. (1984) reinforced the hypothesis that resistance was under the complex control of multiple genes. In these studies, resistant B10.A mice crossed with susceptible A/J strains resulted in F1 hybrids that resembled the resistant B10.A strain, confirming dominance of the resistant characteristic. However, when resistant DBA/2 mice and susceptible A/J mice were crossed, it was found that the offspring resembled the susceptible A/J parent, indicating that, at least in this strain-pairing, resistance in DBA/2 mice was recessive. In further studies, the F1 hybrid of two resistant strains, C57BL/6 and C3H/He, was more resistant than either parent, suggesting to the authors the presence of gene complementarity. Additional evidence was garnered from experiments that showed that back-cross populations did not segregate into resistant and susceptible populations in ratios that would be consistent with clear-cut single-gene control. The absence of a role for the Ir genes that map within the H-2 locus in resistant inbred strains could be concluded from these same studies. To wit, both the susceptible A/J strain and the resistant B10.A strain have the same H-2 haplotype. The authors concluded, however, that these observations did not exclude 'the possibility of minor involvement of H-2 locus genes' in the trait of resistance (Belosevic et al., 1984).

Observations in both resistant and susceptible strains among inbred mice known to be mast cell-deficient and low-producers of IgE have suggested that there may be a role for these components of resistance to *Giardia*. For example, the mast cell-deficient W/W strain developed prolonged infection when exposed to murine *Giardia*. Belosevic et al. (1984) noted that if mast cell degranulation were mediated by IgE, strains which are low IgE producers might be more susceptible in the early phases of infection as manifested by higher cyst excretion. They observed this to be the case in the low IgE producer SJL/J.

Studies of the simultaneous infection of mice with *Giardia* and the intestinal phase of *Trichinella spiralis* suggested a possible role for infection by helminths which resulted in the reduction of pathologic reaction of the host mucosa toward *Giardia* (Roberts-Thomson et al., 1976c). Specifically, the presence of *Trichinella* resulted in reduced intensity of simultaneous *Giardia* infection. Both enhancement of macrophage function and suppression of humoral and cellular immunity were suggested as mechanisms by these authors. Yet they noted that when the most dramatic intestinal mucosal changes induced by *Trichinella* resolved with resolution of the helminthic infection, the effect on *Giardia* receded, thus suggesting that the effect on *Giardia* may be more related to the alteration in intestinal mucosal morphology itself induced by the helminths.

The studies of Underdown et al. (1981) investigated the ability of a resistant strain, BALB/c, and a susceptible strain, C3H/He, to resist a second oral infection after the infected animals were cured of infection by treatment with metronidazole. Both strains were resistant to the second oral challenge. The point for emphasis was that C3H/He mice which failed to clear completely a primary infection, once cured pharmacologically, could resist a second challenge. This implied that the development of immunity took place in this strain even though prolonged infection was observed after the initial oral inoculation. These authors postulated that this inability to completely clear infection by C3H/He mice might be related to some immunosuppressive characteristic of the *Giardia* parasite itself which was effective in the C3H/He strain but might be more readily counteracted by resistant strains such as BALB/c.

Belosevic et al. (1985) postulated a role for the macrophage when they studied resistant B10.A and susceptible A/J inbred strains by measuring the ability of spleen and mesenteric lymph node cells from infected animals to affect in vitro plaque-forming cell responses to sheep red blood cells. They found that cells harvested from mice at various intervals – up to twenty days after infection in B10.A and up to thirty days in A/J mice – suppressed plaque forming cell responses in vitro. Moreover, they found that this immunodepressant effect was associated with adherent sub-populations of cells, that is, the macrophage, and that the effect was greater in mesenteric lymph node cells than in spleen cell populations.

While these and other (Belosevic and Faubert, 1983, 1986) studies suggested a parasite-induced immunodepressant function mediated by the macrophage, these authors did not elucidate the specific difference in macrophage function in resistant strains compared to susceptible strains.

The role for passive immunity via breast milk was evaluated by a series of experiments on suckling newborn mice (Stevens and Frank, 1978). Previously infected, and presumably immunized, females were bred and their offspring were then suckled. If the offspring were inoculated orally with *Giardia* cysts and returned to their mothers they were protected from infection. They were not protected if they were provided wet-nurses that were previously unimmunized. Conversely, if animals from unimmunized mothers were suckled to immunized wet-nurses, they were protected. These observations strongly suggested a role for passive immunization conveyed by the breast milk. Whether the protection was humoral or cellular was unexplained by these experiments.

Immunized mothers that were free of cyst excretion commenced excreting cysts spontaneously when breast feeding began. After weaning, maternal cyst excretion again stopped, implying restoration of protection against intestinal infection in the maternal host. The authors suggested that this may be evidence for migration of gut-associated lymphoid tissue away from intestine to mammary sites.

5. Conclusion

The murine model of giardiasis has permitted the controlled observation of numerous and often apparently unrelated immune phenomena. These observations have provided enlightening but incomplete insights into properties of the host's immune response and the immunopathogenesis of this infection. Better characterization of specific *Giardia* antigens and host mechanisms for antigen processing are needed. Future studies will benefit from evolving technology that better characterizes the genetic control as well as the specific mechanisms of antibody-cell, lymphokine-cell and cell-cell interactions that modulate and enhance the immune response to *Giardia* infection.

References

Anders, R.F., Roberts-Thomson, I.C. and Mitchell, G.F. (1983) Giardiasis in mice: analysis of humoral and cellular immune responses to *Giardia muris*. Parasite Immunol. 4, 47-57.

Belosevic, M. and Faubert, G.M. (1986) Comparative studies of inflammatory responses in susceptible and resistant mice infected with *Giardia muris*. Clin. Exp. Immunol. 65, 622-630.

Belosevic, M. and Faubert, G.M. (1983) *Giardia muris*: Correlation between oral dosage, course of infection and trophozoite distribution in the mouse small intestine. Exp. Parasitol. 56, 93-100.

Belosevic, M., Faubert, G.M. and MacLean, J.D. (1985) *Giardia muris*-induced depression of the primary immune response in spleen and mesenteric lymph node cell cultures to sheep red blood cells. Parasite Immunol. 7, 467-478.

Belosevic, M., Faubert, G.M. and MacLean, J.D. (1986) Mouse-to-mouse transmission of infections with *Giardia muris*. Parasitology 92, 595-598.

Belosevic, M., Faubert, G.M., Skamene, E. and MacLean, J.D. (1984) Susceptibility and resistance of inbred mice to *Giardia muris*. Infect. Immun. 44, 282-286.

Brett, S.J. (1983) Immunodepression in *Giardia muris* and *Spironucleus muris* infections in mice. Parasitology 87, 507.

Carlson, J.R., Heyworth, M.F. and Owen, R.L. (1987) T-lymphocyte subsets in nude mice with *Giardia muris* infection. Thymus 9, 189-196.

Carlson, J.R., Heyworth, M.F. and Owen, R.L. (1986) Response of Peyer's patch lymphocyte subsets to *Giardia muris* infection in BALB/c mice. Cell Immunol. 97, 44-50.

Heyworth, M.F., Owen, R.L. and Jones, A.L. (1985a) Comparison of leukocytes obtained from the intestinal lumen of *Giardia*-infected immunocompetent mice and nude mice. Gastroenterology 89, 1360-1365.

Heyworth, M.F., Owen, R.L., Seaman, W.E., Schaefer, Frank W., III and Jones, A.L. (1985b) Harvesting of leukocytes from intestinal lumen in murine giardiasis and preliminary characterization of these cells. Digest. Dis. Sci. 30, 149-153.

Iwanczuk, I. (1965) Studies on the course of infection with *Lamblia muris* Bensen in albino mice. Acta Parasitol. Polon. 13, 227-258.

Olveda, R.K., Andrews, J.S., Jr. and Hewlett, E.L. (1982) Murine giardiasis: localization of trophozoites and small bowel histopathology during the course of infection. Am. J. Trop. Med. Hyg. 31, 60-66.

Owen, R.L., Allen, C.L. and Stevens, D.P. (1981) Phagocytosis of *Giardia muris* by macrophages in Peyer's patches epithelium in mice. Infect. Immun. 33, 591-601.

Owen, R.L., Nemanic, P.C. and Stevens, D.P. (1979) Ultrastructural observations on giardiasis in a murine model. I. Intestinal distribution, attachment, and relationship to the immune system of *Giardia muris*. Gastroenterology 76, 757-769.

Roberts-Thomson, I.C., Grove, D.I., Stevens, D.P., et al. (1976c) Suppression of giardiasis during the intestinal phase of trichinosis in the mouse. Gut 17, 953-958.

Roberts-Thomson, I.C. and Mitchell, G.F. (1978) Giardiasis in mice: I. Prolonged infections in certain mouse strains and hypothymic (nude) mice. Gastroenterology 75, 42-46.

Roberts-Thomson, I.C. and Mitchell, G.F. (1979) Protection of mice against *Giardia muris* infection. Infect. Immun. 24, 971-973.

Roberts-Thomson, I.C., Mitchell, G.F., Anders, R.F., Tait, B.D., Kerlin, P., Kerr-Grant, A. and Cavanach, P. (1980) Genetic studies in human and murine giardiasis. Gut 21, 397-401.

Roberts-Thomson, I.C., Stevens, D.P., Mahmoud, A.A.F. and Warren, K.S. (1976a) Giardiasis in the mouse: an animal model. Gastroenterology 71, 57-61.

Roberts-Thomson, I.C., Stevens, D.P., Mahmoud, A.A.F. and Warren, K.S. (1976b) Acquired resistance to infection in an animal model of giardiasis. J. Immunol. 117, 2036-2037.

Snider, D.P., Gordon, J., McDermott, M.R. and Underdown, B.J. (1985) Chronic *Giardia muris* infection in anti-IgM-treated mice. J. Immunol. 134, 4153-4162.

Snider, D.P. and Underdown, B.J. (1986) Quantitative and temporal analyses of murine antibody response in serum and gut secretions to infection with *Giardia muris*. Infect. Immun. 52, 271-278.

Stevens, D.P. (1982) Giardiasis: host-pathogen biology. Rev. Infect. Dis. 4, 851-858.

Stevens, D.P. and Frank, D.M. (1978) Local immunity in murine giardiasis: is milk protective at the expense of maternal gut? Trans. Assoc. Am. Phys. 91, 268-272.

Stevens, D.P., Frank, D.M. and Mahmoud, A.A.F. (1978) Thymus dependency of host resistance to *Giardia muris* infection: studies in nude mice. J. Immunol. 120, 680.

Stevens, D.P. and Roberts-Thomson, I.C. (1978) Animal model of human disease: Giardiasis. Am. J. Pathol. 90, 529.

Underdown, B.J., Roberts-Thomson, I.C., Anders, R.F. and Mitchell, G.F. (1981) Giardiasis in mice: studies on the characteristics of chronic infection in C3H/He mice. J. Immunol. 126, 669-672.

Giardiasis (E.A. Meyer, ed.)
© 1990 Elsevier Science Publishers B.V. (Biomedical Division)

6

In vitro cultivation of *Giardia* trophozoites

SIMONA RADULESCU[1] and ERNEST A. MEYER[2]

[1]*Cantacuzino Institute, Bucharest, Romania* and [2]*Department of Microbiology and Immunology, Oregon Health Sciences University, Portland, OR 97201-3098, U.S.A.*

1. Introduction	99
2. Initiation of cultures: intestinal trophozoites as inoculum	101
3. Initiation of cultures: excysted trophozoites as inoculum	103
4. Initiation of cultures: surrogate animal hosts as a source of trophozoites for inoculum	104
5. Inoculum preparation	105
5.1. Trophozoites from the human host	106
5.2. Trophozoites from lower animals	106
5.3. Concentration and purification of *Giardia* trophozoites and cysts from the host	106
6. Induction of excystation of *Giardia* for culture initiation	107
7. Culture management	108
References	109

1. Introduction

Of the amoebic and flagellated protozoa that are common inhabitants of the human intestine, the *Giardia* were the first to be described and the last to be cultured. The medium of Boeck and Drbhlov, introduced in 1925 for the cultivation of *Entamoeba histolytica*, was shown that same year to also support the growth of *Trichomonas hominis* and *Chilomastix mesnili*. In contrast, it was not until 1960 (see below) that reports appeared describing culture of *Giardia* from humans.

Three books by Taylor and Baker (1968, 1978, 1988) are valuable sources of information for those interested in culturing these and other parasites. The recent volume edited by James Jensen (1986) has useful details of in vitro culture of protozoan parasites, and reviews by Meyer (1979) and Meyer and Radulescu (1984) describe the development of *Giardia* culture methods in some detail.

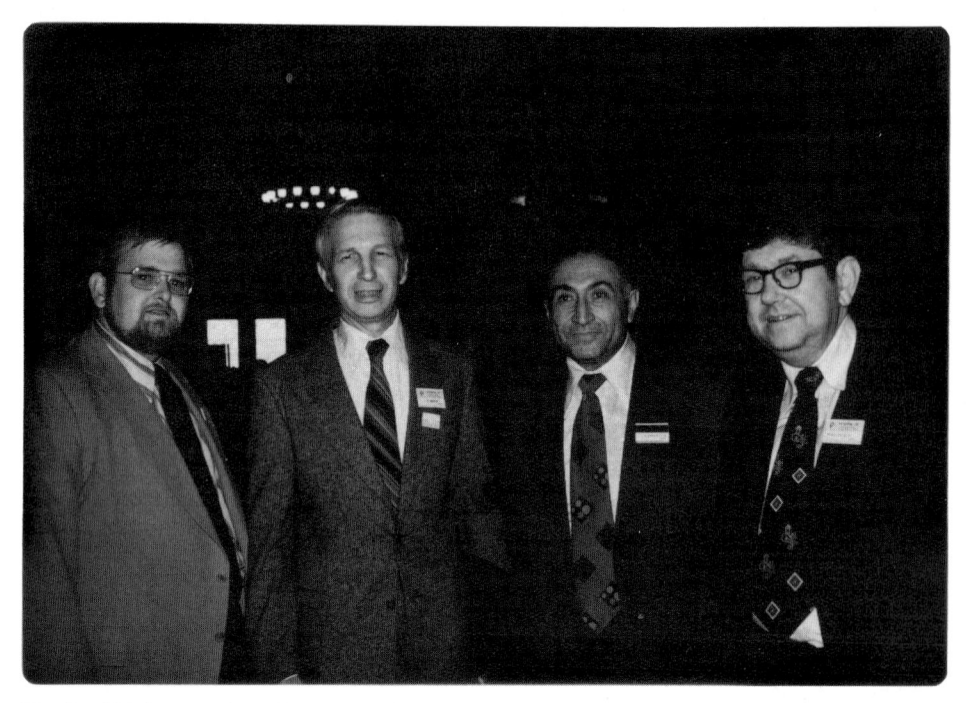

Fig. 1. *Giardia* researchers: East meets West – Warsaw, 1978. From left: E.L. Jarroll, E.A. Meyer, A.E. Karapetyan and (the late) M.M. Soloviev.

The progenitor of *Giardia* culture is A.E. Karapetyan, a researcher in the Soviet Union. Publishing first in Russian in 1960, then in English in 1962, Karapetyan described the methods he had used to culture *Giardia* trophozoites from humans for nine months. His complex medium included serum, chick embryo extract, a tryptic digest of meat, and Earle's or Hanks' solution. Additionally present were living *Candida guillermondi* (obtained with the trophozoites during duodenal intubation) and chick fibroblasts. Culture medium was changed daily, during which time fibroblasts gradually died. Thus the culture system ultimately became monoxenic. Later, Karapetyan (1962) modified the system and maintained human and rabbit *Giardia* for up to five months. In the latter system he deleted fibroblasts and substituted *Saccharomyces cerevisiae* for *Candida*. His efforts to axenically culture these *Giardia* were not successful. The necessity for yeast or yeast-like fungi in *Giardia* culture led Karapetyan to believe that these two organisms existed symbiotically.

During this period we had been attempting, with little success, to culture *Giardia*. When Karapetyan's work became known, we set out to duplicate it. Some trophozoite growth was obtained, then the organisms would die. We found that by modifying the method, our rabbit and chinchilla *Giardia* could be maintained in culture (Meyer and Pope, 1965). The modification involved the daily addition to our culture tubes of the yeast *Saccharomyces cerevisiae*. Layne Gentry described in his thesis the results of his studies of these organisms (1965). Gentry demonstrated that trypticase (a tryptic digest of casein) could substitute for the tryptic digest of meat that Karapetyan had used. He also showed that in our system the human serum used could not be substituted with beef or horse serum, as Karapetyan had observed for his system.

2. Initiation of cultures: intestinal trophozoites as inoculum

In 1970, Meyer reported axenically culturing *Giardia* trophozoites from the rabbit, chinchilla and cat. Yeast extract substituted for living yeast. Axenic culture of *Giardia* from the guinea pig was reported by Fortess and Meyer in 1976, and from a human by Meyer in the same year. Culture medium in both instances contained human serum, Hanks' solution, Phytone peptone (a papaic digest of soybean meal), and cysteine (see Table 1).

TABLE 1

Culture methods employed in obtaining or maintaining *Giardia* cultures

Author(s)	Year	Animal source	Culture medium employed*
Inoculum: trophozoites from naturally-infected host			
Meyer	1970	Cat, rabbit, chinchilla	M3 (Hanks, serum, yeast extract, cysteine)
Fortess and Meyer	1976	Guinea pig	HSP (Hanks, serum, Phytone, cysteine)
Meyer	1976	Human	HSP
Gillin and Diamond	1979	Human	Filtered TYI-S-33, filtered TPS-1
Visvesvara	1980a	Human	Filtered TPS-1
Belosevic et al.	1982	Human	Filtered TYI-S-33 vs. autoclaved TYI-S-33
Smith et al.	1982	Human	Filtered TPS-1, then filtered TYI-S-33
Faubert et al.	1983	Beaver	Filtered TYI-S-33
Keister	1983	Human	Filtered, bile supplemented (FBS) TYI-S-33
Farthing et al.	1983	Human	FBS TYI-S-33
Gordts et al.	1984 1985a,b	Human	Filtered TPS-1 Filtered TPS-1
Kasprzak and Majewska	1985	Human	FBS TPS-1 and FBS TYI-S-33

Author(s)	Year	Animal source	Culture medium employed*
Inoculum: newly excysted trophozoites			
Bingham and Meyer	1979	Human, monkey	HSP
Bhatia and Warhurst	1981	Human	Filtered TPS-1
Kasprzak and Majewska	1983	Human	Filtered TPS-1
Kasprzak and Majewska	1985	Human	Filtered TPS-1 FBS TYI-S-33
Isaac-Renton et al.	1986	Human, beaver	FBS TYI-S-33
Inoculum: trophozoites from surrogate host			
Faubert et al.	1983	Mongolian gerbils orally infected with cysts from beaver	TYI-S-33
Wallis and Wallis	1986	Mongolion gerbils infected with cysts from meadow vole, beaver, dog and human	Filtered TYI-S-33
Nash et al.	1985	Neonatal mice infected (percutaneous, intragastric) with cysts from humans	Modified TYI-S-33
McIntyre et al.	1986	Suckling mice infected intragastrically with trophozoites from humans	Modified TYI-S-33

* See literature reference for detailed description of medium preparation.

Fastidious organisms which must be grown on undefined media present the researcher with a problem not faced by those culturing less demanding organisms. That problem is the organism's varying growth response in different batches of medium. Visvesvara encountered this when he cultured the human *Giardia* (Portland-1 strain) we supplied him. Our culture medium presented Visvesvara an additional problem: he wanted to employ his trophozoites in a indirect immunofluorescent test: the human serum stained the organisms non-specifically. Visvesvara (1980a) succeeded in adapting these *Giardia* to grow in modified TPS-1, a medium introduced by Diamond in 1968 for culturing of *Entamoeba histolytica*. The modifications: (1) the medium was filtered not autoclaved, (2) bovine serum was employed, and (3) tissue culture medium NCTC 109 was used instead of NCTC 107. Using this medium, Visvesvara and Healy were able easily to obtain large numbers of cultured trophozoites which he used in an indirect immunofluorescent test (1979).

The initials TPS (in TPS-1 medium) stand for trypticase, panmede (an ox liver digest) and serum (bovine). Increasing difficulty in obtaining batches of Panmede that would support amoebic growth led Diamond to look for a substitute. In 1978, Diamond et al. introduced TYI-S-33 medium for *Entamoeba histolytica* culture. It is gradually replacing TPS-1 for this purpose. The initials in TYI-S-33 stand for trypticase, yeast extract, iron and serum. In 1979, Gillin and Diamond also reported that the Portland-1 strain of *Giardia* could be grown in a modified TYI-S-33, and that the L-cysteine hydrochloride in this medium, and in TPS-1, was essential for *Giardia* growth.

In the early 1980s, modifications of TPS-1 and TYI-S-33 were being used successfully by *Giardia* researchers. Smith et al. in 1982 isolated and cultured a strain (WB) of *Giardia* from a patient who had apparently acquired the infection in Afghanistan. Started in filter-sterilized TPS-1, the organisms were adapted to modified TYI-S-33 medium.

The 1982 American Type Culture Collection (ATCC) catalog listed two strains of *Giardia*, the Portland-1 strain, and the WB strain; further, the ATCC recommended that both be cultivated on filter-sterilized Diamond's TPS-1 medium.

In 1983, Keister, and Farthing et al., independently noted that mammalian bile promotes the growth of *Giardia* trophozoites in culture in a modified TYI-S-33 medium.

The ATCC then encountered difficulties with medium ingredients for culture of *Giardia* and *Entamoeba*. As a result, for *Giardia* culture, the ATCC recommended a modification of Keister's 1983 medium; in the ATCC medium, trypticase is substituted with either a suitable lot of biosate (a mixture of casein digest and yeast extract-BBL 97580), or casein digest (BBL 97023) and yeast extract. Since 1983, a number of reports have documented successful establishment of *Giardia* cultures initiated with trophozoites from the small intestine of naturally infected hosts; as medium, either a modified TPS-1 or modified TYI-S-33 medium was employed. References to some of these reports are listed in Table 1.

3. Initiation of cultures: excysted trophozoites as inoculum

By the late 1970s, two groups of workers had obtained axenic cultures of *Giardia*. Both groups had used as inocula trophozoites from host intestine. Newly excysted trophozoites had not been used to start cultures because at that time the mechanism of *Giardia* excystation was not known. The U.S. Environmental Protection Agency provided the wherewithal that permitted the study of this phenomenon. Evidence suggested that waterborne cysts were a common cause of outbreaks of giardiasis. The EPA wanted to establish means of inactivating *Giardia* cysts. But how best to determine the viability of these cysts?

At that time, eosin exclusion – the ability of the cyst to exclude a dye – was considered a criterion for viability. Earlier, dye exclusion had been used, and criticized, as a means of determining cyst viability of *Entamoeba histolytica*.

Alan Bingham, a graduate student in Oregon, accepted the task of studying determinants of viability in *Giardia* cysts. The reasoning was that the ability of a cyst to excyst might be a better criterion of viability than its ability to exclude a dye. Bingham set out to study excystation. He considered those factors – digestive fluids, pH, temperature, time – encountered by an ingested cyst in transit from the host's mouth to its excystation in the small intestine. In relatively short order, he succeeded not only in inducing excystation, but in defining the factors involved. Bingham and Meyer reported (1979) that *Giardia* excystation depends on low pH, time of acid exposure, temperature, and composition of the medium after cyst exposure to low pH. They also showed that eosin exclusion consistently indicates greater cyst viability than does excystation (Bingham et al., 1979).

The ability to induce in vitro excystation of *Giardia* offered the possibility of establishing cultures using as inocula trophozoites, obtained as a result of excystation. In fact, Bingham and Meyer (1979) reported starting such cultures from cysts from humans and monkeys. In 1981, Bhatia and Warhurst initiated five cultures from *Giardia* cysts from humans. And Kaspryzak and Majewska in Poland isolated three more such strains from cysts in 1983. Whereas Bingham and Meyer had used HSP medium, the latter two groups of workers employed modified TPS-1 medium.

In an interesting 1985 paper, Kaspryzak and Majewska reported further *Giardia* culture studies. They compared the effectiveness of initiation of cultures of (1) duodenal trophozoites and fecal cysts as inocula, (2) inocula from symptomatic and asymptomatic hosts, (3) TPS-1 versus modified TYI-S-33 medium, and (4) five different animal sera as medium components. The study yielded 17 additional strains of *Giardia*. They concluded: (1) neither trophozoites nor cysts proved clearly superior as inocula, (2) similar culture success was obtained using inocula from symptomatic and asymptomatic donors, (3) modified TYI-S-33 proved superior to TPS-1, and (4) only bovine and calf serum resulted in consistently good growth.

Recently, Isaac-Renton et al. (1986) reported establishing *Giardia* cultures from human and beaver; they used as inocula fecal cysts which were concentrated, exposed to an induction step, then suspended in a modified TYI-S-33 medium.

4. Initiation of cultures: surrogate animal hosts as a source of trophozoites for inoculum

Mongolian gerbils (or jirds) and suckling mice, both of which have been used as animal models for studying *Giardia* infection, also have been used successfully to obtain these protozoa in culture. Advantage is taken of the fact that both of these animals can be infected with *Giardia* from a variety of other animals. If infection proceeds, large numbers of trophozoites may be obtained. Interestingly, cyst production may be sparse or absent (Visvesvara et al., 1988).

Faubert et al. in 1983 demonstrated that oral inoculation of 6 to 10 week old male jirds with *Giardia* cysts from mice, beavers, and humans resulted in infection with varying patterns of cyst release. Trophozoites from jirds initially given cysts from a beaver were inoculated into TYI-S-33 medium and subsequently axenized.

In a similar way, Wallis and Wallis (1986) infected jirds with cysts and trophozoites from meadow voles, dogs, beavers, and humans. While trophozoites were commonly present in the small intestine, fecal cysts were often absent. The exception: jirds infected with *Giardia* from meadow voles consistently excreted cysts. While these animals may not serve as a satisfactory source of cysts, they do provide a continuing supply of trophozoites. Although the efforts of Wallis and Wallis in this study resulted in initial in vitro *Giardia* growth, bacterial contamination prevented their obtaining axenic cultures.

The first report of the use of neonatal mice as a means of propagating *Giardia* for subsequent in vitro isolation was that of Nash et al. in 1985. They reported employing five strains of *Giardia*, all of which were axenized at the National Institutes of Health (Bethesda, MD) by first injecting *Giardia* cysts from humans intragastrically into suckling mice; trophozoites from the intestines of these mice were used to establish cultures. Earlier, Vinayak et al. (1979) and Hill et al. (1983) had shown that suckling mice could be infected with *Giardia* of human origin.

Preliminary passage of *Giardia* trophozoites of human origin through mice to facilitate axenization was studied by McIntyre et al. (1986). Duodenal juices containing trophozoites were given intragastrically to mice younger than 5 days of age. Ten days later, the small intestines were removed, and the trophozoites concentrated by washing, and inoculated into modified TYI-S-33 medium. The success rate at establishing cultures using this method proved greater than that when these human duodenal juices were inoculated directly into culture medium.

In summary, increasing numbers of workers are reporting successful isolation of *Giardia* of the *duodenalis* type in culture. Although organisms from humans have been most frequently isolated, *Giardia* from several other animal species have also been obtained. Inoculum can be trophozoites, or cysts induced to excyst. And while a modified TYI-S-33 medium is presently favored, a variety of other media has been used successfully.

5. Inoculum preparation

Giardia cultures can be initiated with either trophozoites or cysts. Trophozoites from host intestines offer the advantage of being obtained with few if any contaminating miroorganisms. A possible disadvantage is the fact that, unlike cysts, only a single specimen may be obtainable from a given donor. For humans, duodenal intubation as a means of obtaining trophozoites is an unpleasant procedure and donors may not consent to repeated intubations. Additionally, most such human infections are diagnosed in patients whose symptoms were the reason for medical consultation. Once diagnosed, such patients are often unwilling to delay treatment, even in the altruistic name of research. And as far as small animals are concerned, obtaining the duodenal specimen usually involves the death of the animal.

5.1. Trophozoites from the human host

Liquid from the duodenal intubation can be used directly, or concentrated, in the attempt to establish *Giardia* cultures. Any motile trophozoites seen in the duodenal fluid can be concentrated by gentle centrifugation (600 × g, 10 min), most of the supernatant pipetted off and discarded, and the pellet resuspended in the remaining fluid and used as inoculum. After 1/2 hour at 37°C, the culture fluid is decanted and replaced with fresh medium; any toxic components associated with the intestinal contents are thus removed.

5.2. Trophozoites from lower animals

Trophozoites can be obtained for culture by sacrificing any of a variety of infected small mammals. In the laboratory the small intestine of the freshly killed animal is exposed. A 10-15 cm section of small intestine is removed, and the contents gently stripped out and discarded. The segment is opened with a lengthwise cut, then the inner surface scraped with a scalpel and the scraping suspended in 15-20 ml of Hanks' balanced salt solution. The suspension is dispersed by forcing the suspension repeatedly through a Pasteur pipette. The mixture is then filtered through a clean coarse cloth filter. The filtrate is centrifuged at 600 × g for 10 min, most of the supernatant removed and discarded, and the remainder used as inoculum.

Several other methods of obtaining an inoculum of *Giardia* trophozoites have been described. In one (Nash et al., 1985), a segment of small intestine is opened and placed directly into tubes containing medium and antibiotics. Examination with the inverted microscope after 5-10 min at 37°C will establish whether trophozoites are in the medium and attached to the tube surface. At this time, the intestinal segment can be aseptically removed and either discarded or used in an attempt to establish another culture in a second tube. More recently, Wallis and Wallis (1986) have described a similar method.

An alternative approach can be taken if it is desired to make repeated efforts to culture organisms from a particular host. *Giardia* from the animal in question can be used to infect either gerbils or suckling mice. These animals in turn can be the source of organisms for culture. References to this procedure are to be found in Section 4 of this chapter.

5.3. Concentration and purification of Giardia *trophozoites and cysts from hosts*

Feely (1984) has described several methods which have been used to isolate, concentrate and purify trophozoites. These methods are summarized in Table 2.

A simple method of concentrating cysts from human feces was described by Rendtorff in 1954. It involves filtering a fecal slurry through cheesecloth, then repeated centrifugation which results in cysts in the pellet. The resuspended sediment is placed in a watch glass and the cysts allowed to settle. The supernatant is decanted. The residue is repeatedly washed and the supernatant removed. This technique has the advantage that the cysts

TABLE 2

Methods of concentration of *Giardia* trophozoites from host intestine

Reference	Organism	Method
Andrews et al., 1980	G. muris	Density gradient separation, then elution through nylon columns.
Roberts-Thomson and Mitchell, 1979	G. muris	Removal of intestinal trophozoites by vibration, then repeated centrifugation.
Feely and Erlandsen, 1981	G. muris, G. duodenalis	Trophozoites specifically attach to warm surface; detach by cold temperature incubation, then reattach to clean Petri dishes.

are never exposed to the osmotic changes involved when sucrose or zinc sulfate is used.

Sucrose density gradient centrifugation is widely used to concentrate both *G. duodenalis* and *G. muris* cysts. Such methods have been described by Roberts-Thomson et al. (1976), Sheffield and Bjorvatn (1977) and Bingham et al. (1979). All such methods involve most or all of the following steps: (1) Suspending the stools in water and breaking them into a slurry. (2) Removal of large particles by filtration, through cheesecloth, nylon mesh or sieves. (3) Concentrating and washing the cysts by centrifugation. (4) Preparation of a concentrated cyst suspension in water. (5) Gentle layering of the cyst suspension on chilled sucrose (0.85 M or 1.0 M) in a centrifuge tube. (6) Centrifugation for 5 min at $600 \times g$. (7) Removing the sucrose-water interface (which contains the cysts), diluting with water, and washing by centrifugation. (8) Resuspending the pellet in a small volume of water and repeating the sucrose gradient steps.

Do not store cyst suspension in sucrose solution. Ideally, cysts are used on the day they are concentrated. Some cysts in such a suspension will remain viable for 2 weeks or more at refrigerator temperatures; antibacterial and antifungal agents may reduce growth of contaminants.

6. Induction of excystation of Giardia *cysts for culture initiation.*

Bingham and Meyer (1979) made the initial observation that *G. duodenalis* cysts could be induced to excyst, and initiate cultures, if first exposed to low pH values, at 37°C, for relatively short periods. Since then, considerably more information is available regarding *G. duodenalis* (and *G. muris*) excystation. A review of this subject is to be found in Chapter 7 of this volume. Bhatia and Warhurst (1981), Kasprzak and Majewska (1985), and Isaac-Renton et al. (1986) have described the methods they used to successfully establish *Giardia duodenalis*-type organisms. More recently, Schupp et al. (1988) reported the following procedure for initiating *Giardia* cultures from cysts:

Aseptically dilute 6 ml of 100 mM cysteine-ascorbic acid solution in Eagle's minimal essential medium to a total of 50 ml in Hanks' balanced salt solution. Culture tubes (13 × 100 mm) containing 6 ml of the diluted cysteine-ascorbic acid solution are incubated in a water bath at 37°C. Each tube is inoculated with *Giardia* cysts in 0.1 ml water. The tubes are stoppered and incubated for 15 min at 37°C. The pH is adjusted to neutrality by the dropwise addition of N NaHCO$_3$ after incubation. The cysts are immediately centrifuged at 1000 × g for 10 min at 4°C, the supernatant is removed, and the tubes refilled with TYI-S-33 medium. The stoppered tubes are placed in a 37°C incubator and examined periodically for signs of excystation and the presence of trophozoites.

7. Culture management

Giardia cultures are conveniently maintained in 13 × 100 mm screw-capped or rubber-stoppered glass test tubes. TYI-S-33 medium has proven to be consistently more satisfactory than other media.

TYI broth (lacking serum, cysteine and antibiotics) is made up in 1 l amounts, filter sterilized, dispensed in 50 to 100 ml volumes, and stored frozen until used. The complete medium is usually used on the day it is prepared; it can be stored overnight in the refrigerator if necessary. Because medium constituents vary, it is a good idea to make and test a new batch of medium before the old batch is expended.

To initiate cultures, aseptically add about 6 ml of complete TYI-S-33 medium to each tube, and 0.1-0.5 ml of inoculum. Incubate tightly stoppered tubes on a slant at 35-37°C. Examine with an inverted microscope. Medium can be changed when organisms can be seen multiplying and attached to the glass. Tubes containing established cultures should be changed at 48 or 72 h intervals. Tubes that have only a few trophozoites and which are not contaminated may not need changing.

Medium can be changed in either of two ways: (1) All of the culture fluid can be poured out of the tube, and immediately replaced with fresh medium. Alternately, (2) Organisms can be transferred to new tubes by chilling the culture tubes in ice 10-15 min, which causes the trophozoites to detach. Culture tubes are gently inverted, then 1 ml or more of culture fluid is transferred to another tube, which is filled with fresh medium. This method can also be used to initiate large numbers of subcultures.

References

Andrews, J.S., Ellner, J.J. and Stevens, D.P. (1980) Purification of *Giardia muris* trophozoites by using nylon fiber columns. Am. J. Trop. Med. Hyg. 29, 12-15.

Bhatia, V.M. and Warhurst, D.C. (1981) Hatching and subsequent cultivation of cysts of *Giardia intestinalis* in Diamond's medium. J. Trop. Med. Hyg. 84, 45.

Bingham, A.K. and Meyer, E.A. (1979) *Giardia* excystation can be induced in vitro in acidic solutions. Nature (London) 277, 301-302.

Bingham, A., Jarroll, E.L., Meyer, E.A. and Radulescu, S. (1979) Induction of *Giardia* excystation and the effect of temperature on cyst viability as compared by eosin-exclusion and in vitro excystation. In: W. Jakubowski and J.C. Hoff (Eds.), Waterborne Transmission of Giardiasis, pp. 217-229. U.S. Environmental Protection Agency, Cincinnati, Ohio.

Boeck, W.C. and Drbohlav, J. (1925) The cultivation of *Entamoeba histolytica*. Am. J. Hyg. 5, 371-407.

Diamond, L.S., Harlow, D.R. and Cunnick, C.C. (1978) A new medium for the axenic cultivation of *Entamoeba histolytica* and other *Entamoeba*. Trans. R. Soc. Trop. Med. Hyg. 72, 431-432.

Farthing, M.J.G., Varon, S.R. and Keusch, G.G. (1983) Mammalian bile promotes growth of *Giardia lamblia* in axenic culture. Trans. R. Soc. Trop. Med. Hyg. 77, 467-469.

Faubert, G.M., Belosevic, M., Walker, T.S., Maclean, J.D. and Meerovitch, E. (1983) Comparative studies on the pattern of infection with *Giardia* spp. in Mongolian gerbils. J. Parasitol. 69, 802-805.

Feely, D.E. (1984) Methods of Isolating Trophozoites and Cysts. In: S.L. Erlandsen and E.A. Meyer (Eds.), Giardia and Giardiasis. Biology, Pathogenesis and Epidemiology, pp. 89–97. Plenum Press, New York.

Feely, D.E. and Erlandsen, S.L. (1981) Isolation and axenic cultivation of *Giardia* trophozoites from rat intestine. J. Parasitol. 67, 59-64.

Fortess, E. and Meyer, E.A. (1976) Isolation and axenic cultivation of *Giardia* trophozoites from the guinea pig. J. Parasitol. 62, 689.

Gentry, L.O. (1965) Studies of the in vitro growth requirements of *Giardia*. M.S. thesis, University of Oregon Medical School, Portland.

Gillin, F.D. and Diamond, L.S. (1979) Axenically cultivated *Giardia lamblia*: growth, attachment and the role of L-cysteine. In: W. Jakubowski and J.C. Hoff (Eds.), Waterborne Transmission of Giardiasis, pp. 270-272. U.S. Environmental Protection Agency, Cincinnati, Ohio.

Hill, D.R., Guerrant, R.L., Pearson, R.D. and Hewlett, E.L. (1983) *Giardia lamblia* infection in suckling mice. J. Infect. Dis. 147, 217-221.

Isaac-Renton, J., Proctor, E.M., Prameya, R. and Wong, Q. (1986) A method of excystation and culture of *Giardia lamblia*. Trans. R. Soc. Trop. Med. Hyg. 80, 989-990.

Jensen, J.B. (1986) In vitro Cultivation of Protozoan Parasites. CRC Press, Boca Raton, Florida.

Karapetyan, A.E. (1960) Methods of *Lamblia* cultivation. Tsitologiya 2, 379-384.

Karapetyan, A. (1962) In vitro cultivation of *Giardia duodenalis*. J. Parasitol. 48, 337-340.

Kasprzak, W. and Majewska, A.C. (1983) Isolation and axenic growth of fresh *Giardia intestinalis* strains in TPS-1 medium. Trans. R. Soc. Trop. Med. Hyg. 77, 223-224.

Kasprzak, W. and Majewska, A.C. (1985) Improvement in isolation and axenic growth of *Giardia intestinalis* strains. Trans. R. Soc. Trop. Med. Hyg. 79, 551-557.

Keister, D.B. (1983) Axenic culture of *Giardia lamblia* in TYI-S-33 medium supplemented with bile. Trans. R. Soc. Trop. Med. Hyg. 77, 487-488.

McIntyre, P., Boreham, P.F.L., Phillips, R.E. and Shepherd, R.W. (1986) Chemotherapy in giardiasis: clinical responses and in vitro drug sensitivity of human isolates in axenic culture. J. Pediatr. 108, 1005-1010.

Meyer, E.A. (1970) Isolation and axenic cultivation of *Giardia* trophozoites from the rabbit, chinchilla, and cat. Exp. Parasitol. 27, 179-183.

Meyer, E.A. (1976) *Giardia lamblia*: isolation and axenic cultivation. Exp. Parasitol. 39, 101-105.

Meyer, E.A. (1979) The propagation of *Giardia* trophozoites in vitro. In: W. Jakubowski and J.C. Hoff (Eds.),

Waterborne Transmission of Giardiasis, pp. 211-216. U.S. Environmental Protection Agency, Cincinnati, Ohio.

Meyer, E.A. and Pope, B.L. (1965) Culture in vitro of *Giardia* trophozoites from the rabbit and chinchilla. Nature (London) 207, 1417-1418.

Meyer, E.A. and Radulescu, S. (1984) In vitro cultivation of *Giardia* trophozoites. In: S.L. Erlandsen and E.A. Meyer (Eds.), *Giardia* and Giardiasis. Biology, Pathogenesis, and Epidemiology, pp. 99-110. Plenum Press, New York.

Nash, T.E., McCutchan, T., Keister, D., Dame, J.B., Conrad, J.D. and Gillin, F.D. (1985) Restriction-endonuclease analysis of DNA from 15 *Giardia* isolates obtained from humans and animals. J. Infect. Dis. 152, 64-73.

Rendtorff, R.C. (1954) The experimental transmission of human intestinal protozoan parasites. II. *Giardia lamblia* cysts given in capsules. Am. J. Hyg. 59, 209-220.

Roberts-Thomson, E.C. and Mitchell, G.G. (1979) Protection of mice against *Giardia* infection. Infect. Immun. 24, 971-973.

Roberts-Thomson, I.C., Stevens, D.P., Mahmoud, A.A.F. and Warren, K.S. (1976) Giardiasis in the mouse: an animal model. Gastroenterology 71, 57-61.

Schupp, D.G., Januschka, M.M., Sherlock, L.F., Stibbs, H.H., Meyer, E.A., Bemrick, W.J. and Erlandsen, S.L. (1988) Production of viable *Giardia* cysts in vitro: determination by fluorogenic dye staining, excystation, and animal infectivity in the mouse and Mongolian gerbil. Gastroenterology, 95, 1-10.

Sheffield, H.G. and Bjorvatn, B. (1977) Ultrastructure of the cyst of *Giardia lamblia*. Am. J. Trop. Med. Hyg. 26, 23-30.

Smith, P.D., Gillin, F.D., Brown, W.R. and Nash, T.E. (1982) Chronic giardiasis: Studies on drug sensitivity, toxin production, and host immune response. Gastroenterology 83, 797-803.

Soloviev, M.M., Akimova, R.F. and Shmakova, V.I. (1971) Isolation and maintenance of *Lamblia duodenalis* cultures on a modified Karapetyan medium. Med. Parazitol. 40, 75-78.

Taylor, A.E.R. and Baker, J.R. (1968) The Cultivation of Parasites In Vitro. Blackwell, Oxford.

Taylor, A.E.R. and Baker, J.R. (Eds.) (1978) Methods of Cultivating Parasites In Vitro. Academic Press, London.

Taylor, A.E.R. and Baker, J.R. (Eds.) (1988) In Vitro Methods for Parasite Information. Academic Press, London.

Vinayak, V.K., Sharma, G.L. and Naik, S.R. (1979) Experimental *Giardia lamblia* infection in Swiss mice. A preliminary report. Ind. J. Med. Res. 70, 195-198.

Visvesvara, G.S. (1980a) Axenic growth of *Giardia lamblia* in TPS-1 medium. Trans. R. Soc. Trop. Med. Hyg. 74, 213-215.

Visvesvara, G.S. and Healy, G.R. (1979) The possible use of an indirect immunofluorescent test using axenically grown *Giardia lamblia* antigens in diagnosing giardiasis. In: W. Jakubowski and J.C. Hoff (Eds.), Waterborne Transmission of Giardiasis, pp. 53-63. U.S. Environmental Protection Agency, Cincinnati, Ohio.

Visvesvara, G.S., Dickerson, J.W. and Healy, G.R. (1988) Variable infectivity of human-derived *Giardia lamblia* cysts for Mongolian gerbils (*Meriones unguiculatus*). J. Clin. Microbiol. 26, 837-841.

Wallis, P.M. and Wallis, H.M. (1986) Excystation and culturing of human and animal *Giardia* spp. by using gerbils and TYI-S-33 medium. Appl. Env. Microbiol. 51, 647-651.

7

Methods for excystation of *Giardia*

FRANK W. SCHAEFER, III

Health Effects Research Laboratory, United States Environmental Protection Agency, Cincinnati, OH 45268 U.S.A.

1. Introduction	111
2. Excystation	112
2.1. In vivo excystation	112
2.2. In vitro excystation	113
2.2.1. Excystation ultrastructure	113
2.2.2. Quantitation of excystation	114
2.2.3. *Giardia duodenalis* excystation	118
2.2.4. *Giardia muris* excystation	125
2.2.5. Comparison of *G. duodenalis* and *G. muris* excystation	128
3. Comparison of excystation to other viability methods	130
3.1. Vital staining	130
3.2. Fluorescent staining	130
3.3. Morphology	131
3.4. Animal infectivity	132
4. Conclusions	133
References	133

1. Introduction

Giardia species are flagellated protozoan parasites found in the intestinal tract of many vertebrates. The parasite can exist in two forms both of which are usually found within the host's intestinal tract. The trophozoite, which is the active, vegetative form, lives in the upper part of the small intestine. Trophozoites, caught in the luminal flow, are swept down the intestinal tract and transform into cysts. The transformation from trophozoite to immature cyst is usually complete by the time the parasite reaches the distal portion of the small intestine. The cyst is the dormant, transmission form of the parasite. The mature cyst is essentially a rounded trophozoite, which is surrounded by a cyst wall, and has completed karyokinesis, but usually not cytokinesis. A different type of mature cyst from microtine rodents has been described by Boeck (1919). It is composed of two trophozoites which have completed both karyokinesis and cytokinesis enclosed within a cyst wall.

Transmission of the parasite occurs directly via the fecal-oral route. Transmission can occur by ingestion of contaminated food (Barnard and Jackson, 1984; Osterholm et al., 1981), by person to person contact (Black et al., 1977; Keystone et al., 1978; Meyers et al., 1977), and by consumption of contaminated drinking water (Craun, 1986; Lippy, 1981).

Determining trophozoite viability generally is not a problem, because flagellar and caudal movement can be detected by conventional microscopy. In addition to motility, fluorescent dyes can be used to assess the viability of *Giardia* trophozoites easily (Heyworth, 1987). Cyst viability, on the other hand, is not as easily determined, since they do not exhibit easily detected motility. The use of fluorescent dyes on cysts as a method for determining viability at this time is open to question and is being evaluated in various laboratories. Viability information on a cyst population is necessary for cyst disinfection studies and in determining risk assessments for contaminated drinking water supplies.

To date the procedures for determining *Giardia* cyst viability have included in vivo excystation, in vivo infectivity, in vitro excystation, vital stains, and differential interference contrast microscopy. The following discussion will primarily address various aspects of *Giardia* excystation methods. Comparisons between excystation and the other means of determining viability will be made. Excystation procedures have been instrumental in the successful completion of *Giardia* cyst disinfection studies (Hoff et al., 1984; Jarroll et al., 1984; Wickramananyake et al., 1985). A detailed discussion of the initial research on in vitro excystation may be found in the review by Meyer and Schaefer (1984).

2. Excystation

2.1. In vivo excystation

Hegner (1927a, b, c) described in vivo excystation of human source *Giardia* cysts that had been injected into the stomach of, and later removed from, rats. Hegner noted that excystation occurs in the jejunum and ileum and speculated that the factors responsible for excystation include a temperature of 37°C and moisture. He also suggested (1927c) that host digestive juices are unnecessary for excystation.

Armaghan (1937) attempted to determine the site of excystation by placing *G. muris* cyst suspensions in various parts of the rat gastrointestinal tract (stomach, duodenum, ileum, and cecum). The rats were opened surgically so *G. muris* cysts could be injected accurately into the desired portion of the intestinal tract. Excystation was considered positive if cysts could be isolated from the fecal material and/or trophozoites could be isolated from the gastrointestinal tract post exposure. Infections were detected only in those rats injected with cysts either in the stomach or duodenum. Armaghan concluded that in the rat excystation occurred in the section of the small intestine 20 to 70 cm posterior to the stomach.

Wallis and Wallis (1986) obtained trophozoites from cyst preparations by excystation in Mongolian gerbils (*Meriones unguiculatus*). *Giardia duodenalis* cysts were isolated from human, dog (*Canis familiaris*), beaver (*Castor canadensis*), and meadow vole (*Microtus pennsylvanicus*) fecal material. Trophozoites were isolated from the contents of the small intestine of sacrificed gerbils for culture in TYI-S-33. These workers were able to culture isolates from humans, dogs, and beavers, but not the meadow vole. They assumed the trophozoites from the meadow vole were *G. muris* which are not culturable using the technique they used (Meyer and Radulescu, 1984). Although the gerbil was found to be a generally effective way of excysting trophozoites from a variety of hosts, a number of problems were encountered. Large inocula of cysts (1.0×10^4 to 1.5×10^6 cysts/gerbil) were required depending on the source; the cyst preparations had to be freshly prepared; and isolation of the trophozoites aseptically from the gerbil was labor intensive.

2.2. In vitro excystation

2.2.1. Excystation ultrastructure
Excystation of *G. duodenalis* and *G. muris* cysts is an active process on the part of the parasite (Bingham and Meyer, 1979; Coggins and Schaefer, 1984, 1986; Schaefer et al., 1984; Buchel et al., 1987). Initially the caudal flagella and distal ends of the other flagella protrude from one end of the cyst wall. Flagellar movement starts slowly but rapidly increases within the first 5-10 min of their emergence. The rapid flagellar movement seems to help pull and/or break the trophozoite out of the cyst wall, posterior end first. Scanning electron microscopy of this process has shown a tear in the cyst wall of *G. muris* cysts from the polar opening toward the opposite cyst pole (Coggins and Schaefer, 1984). This opening appears to be subsequently enlarged, presumably by flagellar and/or body movements. In their scanning electron microscopy studies of *G. duodenalis* excystation (see Figs. 1-13), Buchel et al. (1987) did not see the subsequent enlargement of the polar cyst opening. Unlike Bingham and Meyer (1979) and Coggins and Schaefer (1984), Buchel et al. (1987) were unable to detect mucus-like material secreted from the polar cyst opening during *G. duodenalis* excystation.

Transmission electron microscopy of induced *G. muris* cysts by Coggins and Schaefer (1986) has shown a cytoplasm devoid of endoplasmic reticulum, Golgi bodies, and mitochondria (see Figs. 14-23). In uninduced cysts (Figs. 14-16), large membrane bound ectoplasmic vacuoles are seen. After induction (Figs. 18-20), these ectoplasmic vacuoles appear to dump their contents into the peritrophic space. Speculation (Coggins and Schaefer, 1986) that the contents of these vacuoles are enzymatic is supported indirectly by the demonstration of lysosomal enzymes (Feely, 1982; Lindmark, 1980) along with evidence for mucus-like material secreted during excystation (Bingham and Meyer, 1979; Coggins and Schaefer, 1984). More conclusive evidence was recently reported by Feely and Dyer (1987) who demonstrated acid phosphatase activity in the ectoplasmic (peripheral) vacuoles of *G. duodenalis* and *G. muris* trophozoites by cytochemical light and electron microscopy. However, according to Coggins and Schaefer (1986), the characteristic ectoplasmic vacuoles documented in mature *G. muris* cysts and trophozoites still are rare in excysted trophozoites undergoing cytokinesis and in daughter trophozoites 30 min after excysting (Figs. 22 and 23). These observations are consistent with the suggestion that these ectoplasmic vacuoles play a role in excystation.

Newly emerged trophozoites appear disorganized (Coggins and Schaefer, 1984; Buchel et al., 1987) and oval in shape. Quadrinucleate trophozoites quickly begin to flatten, elongate, and undergo cytokinesis (Figs. 9-13, 22, 23) within 30 min of emergence to form binucleate trophozoites with completely organized adhesive disks.

2.2.2. Quantitation of excystation

The development of in vitro excystation facilitated the application of quantitative procedures for assessing survival of *Giardia* cysts exposed to chemicals. Excystation has been quantified two ways depending on whether *G. duodenalis* or *G. muris* cysts were being excysted. Bingham et al. (1979) and Rice and Schaefer (1981) determined the percentage excystation of *G. duodenalis* cysts by counting the number of intact cysts (IC), partially excysted trophozoites (PET, a cyst which has started the excystation process and progressed to the point where the trophozoite has either started to emerge or has completely emerged and is still attached to the cyst wall), and totally excysted trophozoites (TET) and applying the following formula:

$$\% \text{ excystation} = \frac{\text{TET}/2 + \text{PET}}{\text{TET}/2 + \text{PET} + \text{IC}} \times 100. \tag{1}$$

The number of totally excysted trophozoites was divided by 2 in this formula, because each excysted organism yielded a pair of trophozoites. Empty cyst walls were not counted, because they were difficult to detect. Each excystation percentage derived by Bingham et al. (1979) involved 3 to 5 separate counts in which an average of 708 cysts were counted to obtain each value. Hudson et al. (1987) and Feely (1986) have used this formula for *G. muris* excystation as well. On the other hand, Schaefer et al. (1984) counted full (unexcysted) and empty (excysted) *G. muris* cyst walls rather than totally excysted trophozoites, because empty cyst walls were easier to count than swimming trophozoites. They calculated percentage excystation using the following equation:

$$\% \text{ excystation} = \frac{\text{ECW} + \text{PET}}{\text{ECW} + \text{PET} + \text{IC}} \times 100. \tag{2}$$

where ECW is the number of empty cyst walls, PET is the number of partially excysted trophozoites, and IC is the number of intact cysts. Examples of *G. muris* ECWs, ICs,

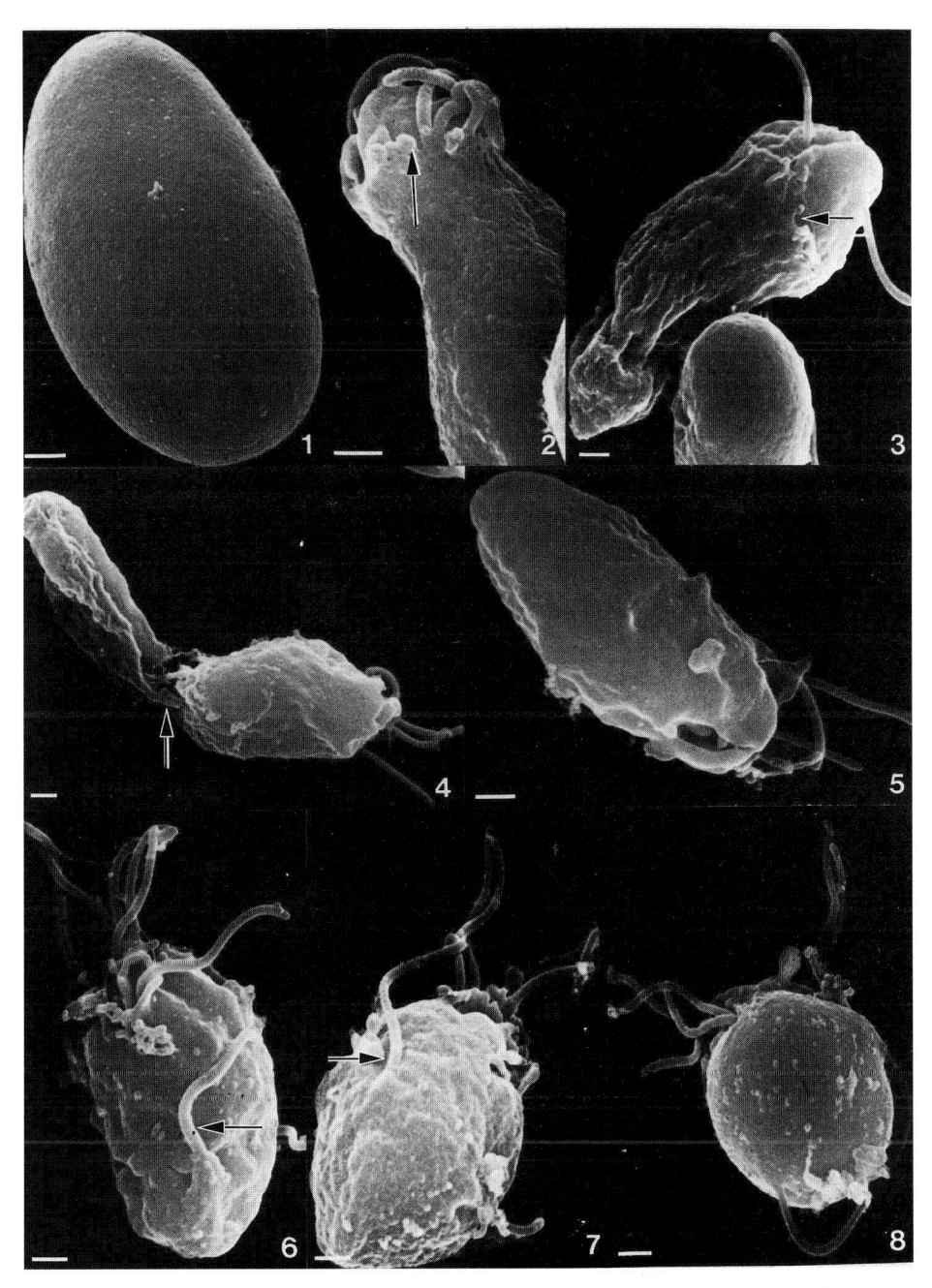

Figs. 1-8. Scale bars, 1 μm. 1. Untreated human *Giardia* cysts. 2. Opening of the cyst wall and appearance of the first emerging flagella corresponding to the first step of excystation. The limit of the opening is quite distinct and is bordered by microspherules (arrow). 3. Emergence of the smooth cell body: it appears with unfolded flagella. The border-line between the newly emerging parasite and the cyst wall is perfectly visible (arrow). 4. Newly emerged trophozoite; a flattened empty cyst in the background still slightly attached to the parasite (arrow). 5. Newly emerged trophozoite still oval in shape. It seems molded by the cyst and the flagella can be seen. 6, 7. Change in shape, becoming progressively rounded, lateral flagella are visible (arrows). 8. Round shape of the cell body with 8 flagella. From Buchel et al. (1987), courtesy of the authors and the Journal of Parasitology.

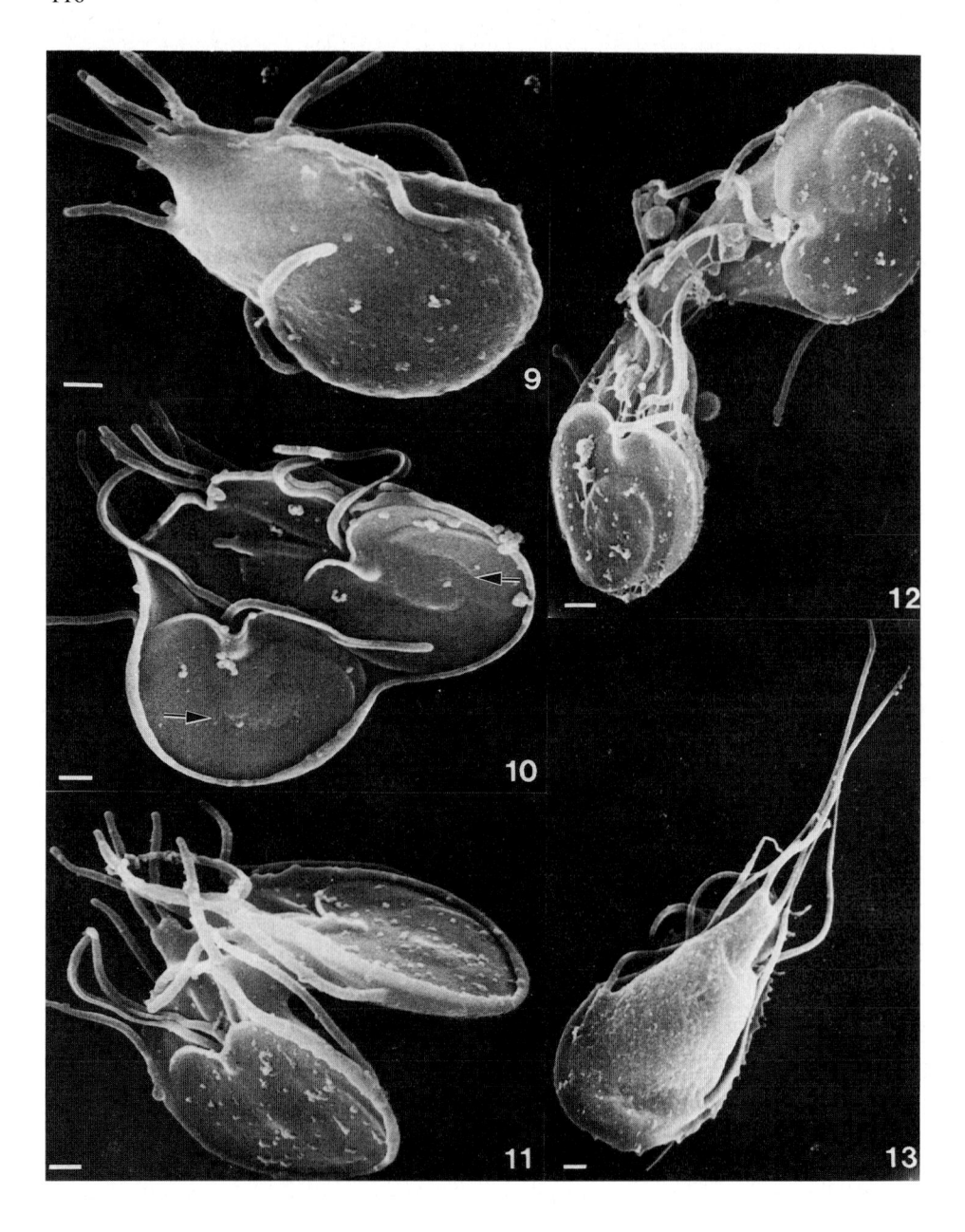

Figs. 9-13. Scale bars, 1 μm. 9. The trophozoite begins to elongate, flattens, and undergoes cytokinesis. 10. The daughter trophozoites acquire their typical features in the anterior area: adhesive discs are now visible on the ventral surface (arrows). 11, 12. Differentiation of the posterior region with 2 sets of 8 flagella before the final separation of the daughter trophozoites. 13. Free trophozoite attached to the substrate showing its dorsal surface. From Buchel et al. (1987), courtesy of the authors and the Journal of Parasitology.

117

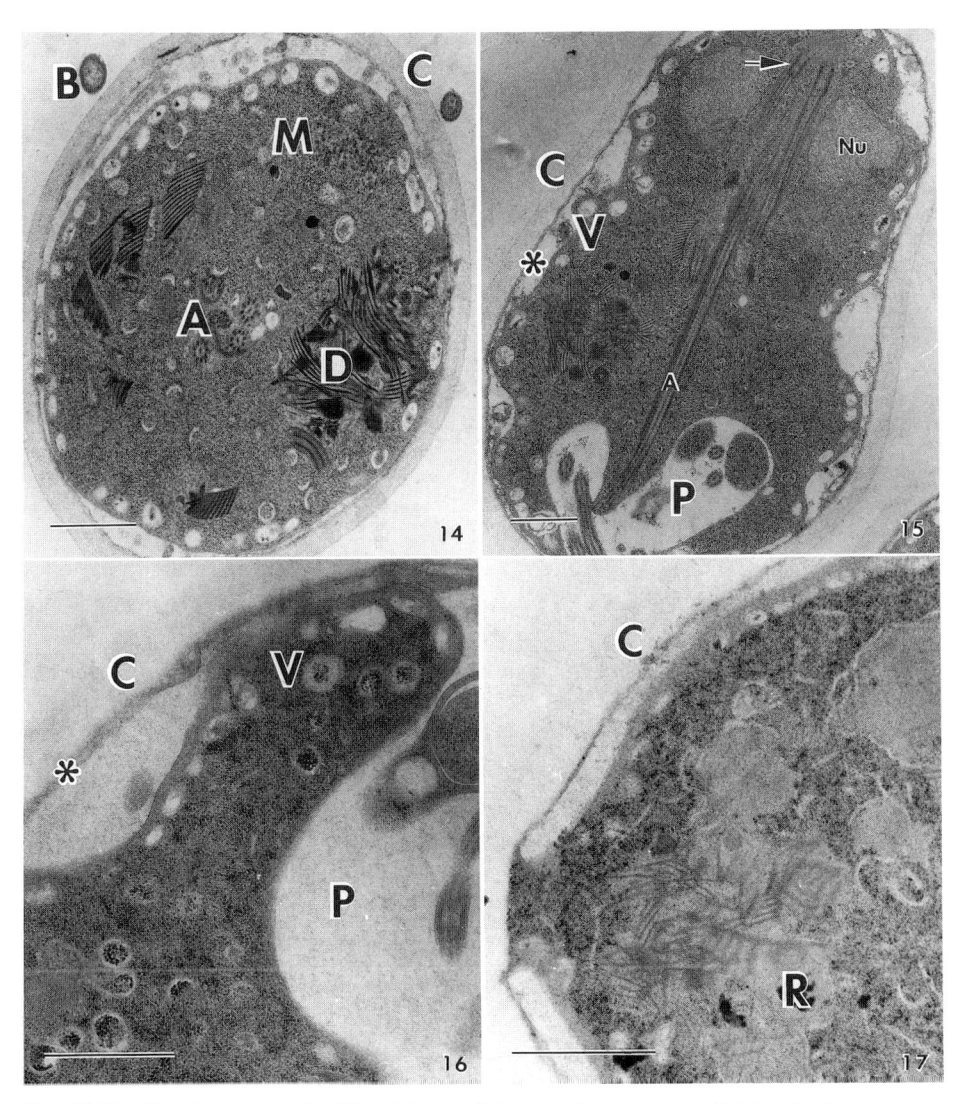

Figs. 14-17. Scale bars, 1 μm. 14. Untreated cyst of *G. muris* showing cyst wall (C) with adherent bacteria (B). Dense ribbons represent precursors of the adhesive disk (D); the unordered series of microtubules represents the median body (M). Flagellar axonemes (A) occupy the medullary cell region. 15. Longitudinal section of untreated *G. muris*. The outer cyst wall (C) is bounded closely on the interior by a dense inner membrane (asterisk). The peritrophic space (P) is visible at several areas around the organism but is most pronounced at the posterior region of the cyst. Note the large number of ectoplasmic vacuoles (V). Also seen are nuclei (Nu), axonemes (A), kinetosome (arrow). 16. Untreated *G. muris* cyst. The dense inner membrane (asterisk) is closely applied to the outer cyst wall (C). An extensive peritrophic space (P) is present. The ectoplasmic cytoplasm contains large numbers of vacuoles (V) but is devoid of other cellular organelles. 17. *G. muris* after induction. Cytoplasm of the enclosed trophozoite directly abuts the outer cyst wall (C). The continuity of the trophozoite plasma membrane with the inner membrane of the cyst wall is apparent. Note the microtubular ribbons (R) within the cytoplasm. From Coggins and Schaefer (1986), courtesy of the authors and Experimental Parasitology.

PETs, and TETs are shown in Figs. 24-30. Each excystation percentage determination involved a total of 100 cyst types. When viability was less than 1%, however, no empty cyst walls were found on counting 100 cysts. If the entire slide which held approximately 100 000 cysts was scanned for motile trophozoites, some were found. This indicated that counting only 100 cysts does not sample a large enough portion of the population to distinguish percentages of less than 1. In a later work (Hoff et al., 1985), this same research group, in comparing animal infectivity and excystation of chlorine-inactivated *G. muris* cysts, increased the number of cyst forms scored from 200 to 1000 in individual experiments. In determining percentage excystation by either quantitative procedure, there is no universally accepted minimum number of cysts that must be counted to insure precision and accuracy of the result. Further research on this point is needed to eliminate the arbitrary way in which excystation has been quantified to this point.

2.2.3. Giardia duodenalis *excystation*

Bingham and Meyer (1979) reported the first successful in vitro excystation of *Giardia* cysts from humans, monkeys, and dogs, and *G. muris* cysts from rats and mice. Their procedure, which was carried out at 37°C, consists of three steps: a low pH induction step for 1 h, a wash step to remove the acid, and an incubation step for 1 h in a nutrient medium to complete the excystation process. Synthetic gastric juice (pepsin and hydrochloric acid), aqueous acids, and water were tried as induction solutions. For incubation media, they used water and HSP-3 (Hanks' balanced salt solution, serum, phytone, and NCTC-135; Meyer, 1976). Excystation occurred when the induction solution was synthetic gastric juice or aqueous acid, and the incubation medium was HSP-3. Salts and pepsin in the synthetic gastric juice did not significantly alter the excystation level indicating that the acid alone was critical to the process. Although a number of inorganic acids were

---

Figs. 18-23. 18. *Giardia muris* trophozoite, initial incubation. Note the lack of an intact cyst wall. Few vacuoles (V) occur within the cytoplasm. A number of vesicles (Vs) surround the parasite. Cellular constituents include an extensive network of granular endoplasmic reticulum (er), nucleus (Nu), and flagellar axonemes (A). The adhesive disk and lateral flange (F) appear partially organized at this point in the excystation process. Scale bar, 1 μm. 19. *Giardia muris* trophozoite 15 min after incubation. A network of loosely packed fibers (W) representing remnants of the cyst wall surround the organism. Note the lack of a cyst wall inner membrane and the large number of vesicles (Vs) on the cell surface. The lateral flange (F) appears well organized. Scale bar, 1 μm. 20. *Giardia muris* trophozoite 15 min after incubation. Several vesicles (Vs) in the process of exocytosis are shown while others line the cell surface. Note the profiles of endoplasmic reticulum (er). Scale bar, 0.5 μm. 21. *Giardia muris* trophozoite 15 min after incubation. An apparently well organized adhesive disk is composed of a regular series of microtubules (asterisk) located just beneath the plasma membrane with attached, dorsally oriented dense ribbons (R). Scale bar, 0.25 μm. 22. *Giardia muris* trophozoite 30 min after incubation. Few vacuoles or cellular organelles are present except for endoplasmic reticulum (er) and the nucleus (Nu). Note the absence of any surrounding fibers. Concentric ring arrangement of the adhesive disk (D) is shown. Scale bar, 1 μm. 23. *Giardia muris* 30 min after incubation. Formation of daughter trophozoites by cytokinesis is shown. Adhesive disk (D), lateral flange (F), nuclei (Nu), and axonemes are present. Few vacuoles are noted at this stage. Scale bar, 1 μm. From Coggins and Schaefer (1986), courtesy of the authors and Experimental Parasitology.

119

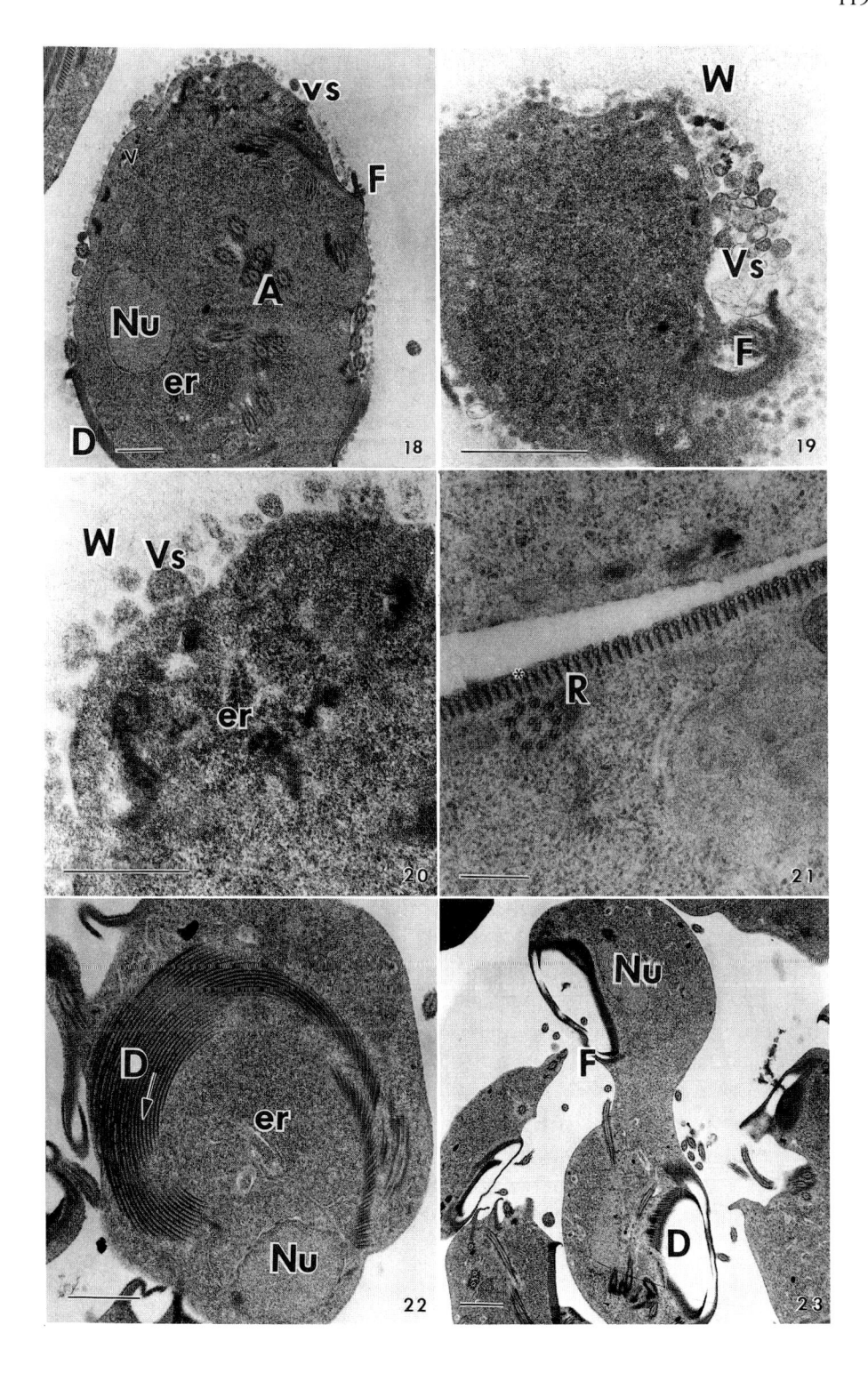

tested in induction solutions and were found effective, hydrochloric acid was selected for routine use. Peak excystation (22-26%) occurred when the pH was between 1.3 and 2.7 in the induction solution and the incubation medium was HSP-3.

Using *Giardia* cysts isolated from a single human donor, Bingham et al. (1979) studied other factors in the excystation process. Of all factors tested, time, temperature, pH, and incubation medium were shown to affect excystation levels. The exposure time in the induction solution decreased as the pH decreased. For example, a hydrochloric acid induction solution at pH 2.0 only required an exposure time between 10 and 30 min, whereas a hydrochloric acid induction solution at pH 6.2 required an exposure time between 60 and 120 min. Even though excystation occurred at the longer exposure time at pH 6.2, it was never as high as the excystation that occurred at pH 2. The highest excystation levels always occurred when both the induction solution and the incubation medium were at 37°C. The pH of the HSP-3 incubation medium was critical, too. No excystation occurred when the HSP-3 pH was in the 0.5 to 4.0 range; excystation started at pH 6.2 but was best at pH 6.8.

A comparison of HSP-3 medium components with complete HSP-3 medium was carried out using acid-induced cysts (Bingham, 1979). Significantly lower excystation levels occurred in Hanks' phytone broth than occurred in either Hanks' phytone broth plus serum or complete HSP-3 medium. The factors Bingham and Meyer (1979) found favoring in vitro excystation (Table 1) closely approximated the host's in vivo environment in the stomach (induction step) and the duodenum (incubation step). They also reported that a period of cyst maturation at 4°C varying from 2 to 7 days following isolation from feces was required to ensure maximal excystation.

Rice and Schaefer (1981) devised a modification of the Bingham-Meyer procedure for excysting *G. duodenalis* cysts isolated from human donors. Initial attempts to use the Bingham-Meyer procedure on *G. duodenalis* and *G. muris* cysts resulted in excystations of only 2-3%. The Rice-Schaefer modification of *G. duodenalis* cysts includes induction, wash, and incubation steps as does the Bingham-Meyer procedure. However, the induction step involves the addition of hydrochloric acid (pH 2), Hanks' balanced salt solution supplemented with 1-cysteine hydrochloride and glutathione, and sodium bicarbonate to the cyst preparation in that order. Immediately thereafter, the tube containing the cysts is capped tightly, mixed, and incubated for 30 min at 37°C. The cysts are washed by centrifugation and resuspended in trypsin-Tyrode's incubation medium (pH adjusted to 8.0 with sodium bicarbonate). This suspension is incubated 1 h at 37°C.

Rice and Schaefer (1981) tested their modified excystation procedure on *G. duodenalis* cysts from 5 human donors. They used cysts from two symptomatic donors in 10

Figs. 24-30. Scale bars, 10 μm. 24. *Giardia muris* intact cysts (IC). 25-27. Successive stages of *Giardia muris* excystation; C = cyst wall, T = trophozoite, and pet = partially excysted trophozoite which is still attached to the cyst wall. 28. *Giardia muris* totally excysted trophozoite (tet), no longer attached to the cyst wall, undergoing cytokinesis; dart points to the ventral sucking disk on a totally excysted trophozoite. 29. *Giardia muris* empty cyst walls (ECW) seen from the side. 30. *Giardia muris* empty cyst walls seen on end; darts point to scalloped polar openings through which trophozoites emerged.

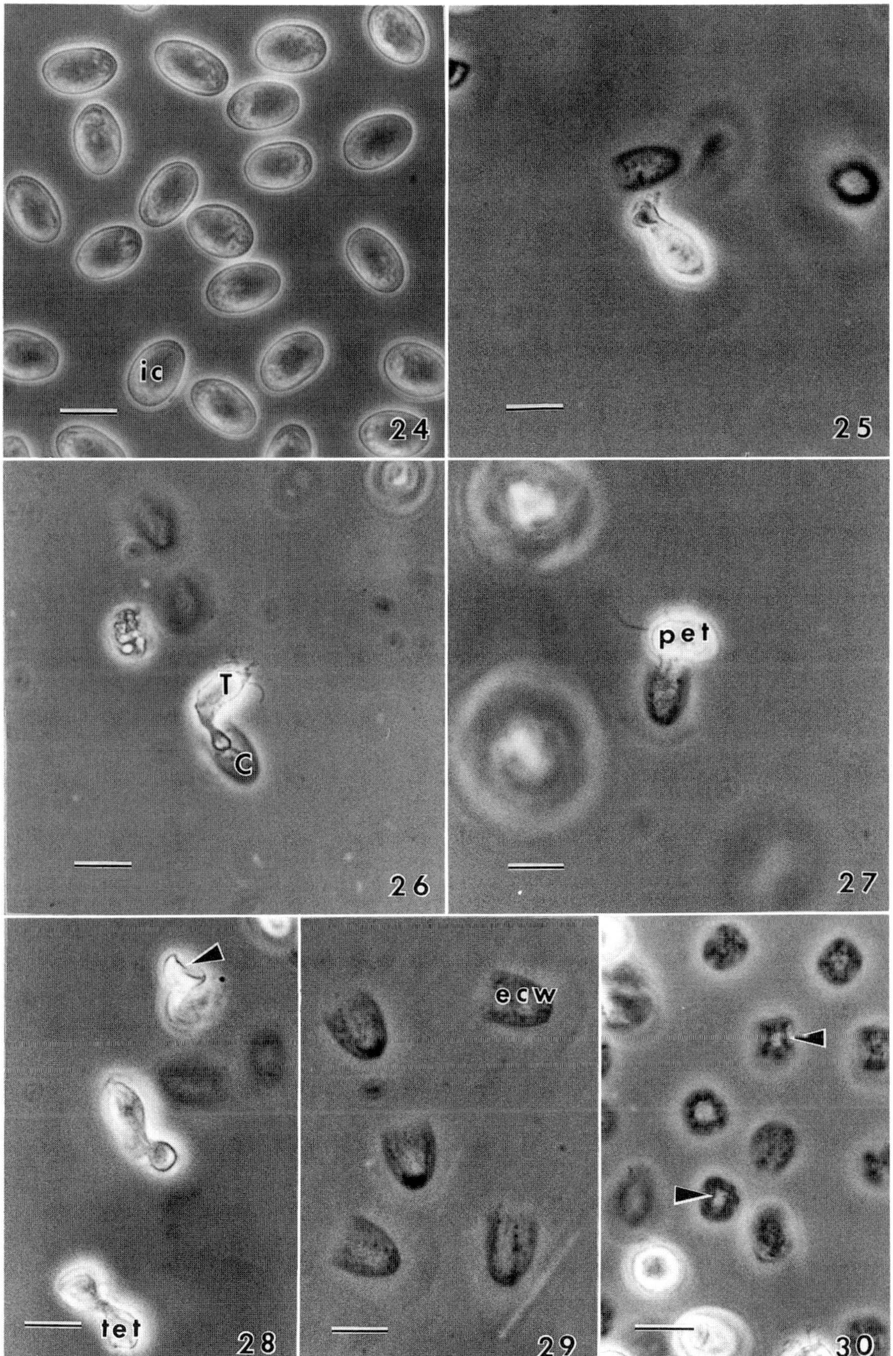
ic
24
25
T
C
26
pet
27
tet
28
ecw
29
30

TABLE 1
Factors used to excyst *Giardia lamblia* cysts in vitro

Induction step				Wash step	Incubation step			Reference
Medium	pH	Temp. (°C)	Gas	Medium	Medium	pH	Temp. (°C)	
HCl	1.3-2.7 (10-30 min)	37	—	H_2O	HSP-3	6.2-6.8 (60 min)	37	Bingham and Meyer (1979)
HCl Reducing Soln. Bicarbonate	2.0 (30 min)	37	C_2	trypsin-Tyrode's	trypsin-Tyrode's	8.0 (60 min)	37	Rice and Schaefer (1981)
HCl	2.0 (5-30 min)	37	—	H_2O	TPS-1	7.0 (30 min-1 week)	37	Bhatia and Warhurst (1981)
1% pepsin-saline	2.0 (30 min)	?	—	H_2O	TPS-1[a]	7.0	37	Kasprzak and Majewska (1983)
HCl Hanks' BSS Bicarbonate	2.0 (30 min)	37	CO_2	50% bovine bile 50% Tyrode's	TPS-1[b]	7.0 (6-48 h)	37	Isaac-Renton et al. (1986)

TABLE 1 (continued)

	Induction step				Wash step	Incubation step			Reference
Medium	pH	Temp. (°C)	Gas		Medium	Medium	pH	Temp. (°C)	
HCl	2.0 (30 min)	37	—		H$_2$O	TPS-1	7.0 (30 min-7 days)	37	Kaur et al. (1986)
HCl Reducing Soln. Bicarbonate	2.0 (45 min)	37	CO$_2$		0.85% saline	2% phytone Hanks' BSS l-cysteine	7.1 (30 min)	37	Sauch (1987)
Pepsin Salts HCl Bicarbonate	2.0 (1 h)	37	CO$_2$		H$_2$O	Buffered NaCl Hanks'-glucose, or HSP-3	7.0 (15 min)	37	Chochillon et al. (1987)

a   0.2% l-cysteine supplement
b   0.1% l-cysteine + 0.1% dried bovine bile supplement
c   osmolarity adjusted to between 50 and 500 mosmol/liter
—   not used
?   data not available in reference
( )   exposure time

trials and cysts from three asymptomatic donors in 18 trials. The lowest observed percent excystation (40%) occurred with cysts from an asymptomatic donor; the highest percentage (95%) occurred with cysts from both symptomatic and asymptomatic donors. The mean percentage excystation from the symptomatic donors (87%) was higher than that from the asymptomatic donors (70%). The lowest percentage excystation Rice and Schaefer observed (40%) was 10% higher than the maximum reported by Jarroll et al. (1981) using the Bingham-Meyer procedure.

These data indicate that the Rice-Schaefer method may be successfully used to excyst *G. duodenalis* cysts from both asymptomatic and symptomatic donors, and that higher percentages of excystation may be expected from symptomatic donors. They also confirmed Bingham et al.'s (1979) observation that *G. duodenalis* cysts exhibited higher excystation rates after 7 days maturation at 4°C.

A method for excysting *G. duodenalis* in enzyme-free media was reported recently by Sauch (1988). The induction solution for *G. duodenalis* cysts was the same as Rice and Schaefer's (1981); however, exposure to the induction solution at 37°C was increased from 30 to 45 min. Trypsin-Tyrode's solution was replaced with Hanks' balanced salt solution supplemented with cysteine, sodium bicarbonate, and 2% boiled phytone peptone. Comparison of her method with that of Rice and Schaefer (1981) for *G. duodenalis* cysts isolated from 2 asymptomatic donors showed no significant differences in percent excystation. Excystation trials using cysts from 2 asymptomatic and 13 symptomatic donors showed an average of 56% (1-96%) and 50% (8-85%), respectively. This demonstrates that *G. duodenalis* excystation can be completed in the absence of exogenous enzymes. The excystation results of Sauch and of Rice and Schaefer indicate that great variability is to be expected with the currently developed procedures for *G. duodenalis*.

Chochillon et al. (1987) studied the effect of incubation medium composition and osmolarity on excystation. Human-derived cysts were exposed to induction medium (pepsin, HCl, salts, and bicarbonate) for 1 h at 37°C. Cysts were washed in distilled water and were resuspended in various incubation media. Buffered saline, Hanks' balanced salt solution supplemented with glucose, or HSP-3 were the incubation media. In addition, the osmolarity of these incubation media was adjusted for various experiments to between 50 and 500 mosmol/l. Although excystation was observed in incubation solutions between 100 and 450 mosmol/l, the best excystation percentages were obtained between 250 and 350 mosmol/l. Viability of the excysted trophozoites was dependent upon the nutritive quality of the medium. Survival of the trophozoites was prolonged by the addition of glucose to Hanks' balanced salt solution. Under their best excystation conditions, the percent excystation was between 27 and 37%. These excystation percentages might have been higher if reducing agents and more bicarbonate had been used in the induction solution. However, these results do suggest the presence of a carbon source in an incubation medium with the appropriate osmotic strength is important in obtaining optimal *G. duodenalis* excystation and trophozoite survival.

A number of researchers have used in vitro excystation as a way of obtaining *G.*

duodenalis trophozoites for in vitro culture. Their overall approach has been to use HCl or pepsin-saline at pH 2.0 for induction, a wash step to remove the acid, and resuspension into culture medium to initiate serial subcultivation. The basic variation in these procedures is in the type of culture medium that was used to initiate the cultures. Bhatia and Warhurst (1981), using TPS-1, were able to establish 5 cultures from human cyst isolates. Similarly, Kaur et al. (1986) were able to obtain excystation percentages as high as 25% using HCl induction and TPS-1 incubation medium. Unlike Bhatia and Warhurst, however, Kaur et al. were unable to perpetuate their excysted trophozoites in culture. After supplementing TPS-1 with l-cysteine, Kasprzak and Majewska (1983a) were able to establish 3 cultures from human cyst isolates. Excystation percentages were reported to be 4.0, 14.5, and 64.0%, respectively, for these 3 isolates. Isaac-Renton et al. (1986) modified TPS-1 with l-cysteine and bovine bile. Although no excystation percentages were reported by these researchers, they were able to use their procedure to successfully establish cultures from 3 of 12 human source and 2 of 2 beaver source cyst preparations.

It can be seen from the studies mentioned above that there is little agreement on what constitutes a good incubation medium for *G. duodenalis*. The incubation media used to date include HSP-3 medium, trypsin-Tyrode's solution, TPS-1 with and without bile, and Hanks' balanced salt solution with either glucose or phytone. About the only conclusions that can be drawn are that (1) these media are complex and undefined, (2) a carbon source may be beneficial, (3) medium osmolarity is an important consideration for excystation and trophozoite survival, and (4) exogenous enzymes are not required. Trypsin-Tyrode's solution, and Hanks' balanced salt solution with phytone appear to be the best choices in the author's opinion, because they have produced the highest excystation percentages and have the shortest incubation exposure times.

2.2.4. Giardia muris excystation

Schaefer et al. (1984) reported the results of excystation experiments employing *G. muris* cysts isolated from mouse feces. They obtained excystation levels consistently greater than 90% compared to levels less than 5% with the Bingham-Meyer procedure. All of the *G. muris* excystation procedures consist of the same steps: induction, wash, and incubation (Table 2). In the Schaefer et al. procedure, induction was promoted by exposure of *G. muris* cysts to an induction solution consisting of 1 part reducing solution (Hanks' balanced salt solution supplemented with glutathione and l-cysteine hydrochloride; Meyer, 1976) and 1 part 0.1 M sodium bicarbonate for 30 min at 37°C in a sealed test tube. In this case, no inorganic acid is used. When the induction components are mixed, carbon dioxide is evolved, the pH is 2, and the oxidation-reduction potential is 120 mV. A gradual decline in excystation to 2% or less occurred as the pH and the oxidation-reduction potential were changed to 7 and 57 mV, respectively. The induction step was followed by a wash and incubation step both carried out in trypsin-Tyrode's solution (Rice and Schaefer, 1981). The trypsin-Tyrode's solution is reported by these investigators to be crude and tedious to make. The trypsin they used was an impure

TABLE 2
Factors used to excyst *Giardia muris* cysts in vitro

Medium	Induction step pH	Temp. (°C)	Gas	Wash step Medium	Incubation step Medium	pH	Temp. (°C)	Reference
Reducing soln. + bicarbonate	2.0	37 (30 min)	CO_2	trypsin-Tyrode's	trypsin-Tyrode's (30 min)	8.0	37	Schaefer et al. (1984)
Hanks' BSS	2.0	37 (30 min)	CO_2	Hanks' BSS pH 7.2	TYI-S-33[a] (30 min)	7.2-7.4	37	Feely (1986)
HCl 1% pepsin[b]	1.2	37 (30 min)	–	Hanks' BSS pH 7.2	TC-199	?	37	Gonzalez-Castro et al. (1986)
Phosphate buffer	6.4	37 (10 min)	CO_2	TYI-S-33	TYI-S-33 (5-30 min)	7.2	37	Feely (1987)
Reducing soln. +bicarbonate	4.7	37 (30 min)	CO_2	0.5% proteose peptone	0.5% proteose peptone (30 min)	7.2	37	Sauch (1987)

[a] supplemented with bile as described by Keister (1983)
[b] pretreated with 3.3% hypochlorite
? data not available in reference
– not used

lyophilized extract of hog pancreas which does not completely dissolve after vigorous mixing in 1 × Tyrode's salt solution for 30 min at ambient temperature. The undissolved trypsin was always removed by high speed centrifugation followed by positive pressure filtration. When the trypsin-Tyrode's solution was boiled, *G. muris* excystations declined to the 70th percentile, indicating the enzymatic activity of the solution is not crucial for *G. muris* excystation. This result is similar to those of Hegner (1927c), Bingham and Meyer (1979), and Sauch (1979) who have shown digestive enzymes are not obligatory for *G. duodenalis* excystation. Attempts by Schaefer et al. (1984) to make trypsin-Tyrode's solution with purified pancreatin resulted in little if any *G. muris* excystation. Similar results were obtained by Marchin (personal communication, 1982) when he used purified trypsin in his trypsin-Tyrode's solution. Only when he substituted crude trypsin for purified trypsin was he able to obtain *G. muris* excystations in the 90th percentile. These results suggest nutrients were supplied by the complex trypsin-Tyrode's incubation medium that were not supplied by the highly purified solutions. The factors in trypsin-Tyrode's solution responsible for good *G. muris* excystation are still in need of definition.

Feely (1986) published a procedure for *G. muris* excystation which eliminated the reducing agents in the induction solution. *Giardia muris* cysts were suspended in Hanks' balanced salt solution at pH 2 for 30 min at 37°C. However, this procedure specifies that the Hanks' balanced salt solution must be prepared fresh daily and the pH adjusted to neutrality with sodium bicarbonate before being acidified to pH 2 with 2 N hydrochloric acid. This allows liberation of carbon dioxide from the induction medium during the incubation step as in the Rice and Schaefer (1981) and Schaefer et al. (1984) methods. Cysts were washed in Hanks' balanced salt solution at pH 7.2, followed by incubation in TYI-S-33 (salts, trypticase, yeast extract, glucose, cysteine hydrochloride, ascorbic acid, ferric ammonium citrate, bovine bile, and serum; Keister, 1983) at 37°C for 30 min. The excystation rates reported for this procedure were always greater than 90%. Recently, Feely (1987) further modified his excystation procedure for *G. muris* cysts by changing the induction solution. In this case, the induction solution was 0.1 M sodium phosphate buffer through which 100% CO_2 had been passed. The resultant pH was 6.4. After incubation in TYI-S-33 for only 5 min at 37°C the percent excystation was 92%. These results suggest that CO_2 in only a slightly acid medium is sufficient to induce excystation; reducing agents and low pH appear unnecessary for optimal *G. muris* excystation.

Sauch (1987) reported a procedure for excysting *G. muris* cysts in an enzyme-free medium. Her induction solution for *G. muris* cysts was the same as Schaefer et al.'s (1984). In her procedure, trypsin-Tyrode's solution was replaced with Hanks' balanced salt solution supplemented with cysteine, sodium bicarbonate, and boiled proteose peptone. Comparison of her method with that of Schaefer et al. (1984) for *G. muris* cysts showed no significant differences in percent excystation, which was 89% or higher. These results indicate, as for *G. duodenalis*, that exogenous enzymes are not necessary for *G. muris* excystation and confirm the experiments of Schaefer et al. (1984).

Until recently, no one has been able to culture *G. muris* in vitro successfully (Meyer and Radulescu, 1984). In 1986, Gonzalez-Castro et al. reported excystation and subsequent culture of *G. muris* isolated from laboratory rats. The cysts were initially exposed to 3.3% hypochlorite; inducted with pepsin saline (pH 1.2, 37°C, 50 min); washed in Hanks' balanced salt solution (pH 7.2), resuspended in tissue culture medium-199 for 15 min at 37°C, and finally transferred to culture medium. While excystation percentages were not listed, growth of excysted *G. muris* trophozoites was claimed in five different media. Growth curves indicated normal growth phases in all media, but whether transfers were made and serial subcultivation was possible was not mentioned. Since neither cyst dimensions nor morphology of the median body was stated, this work is subject to question. Was this work done with *G. muris* or was the organism actually *G. simoni*, a *duodenalis* type (Filice, 1952), like *G. duodenalis*? Further information and work is needed to substantiate this report.

2.2.5. Comparison of G. duodenalis *and* G. muris *excystation*
A number of conclusions may be drawn from the excystation studies done to date on *G. duodenalis* and *G. muris* cysts (Table 3): (1) the induction and incubation temperature should be 37°C; (2) the induction medium should have a pH of approximately 2 and evolve carbon dioxide for *G. duodenalis*; (3) for *G. muris*, the induction medium should have a pH ranging between 2 and 6.4, and evolve CO_2; (4) the wash step should neutralize the acidity from the induction step; (5) the incubation medium should contain nutrients but need not contain serum, bile, or exogenous enzymes; (6) a period of cyst maturation is not needed for *G. muris* cysts; (7) a maturation period of 2 to 7 days for cysts of *G. duodenalis* before excystation has been indicated; (8) *G. muris* cysts can be routinely excysted with efficiencies in the 90th percentile; (9) *G. duodenalis* excystation efficiencies are erratic and usually much less than 90%; and (10) excystation is a process requiring active participation by the parasite.

Giardia duodenalis and *G. muris* exhibit different responses to the same excystation procedure. One might conclude (a) that cysts of *G. duodenalis* require greater stimulation to excyst than cysts of *G. muris*, or (b) that fundamental differences exist between these two organisms. According to Filice (1952) *G. duodenalis* and *G. muris* belong to distinct morphological groups based on size and median body morphology. The ability to culture *duodenalis* and not *muris* group trophozoites is another difference (Meyer and Radulescu, 1984). Cyst maturation has been indicated for *G. duodenalis* but not *G. muris* cysts. Empty *G. muris* cyst walls are easily visualized by phase contrast microscopy, but empty *G. duodenalis* cysts walls are not. Sauch and Mormile (1986) have shown that *G. duodenalis* cysts, isolated from Mongolian gerbils and humans, have similar buoyant densities which differ from *G. muris* cysts isolated from mice. In Mongolian gerbil and human hosts, *G. duodenalis* causes an infection characterized by intermittent cyst passage. On the other hand, *G. muris* infections in mice and Mongolian gerbils are characterized by continuous cyst passage (Faubert et al., 1983). It is obvious from these observations that fundamental physiological and morphological differences exist between *G. duodenalis* and *G. muris*. The most obvious conclusion of all is that we do not as yet know the optimal conditions for repeatable, maximal excystation of *G. duodenalis* cysts.

TABLE 3
Factors common to all *Giardia* sp. excystation methods

Organism	Induction step				Wash step	Incubation step		
	Medium	pH	Temp. (°C)	Gas	Medium	Medium	pH	Temp. (°C)
Giardia duodenalis	HCl Reducing soln. Bicarbonate	2.0	37	CO_2	H_2O or 0.85% saline	Culture medium	7.0-8.0	37
		(30 min)				(30-60 min)		
Giardia muris	Reducing soln. Bicarbonate	2.0-6.4	37	CO_2	Salt solution or culture medium	Culture medium	7.2-8.0	37
		(10-30 min)				(5-30 min)		

( ) exposure time

3. Comparison of excystation to other viability methods

Giardia cyst densities in surface waters have not been reported to any great extent. One study from the states of Oregon, Idaho, Wyoming, and Pennsylvania reported densities ranging from 0.05 to 680 *Giardia* cysts per 380 l (Craun and Jakubowski, 1987). This indicates that *Giardia* cyst densities are usually lower than a thousand cysts per 380 l of sample.

Even if all the *Giardia* cysts could be recovered efficiently from the sample, there would be insufficient cyst numbers to determine viability by current excystation procedures which require between 1 and 5×10^5 cysts. In addition, the specialized procedures for excysting *Giardia* cysts require several hours to complete and are not equally successful in every laboratory. These problems have forced the development of other methods to assay viability which can be used with small numbers of cysts. Among these alternate methods are vital dyes, fluorogenic dyes, differential interference contrast microscopy, and infectivity for animals.

3.1. Vital staining

Several studies have been done which compared dye exclusion with excystation. Cysts that excluded dye were considered viable. Bingham et al. (1979) compared the Bingham-Meyer (1979) procedure for excysting *G. duodenalis* cysts with eosin dye exclusion and found that there was no correlation between the two techniques. The eosin dye exclusion technique always indicated greater viability in the cyst population than excystation did. Kasprzak and Majewska (1983b, 1987) compared excystation with eosin exclusion using *G. muris* cysts isolated from Wistar rats and *G. duodenalis* cysts isolated from humans. Like Bingham et al. (1979), they found eosin exclusion always gave higher viability values than excystation. A comparison of trypan blue exclusion with excystation using *G. duodenalis* cysts from humans was reported by Kaur et al. (1986). Similarly, they found trypan blue exclusion always indicated a much higher degree of viability than excystation. These disparate results could have been for various reasons. The excystation technique may not have been optimal. It is also possible that there were cysts in the population that were alive but could not excyst, or there were dead cysts which excluded the dye. It is also unclear what effect the cyst source and age may have had on these results.

3.2. Fluorescent staining

Hudson et al. (1987) reported fluorescent dye exclusion as a method for determining *Giardia* cyst viability. In this procedure, as in the eosin and trypan blue procedures, live cysts exclude the dye. These workers utilized FluoraBora I (3-(dansylamido)-phenylboronic acid) in *G. muris* and *G. duodenalis* cyst suspensions and compared the results with excystation. They found a high degree of correlation between the dye exclusion and excystation methods in the case of *G. muris* cysts. In the case of *G. duodenalis* cysts, however, the correlation was low. This again suggests that viability as determined by excystation of *G. duodenalis* cysts is being either overestimated or underestimated.

Schupp and Erlandsen (1987a) have developed a method of determining *G. muris* cyst viability which employs fluorescein diacetate (FDA) and propidium iodide (PI) stains. Presumably-viable cysts exposed to FDA fluoresce green resulting from uptake and metabolic conversion of the stain to fluorescein, whereas dead cysts exposed to PI fluoresce orange to bright red depending on the excitation wavelength, resulting from staining by PI. Their results with freshly isolated cysts revealed greater than 85 to 90% of the cyst population stained green and less than 15% of the population stained orange/red. Usually less than 10% of the cysts did not stain at all. Freshly isolated FDA-positive cysts, and cysts that did not stain with either dye, were inoculated into separate groups of mice. Similarly, heat-killed PI stained cysts were inoculated into another group of mice. Infections occurred in those mice receiving either FDA stained or unstained cysts but did not occur in those mice receiving the PI stained cysts. Necropsies of the mice exposed to either FDA or to PI stained cysts always revealed trophozoites in the FDA exposed mice but never in the mice receiving PI stained cysts. These investigators have said that FDA stained cysts are capable of excystation, but they did not provide details. These data demonstrate that fluorescein stained cysts were viable as determined both by staining and infectivity; and also possibly by excystation as well. Rotman and Papermaster (1966) reported that enzymatic hydrolysis of fluorogenic esters in tissue culture cells varied as much as 80 fluorimeter units. Some variability in the fluorescence of FDA stained *G. muris* cysts also has been noted by Schupp and Erlandsen.

Recently, Sauch et al. (1988) compared PI staining with excystation using *G. muris* cyst preparations that had been exposed to varying amounts of either heat or chemical killing. Preliminary results indicate that PI may not be a satisfactory viability test for chemically killed cysts.

Both the FDA-PI and the FluoroBora I viability staining procedures do not stain *Giardia* selectively. These methods are easily used with pure or highly concentrated *Giardia* cyst suspensions. However, in cyst suspensions containing other macro- and microorganisms, the reaction of the *Giardia* cysts could easily be masked by other organisms. There is a need to link selective identification methods with these viability methods.

3.3. Morphology

Schupp and Erlandsen (1987b) and Schupp et al. (1987) compared the light microscopic morphology of FDA-stained *G. muris* cysts to PI-stained *G. muris* cysts. Viable, fluorescein-positive cysts had clearly defined cyst walls, a peritrophic space, and flagella at one pole. Occasionally axonemes were also observed, but no other cytoplasmic organelles were seen in these viable cysts. On the other hand, in nonviable, PI-stained cysts the cytoplasmic organelles (axonemes, median bodies, portions of the adhesive disk, and nuclei) were seen. The peritrophic space in non-viable cysts was not observed, because the cytoplasm appeared to be closely adherent to the cyst wall. These differences were observed with both differential interference contrast and bright field microscopy. Such observations suggest structural differences exist between these two types of *G. muris* cysts and may be a useful way to assess viability.

3.4. Animal infectivity

Animal models of giardiasis have been developed in the Mongolian gerbil, *Meriones unguiculatus*, (Belosevic et al., 1983) and the mouse (Roberts-Thomson et al., 1976). Both models have been successfully used to determine cyst viability and infectivity; however, both have several unsatisfactory aspects. Neither model manifests overt pathology like that seen in some humans. The mouse model produces *G. muris* cysts continuously for several weeks post exposure, unlike the human infection, which can be quite variable in cyst production. Although the Mongolian gerbil intermittently passes cysts for several weeks post exposure, as is common in human infections, not all human-derived *G. duodenalis* cysts will infect gerbils (Visvesvara et al., 1988). Some human-derived *G. duodenalis* cysts infect the gerbil, as evidenced by the production of trophozoites; however, cysts are not produced in some of these infections.

The number of cysts required to produce an infection in the mouse is very low compared to the number required for the Mongolian gerbil. Between 1 and 15 cysts are necessary to infect a mouse with *G. muris* cysts (Hoff et al., 1985). Using *G. muris* cysts which either had or had not been exposed to chlorine, these workers compared in vitro excystation to mouse infectivity. Although their results could not be evaluated on a strict statistical basis, their data suggested in vitro excystation is an adequate indication of *G. muris* cyst infectivity for the mouse. As few as 10 cysts administered in capsules were required to infect human volunteers with *G. duodenalis* cysts (Rendtorff, 1954). With Mongolian gerbils, the probability of infection is directly related to the dosage (Visvesvara et al., 1988); cyst dosages should be greater than 100 cysts per gerbil to insure 70% of the gerbils become infected, when *G. duodenalis* cysts are used. Similar results have recently been obtained when *G. duodenalis* cysts from humans were given to beavers (Erlandsen et al., 1988). Wallis and Wallis (1986) recently were successful in infecting gerbils with *Giardia* cysts isolated from meadow voles, humans, dogs, and beavers. Both cysts and trophozoites were capable of infecting gerbils. Overall rates of infection were 89% for meadow voles, 46% for human isolates, 50% for dog isolates, and 91% for beaver isolates. Cyst dosages ranged between 4000 and 1.5 million cysts per animal. To date the Mongolian gerbil has proven to be the best experimental host for *G. duodenalis*, but the system is subject to errors. Even if an infection did not take in the gerbil, one can not conclude that the cysts used were not alive or infective to humans. The ideal nonhuman model with which to study *G. duodenalis* infection has yet to be described.

4. Conclusions

Excystation, animal infectivity, dye exclusion, and fluorogenic dyes have all been used to determine *Giardia* cyst viability. There are disadvantages to each of these methods. Excystation requires large numbers of cysts and 2 to 3 hours to complete. *Giardia duodenalis* cysts do not excyst routinely at high levels with available methods. Animal infectivity studies require weeks to complete. Furthermore, animals are expensive to buy, feed, and house. Also, only positive results can be conclusively used in animal infectivity studies. Eosin dye exclusion does not correlate well with excystation. Fluorogenic dyes seem to correlate well with *G. muris* excystation. The data on fluorogenic dyes and *G. duodenalis* excystation is presently inconclusive. Preliminary indications are that fluorogenic dyes may not be satisfactory indicators of cyst viability, after cysts have been exposed to chemical disinfectants. Morphological disparity between living and dead cysts correlates well with infectivity in *G. muris* cysts. To date, however, this technique has not been reported for *G. duodenalis* cysts. If differential interference contrast microscopy is used to differentiate living from dead cysts, a large investment is required for the optics. While fluorogenic dyes and differential interference contrast microscopy are promising techniques, they require further evaluation. Clearly, there is a great need for further study in this interesting area of *Giardia* research.

There are varying degrees of *Giardia* cyst viability, when viability is considered in conjunction with the life cycle of the parasite. The ability of the parasite to excyst cannot automatically be inferred from a fluorochrome or morphologic determination that the cyst is alive. Similarly, the ability to infect the host cannot be assumed reliably from a positive excystation determination. An infection of Mongolian gerbils with *Giardia* cysts of unknown origin does not prove the cysts were infective for humans. All of these concepts must be kept in mind when interpreting viability data.

Notice. This document has been reviewed in accordance with U.S. Environmental Protection Agency policy and approved for publication. Mention of trade names or commercial products does not constitute endorsement or recommendation for use.

References

Armaghan, V. (1937) Biological studies on the *Giardia* of rats. Am. J. Hyg. 26, 236-258.
Barnard, R.J. and Jackson, G.J. (1984) *Giardia lamblia*: the transfer of human infections by foods. In: S.L. Erlandsen and E.A. Meyer (Eds.), *Giardia* and Giardiasis, Plenum Press, New York, pp. 365-378.
Belosevic, M., Faubert, G.M., MacLean, J.D., Lau, C. and Croll, N.A. (1983) *Giardia lamblia* infections in Mongolian gerbils: an animal model. J. Infect. Dis. 147, 222-226.
Bhatia, V.N. and Warhurst, D.C. (1981) Hatching and subsequent cultivation of cysts of *Giardia intestinalis* in Diamond's medium. J. Trop. Med. Hyg. 84, 45.
Bingham, A.K. (1979) Studies on excystation of *Giardia*. M.S. thesis, Oregon Health Sciences University, Portland.

Bingham, A.K., Jarroll, Jr., E.L., Meyer, E.A. and Radulescu, S. (1979) *Giardia* sp.: physical factors of excystation in vitro, and excystation vs eosin exclusion as determinants of viability. Exp. Parasitol. 47, 284-291.

Bingham, A.K. and Meyer, E.A. (1979) *Giardia* excystation can be induced in vitro in acidic solutions. Nature (London) 277, 301-302.

Black, R.E., Dykes, A.C., Sinclair, S.P. and Wells, J.G. (1977) Giardiasis in day-care centers: evidence of person to person transmission. Pediatrics 60, 486-491.

Boeck, W.C. (1919) Studies on *Giardia microti*. Univ. Calif. Publ. Zool. 19, 85-134.

Buchel, L.A., Gorenflot, A., Chochillon, C., Savel, J. and Gorbert, J.G. (1987) In vitro excystation of *Giardia* from humans: a scanning electron microscopy study. J. Parasitol. 73, 487-493.

Chochillon, C., Buchel, L.A., Gobert, J.G. and Savel, J. (1987) *Giardia intestinalis*: influence de la composition et de l'osmolarité du milieu sur le dekystement in vitro. C. R. Seances Soc. Biol. Fil. 181, 287-293.

Coggins, J.R. and Schaefer, III, F.W. (1984) *Giardia muris*: scanning electron microscopy of in vitro excystation. Exp. Parasitol. 57, 62-67.

Coggins, J.R. and Schaefer, III, F.W. (1986) *Giardia muris*: ultrastructural analysis of in vitro excystation. Exp. Parasitol. 61, 219-228.

Craun, G.F. (1986) Waterborne giardiasis in the United States, 1965 – 1984. Lancet 2, 513-514.

Craun, G.F. and Jakubowski, W. (1987) Status of waterborne giardiasis outbreaks and monitoring methods. In: C.L. Tate, Jr. (Ed.), Proceedings of the International Symposium on Water-Related Health Issues. American Water Resources Association, Bethesda, Maryland, pp. 167-174.

Erlandsen, S.L., Sherlock, L.A., Januschka, M., Schupp, D.G., Schaefer, III, F.W., Jakubowski, W. and Bemrick, W.J. (1988) Cross-species transmission of *Giardia* spp.; inoculation of beavers and muskrats with cysts of human, beaver, mouse and muskrat origin. Appl. Environ. Microbiol. 54, 2777-2785.

Faubert, G.M., Belosevic, M., Walker, T.S., MacLean, J.D. and Meerovitch, E. (1983) Comparative studies on the pattern of infection with *Giardia* spp. in Mongolian gerbils. J. Parasitol. 69, 802-805.

Feely, D.E. (1982) Histochemical localization of acid phosphatase in *Giardia*. Anat. Rec. 202, 54A.

Feely, D.E. (1986) A simplified method for in vitro excystation of *Giardia muris*. J. Parasitol. 72, 474-475.

Feely, D.E. (1987) Induction of excystation of *Giardia muris* by CO_2. 62nd Annual Meeting of the American Society of Parasitologists, Lincoln, Abstract No. 91.

Feely, D.E. and Dyer, J.K. (1987) Localization of acid phosphatase activity in *Giardia lamblia* and *Giardia muris* trophozoites. J. Protozool. 34, 80-83.

Filice, F.P. (1952) Studies on the cytology and life history of a *Giardia* from the laboratory rat. Univ. Calif. Publ. Zool. 57, 53-146.

Gonzalez-Castro, J., Bermejo-Vicedo, M.T. and Palacios-Gonzalez, F. (1986) Desenquistamiento y cultivo de *Giardia muris*. Rev. Iber. Parasitol. 46, 21-25.

Hegner, R. (1927a) Excystation and infection in the rat with *Giardia lamblia* from man. Am. J. Hyg. 7, 433-447.

Hegner, R. (1927b) The viability of cysts of *Giardia lamblia* from man in the stomach of the rat. Am. J. Hyg. 7, 782-785.

Hegner, R. (1927c) Excystation in vitro of human intestinal protozoa. Science 65, 577-578.

Heyworth, M.F. (1987) Use of fluorescent dyes to assess viability of *Giardia muris* trophozoites. Gastroenterology 92, 1435.

Hoff, J.C., Rice, E.W. and Schaefer, III, F.W. (1984) Disinfection and the control of waterborne giardiasis. In: M. Pirbazari and J.S. Devinny (Eds.), Environmental Engineering. American Society of Civil Engineers, New York, pp. 239-244.

Hoff, J.C., Rice, E.W. and Schaefer, III, F.W. (1985) Comparison of animal infectivity and excystation as measures of *Giardia muris* cyst inactivation by chlorine. Appl. Environ. Microbiol. 50, 1115-1117.

Hudson, S.J., Sauch, J.F. and Lindmark, D.G. (1987) Fluorescent dye exclusion as a method for determining *Giardia* cyst viability. In: P. Wallis (Ed.), Proceedings of the Calgary *Giardia* Conference. University of Calgary, Calgary, pp. 265-269.

Isaac-Renton, J., Proctor, E.M., Prameya, R. and Wong, Q. (1986) A method of excystation and culture of

Giardia lamblia. Trans. R. Soc. Trop. Med. Hyg. 80, 989-990.

Jarroll, E.L., Bingham, A.K. and Meyer, E.A. (1981) Effect of chlorine on cyst viability. Appl. Environ. Microbiol. 41, 483-487.

Jarroll, E.L., Hoff, J.C. and Meyer, E.A. (1984) Resistance of cysts to disinfection agents. In: S.L. Erlandsen and E.A. Meyer (Eds.), *Giardia* and Giardiasis, Plenum Press, New York, pp. 311-328.

Kasprzak, W. and Majewska, A.C. (1983a) Isolation and axenic growth of fresh *Giardia intestinalis* strains in TPS-1 medium. Trans. R. Soc. Trop. Med. Hyg. 77, 223-224.

Kasprzak, W. and Majewska, A.C. (1983b) Infectivity of *Giardia* sp. cysts in relation to eosin exclusion and excystation in vitro. Tropenmed. Parasitol. 34, 70-72.

Kasprzak, W. and Majewska, A.C. (1987) Efficacy of methods for assessing *Giardia* cyst viability. Wiad. Parazytol. 33, 147-155.

Kaur, M., Baveja, U.K., Jyothi, A.S. and Anand, B.S. (1986) Axenic cultures from excysted trophozoites of *Giardia lamblia* and their viability. Indian J. Med. Res. 83, 265-267.

Keister, D.B. (1983) Axenic culture of *Giardia lamblia* in TYI-S-33 medium supplemented with bile. Trans. R. Soc. Trop. Med. Hyg. 77, 487-488.

Keystone, J.S., Krajden, S. and Warren, M.R. (1978) Person to person transmission of *Giardia lamblia* in day care nurseries. Can. Med. Assoc. J. 119, 241-248.

Lindmark, D.G. (1980) Energy metabolism of the anaerobic protozoan *Giardia lamblia*. Mol. Biochem. Parasitol. 1, 1-12.

Lippy, E.C. (1981) Waterborne giardiasis. In: The Proceedings of the International Conference on Lake Management and Restoration. E.P.A. 440/5-81-010. Environmental Protection Agency, pp. 386-389.

Meyer, E.A. (1976) *Giardia lamblia*: isolation and axenic cultivation. Exp. Parasitol. 39, 101-105.

Meyer, E.A. and Radulescu, S. (1984) In vitro cultivation of *Giardia* trophozoites. In: S.L. Erlandsen and E.A. Meyer (Eds.), *Giardia* and Giardiasis. Plenum Press, New York, pp. 99-109.

Meyer, E.A. and Schaefer, III, F.W. (1984) Models for excystation. In: S.L. Erlandsen and E.A. Meyer (Eds.), *Giardia* and Giardiasis. Plenum Press, New York, pp. 131-144.

Meyers, J.D., Kuharic, H.A. and Holmes, K.K. (1977) *Giardia lamblia* infection in homosexual men. Br. J. Vener. Dis. 53, 54-55.

Osterholm, M.T., Forfang, J.C., Ristinen, T.L., Dean, A.G., Washburn, J.W., Godes, J.R., Rude, R.A. and McCullough, J.G. (1981) An outbreak of foodborne giardiasis. N. Engl. J. Med. 304, 24-28.

Rendtorff, R.C. (1954) The experimental transmission of human intestinal protozoan parasites. II. *Giardia lamblia* cysts given in capsules. Am. J. Hyg. 59, 209-220.

Rice, E.W. and Schaefer, III, F.W. (1981) Improved in vitro excystation procedure for *Giardia lamblia* cysts. J. Clin. Microbiol. 14, 709-710.

Roberts-Thomson, I.C., Stevens, D.P., Mahmoud, A.A.F. and Warren, K.S. (1976) Giardiasis in the mouse: an animal model. Gastroenterology 71, 57-61.

Rotman, B. and Papermaster, B.W. (1966) Membrane properties of living mammalian cells as studied by enzymatic hydrolysis of fluorogenic esters. Proc. Natl. Acad. Sci. USA 55, 134-141.

Sauch, J.F. (1987) A new method for excystation of *Giardia*. In: P. Wallis (Ed.), Proceedings of the Calgary *Giardia* Conference. University of Calgary, Calgary, pp. 271-274.

Sauch, J., Flanigan, D., Galvin, M. and Berman, D. (1988) Propidium iodide as an indicator of *Giardia* cyst viability. American Society for Microbiology Annual Meeting, Miami Beach, Florida, Abstract No. Q48.

Sauch, J.F. and Mormile, M. (1986) Buoyant density profiles of *Giardia lamblia* cysts from Mongolian gerbils: comparison to human *Giardia* and *G. muris* cysts. American Society for Microbiology Annual Meeting, Washington, D.C., Abstract No. Q57.

Schaefer, III, F.W., Rice, E.W. and Hoff, J.C. (1984) Factors promoting in vitro excystation of *Giardia muris* cysts. Trans. R. Soc. Trop. Med. Hyg. 78, 795-800.

Schupp, D.G. and Erlandsen, S.L. (1987a) A new method to determine *Giardia* cyst viability: correlation of fluorescein diacetate and propidium iodide staining with animal infectivity. Appl. Environ. Microbiol. 53, 704-707.

Schupp, D.G. and Erlandsen, S.L. (1987b) Determination of *Giardia muris* cysts viability by differential interference contrast, phase, or brightfield microscopy. J. Parasitol. 73, 723-729.

Schupp, D.G., Januschka, M.M. and Erlandsen, S.L. (1987) Assessing *Giardia* cyst viability with fluorogenic dyes: comparisons to animal infectivity and cyst morphology by light and electron microscopy. In: P. Wallis (Ed.), Proceedings of the Calgary *Giardia* Conference. University of Calgary, Calgary pp. 265–269.

Visvesvara, G.S., Dickerson, J.W. and Healy, G.R. (1988) Variable infectivity of human-derived *Giardia lamblia* cysts for Mongolian gerbils (*Meriones unguiculatus*). J. Clin. Microbiol. 26, 837-841.

Wallis, P.M. and Wallis, H.M. (1986) Excystation and culturing of human and animal *Giardia* spp. by using gerbils and TYI-S-33 medium. Appl. Environ. Microbiol. 41, 483-487.

Wickramanayake, G.B., Ruben, A.J. and Sproul, O.J. (1985) Effect of ozone and storage temperature on *Giardia* cysts. J. Am. Water Works Assoc. 77, 74-77.

Giardiasis (E.A. Meyer, ed.)
© *1990 Elsevier Science Publishers B.V. (Biomedical Division)*

8

In vitro encystation of *Giardia*

DANIEL G. SCHUPP[1], DAVID S. REINER[2], FRANCES D. GILLIN[2] and STANLEY L. ERLANDSEN[1]

[1]*Department of Cell Biology and Neuroanatomy, University of Minnesota, Minneapolis, MN, 55455, U.S.A., and* [2]*Department of Pathology H811F, University of California, San Diego, CA 92103, U.S.A.*

1. Introduction	137
2. Induction of *Giardia* spp. cysts in vitro	138
2.1. *Giardia* trophozoites of human origin (WB strain) (Gillin et al., 1986, 1987, 1988a,b)	138
2.2. *Giardia* trophozoites of human, beaver and muskrat origin (Schupp et al., 1988a,b)	142
2.3. *Giardia* trophozoites of human origin (Peruvian isolate) (Sterling et al., 1988)	143
3. Cyst morphology	144
3.1. Light and electron microscopic comparisons of in vivo and in vitro produced cysts	145
4. Viability of in vitro produced cysts	146
4.1. Fluorogenic dyes	147
4.2. Excystation	147
4.3. Animal models	147
5. Biochemical evidence for in vitro cyst wall formation	148
5.1. Identification of *Giardia* cyst wall-specific components with Western blots	148
5.2. Isotope incorporation	151
5.3. Carbohydrate analysis of cyst wall components	151
6. Summary	152
References	152

1. Introduction

The parasitic protozoan *Giardia* has been observed and studied microscopically for over three centuries; however, it was not until the last two decades that axenic cultures of *Giardia* trophozoites have been established. This has led to numerous well-controlled studies of the cellular and molecular biology of this parasite, including metabolism of the trophozoites, biochemical and antigenic analysis, cytoskeletal characterization, contractile proteins and mechanism of adhesion of trophozoites.

Unfortunately, corresponding studies on *Giardia* cysts have been hampered, until recently, because the in vitro cultivation technique for trophozoites does not duplicate the entire life cycle of *Giardia*, since no observable cyst stage appears. The only previously documented observations on the encystment process were on in vivo preparations. Early encystation studies by Perroncito (1887) and Lavier (1942) used fresh mucosal smears from the colon of infected mammals and amphibians.

The cyst is commonly the infective form of the organism and may survive for long periods in the environment, particularly in cold water. Studies on the biochemistry and assembly of the cyst wall could offer insights into how the cyst survives and may lead to new means of control of this ubiquitous parasite. In vitro encystation provides a source of pure cysts and a model system that could provide basic information on parasite differentiation. In addition, such a model allows investigation of secretion and assembly of the filamentous cyst wall, a remarkable process for a cell reported to lack a Golgi apparatus and containing a scant network of rough endoplasmic reticulum.

Breakthroughs by three separate groups occurred when Gillin et al. (1986, 1987, 1988a,b), Sterling et al. (1988a,b) and Schupp et al. (1988b,c) reported methods for in vitro encystation. Because of the success of Bingham and Meyer (1979) with the excystation model, which requires gastric conditions for the activation of the dormant cyst, similar 'host factors' were investigated for the signal or stimulus to encyst. Two of the techniques (Gillin et al., 1986, 1987, 1988a,b; Schupp et al., 1988a–c) reported the use of bile-enriched growth media, whereas the technique of Sterling et al. (1988) was based on changing gas mixtures during incubation in the absence of bile-enriched media. The technique of Gillin et al. utilizes primary bile salts with a human strain of *Giardia* (WB, ATCC No. 30957, Bethesda, MD), whereas the procedure of Schupp et al. involves a crude bile fraction. They employed six different isolates with the best results obtained from a *Giardia duodenalis* type organism that was isolated from a muskrat (MR4, Dr. P. Wallis) but did not have the morphologic or immunologic characteristics of *Giardia ondatrae* (Erlandsen and Bemrick, 1987).

2. Induction of Giardia *spp. cysts in vitro*

2.1. Giardia *trophozoites of human origin (WB strain) (Gillin et al., 1986, 1987, 1988a,b)*

In humans, *Giardia* trophozoites colonize the upper small intestine below the entry of the common bile duct. In this location, they are exposed to complex mixtures of biliary, pancreatic, and gastrointestinal secretions which interact to form new physical structures and compounds. For example, bile salts form micelles with products of lipolysis released from dietary lipids by pancreatic lipases. Trophozoites penetrate the mucus layer and attach to the epithelium where they may be sequestered from the intestinal fluid. Alternatively, if they enter the lumenal compartment and are swept 'downstream', they must encyst or die, because trophozoites do not naturally survive long in feces or outside the host.

Accordingly, Gillin et al. (1986, 1987) proposed that specific conditions in the human small intestine might promote in vitro encystation of human-source *Giardia*. To test this hypothesis, they first determined the location of trophozoites and cysts in the intestinal tract of suckling mice infected with axenically cultured trophozoites of *Giardia* strain WB (Gillin et al., 1987). Through day 16 of infection, large numbers of cysts were found in the mid- to lower jejunum. Cysts are not motile and can only move 'downstream' passively, thus this established a major site of encystation.

Because bile salts and products of lipolysis are major specific components of the small intestinal milieu, the next series of experiments tested the ability of individual bile salts to promote encystation in vitro when added to TYI-S-33 growth medium (see Chapter 6) without bovine bile (Gillin et al., 1987). Of the six major bile salts of human bile, the primary bile salts induced higher levels and more rapid encystation of strain WB trophozoites than did the secondary bile salts. The four primary bile salts (the glycine- and taurine-conjugates of cholate and chenodeoxycholate) are synthesized in the liver from cholesterol. In contrast, deoxycholate is formed by bacterial dehydroxylation of cholate in the lower intestine followed by absorption and conjugation in the liver. Bile salts are actively reabsorbed in the terminal ileum and secreted into the bile where primary bile salts predominate 3:1 (Hofmann, 1984). Therefore, bile salt concentrations remain high throughout the small intestine.

Because these initial experiments supported the idea that small intestinal factors were important triggers of encystation, it was important to examine their role under local physiologic conditions. When the acidic gastric chyme enters the duodenum, it is rapidly neutralized by bicarbonate secretion. Although the fluid in the upper portion of the duodenum tends to be acidic, the pH gradually increases distally and may reach 7.6 to 8.0 in the lower jejunum (Fordtran and Locklear, 1966). This slightly alkaline pH promotes the ionization of fatty acids, increases their tendency to associate with bile salts in mixed micelles (Hofmann and Roda, 1984), and decreases their toxicity to *Giardia* in vitro (Reiner et al., 1986).

The ability to resist hypotonic lysis is a hallmark of cysts from human feces and a rigorous criterion for quantitation of in vitro encystation. The next series of experiments (Gillin et al., 1988a) showed that raising the pH to 7.8 greatly increased the numbers of water-resistant human-source *Giardia* cysts induced by a primary bile salt (Na glycocholate) and a fatty acid (myristic acid) (Fig. 1). The stimulatory activity of the fatty acids was not specific, because all fatty acids tested (from C8 to C18) in combination with glycocholate induced encystation at pH 7.8. Bile salts may stimulate encystation indirectly because of their capacity to bind fatty acids, and because excess fatty acids can induce encystation without added bile salt.

More recent experiments (Gillin, Boucher, Reiner, unpublished data) have extended these studies to human bile. Hepatic bile from a human patient, as well as bile from certain lower mammals, stimulated encystation of strain WB at pH 7.8. In contrast to

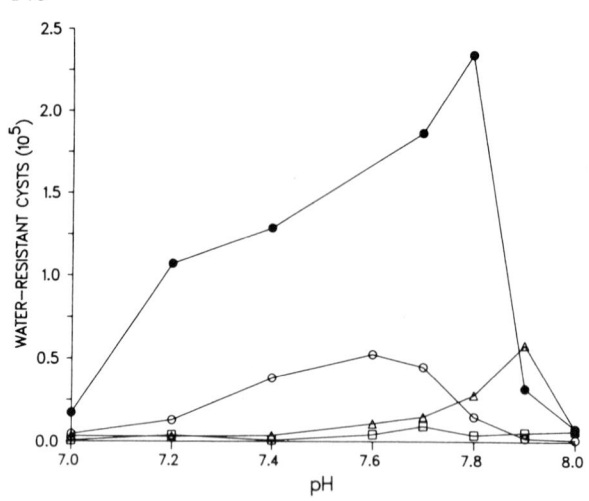

Fig. 1. The effects of pH on encystation human-source *Giardia* in the presence and absence of glycocholate and myristic acid. Trophozoites were incubated as described (Gillin et al., 1988) in TYI-S-33 medium without bovine bile containing glycocholate alone (8 mM, (○), myristic acid alone (0.5 mM, (△) or together (●) or with no additions (□), control). The pH refers to the initial pH; the number of water resistant cysts is per 4 ml vial (From Gillin et al., 1988).

the observations of Schupp et al. (1988) with the muskrat strain MR4, bovine bile at concentrations from 0.5 to 20 mg/ml and pH 7.0 did not induce encystation of the human strain WB ($<10^3$ cysts/ml).

Currently, in Gillin's laboratory, 5 to 150×10^3 water-resistant fecal-type cysts/ml are recovered in 48 h at pH 7.8 with a number of defined (A: 8 mM natrium glycocholate, 0.5 mM myristic acid, plus 0.1 mM oleic acid or B: 2 mM myristic acid plus 0.1 mM oleic acid) or undefined (human or lower mammalian bile) stimuli. Their morphology by Nomarski differential interference contrast optics is like that of cysts from human feces: 6×10 μm, oval, with characteristic cyst wall, nucleic, median bodies, and axostyles. Most fecal-type cysts are viable because they take up fluorescein diacetate and exclude propidium iodide by the method of Schupp and Erlandsen (1987a, see below). Ultrastructure of in vitro-derived strain WB cysts has been confirmed by transmission electron microscopy, and the presence of four nuclei has been shown by ethidium bromide staining of fixed, permeabilized cysts (Fig. 2; Gillin et al., 1987). Biological activity of induced cysts was demonstrated (Gillin, 1988) by infection of suckling mice using the model of Hill et al. (1983), and by excystation in vitro. Excystation efficiencies of 3 to 10% are observed by Gillin's group. Trophozoites which emerged from in vitro-induced WB cysts following either excystation or infection of suckling mice have been re-cultured and induced to undergo a subsequent round of encystation in vitro, thus completing the life cycle of *Giardia* from humans in vitro.

Excretion of *Giardia* cysts by human patients and experimentally infected gerbils is highly irregular. The studies summarized here suggest that local fluctuations in pH and, concentrations of bile salts and fatty acids may affect the efficiency of such *Giardia* encystation in vivo.

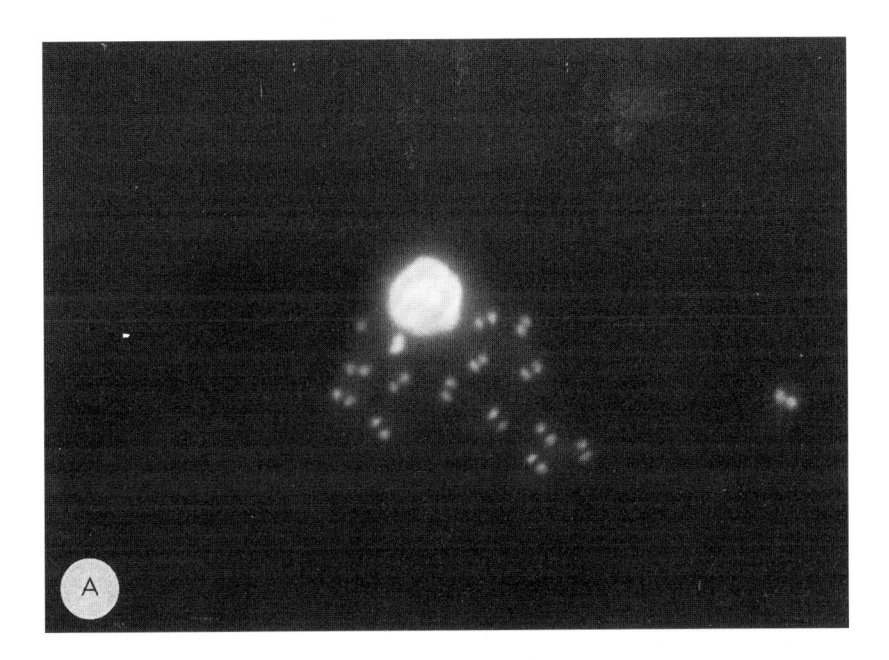

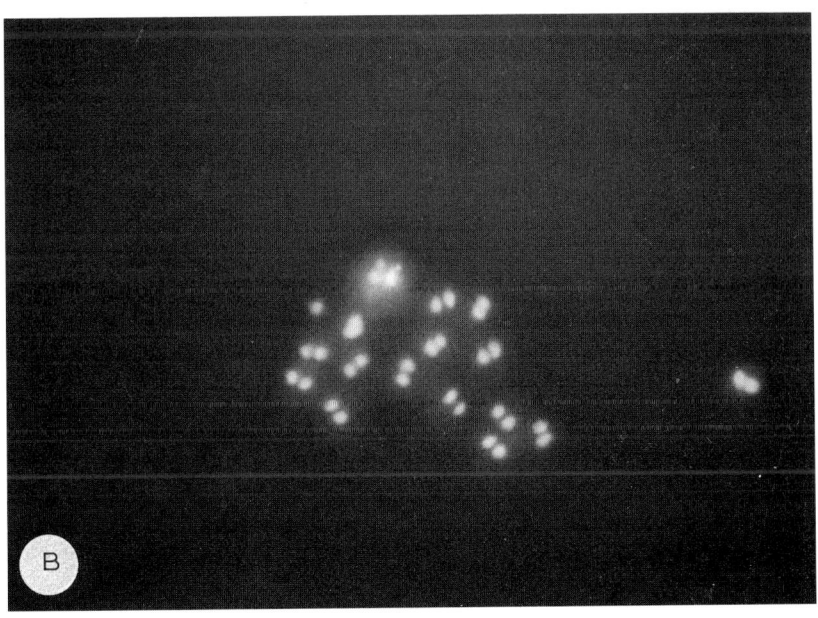

Fig. 2. An in vitro derived quadrinucleate cyst and binucleate trophozoites. Parasites were harvested, fixed, and reacted with rabbit antibody to cysts and then FITC-goat antirabbit antiserum as described (Gillin et al., 1987a). Nuclei are stained with ethidium bromide. (A) Photographed with filters for fluorescein. The binucleate trophozoites do not react with the cyst-specific serum. (B) Photographed with filters for rhodamine (original magnification ×1000).

2.2. Giardia trophozoites of human, beaver and muskrat origin (Schupp et al., 1988b,c)

Six different isolates of *Giardia* including the WB strain isolated from humans (Smith et al., 1982b) (American Type Culture Collection No. 30957, Bethesda, MD), four beaver isolates (IP-0482:1 and IP-0583:1 from Dr L. Diamond; PB-1 and B-5 from H. Stibbs), and one muskrat isolate (MR4 from Dr H. Stibbs and Dr P. Wallace) were grown axenically and shown to be capable of forming cysts in vitro (see Fig. 3). Trophozoites grown in TYI-S-33 medium that had 2.5 mg/ml or less of bovine bile did not form cysts, but the trophozoites exhibited typical growth and reproduction. When the culture medium was replaced with fresh TYI-S-33 containing 5 mg/ml bile, encystation occurred at rates ranging from 5 to 50%, depending on the isolate. Increasing the bile content to

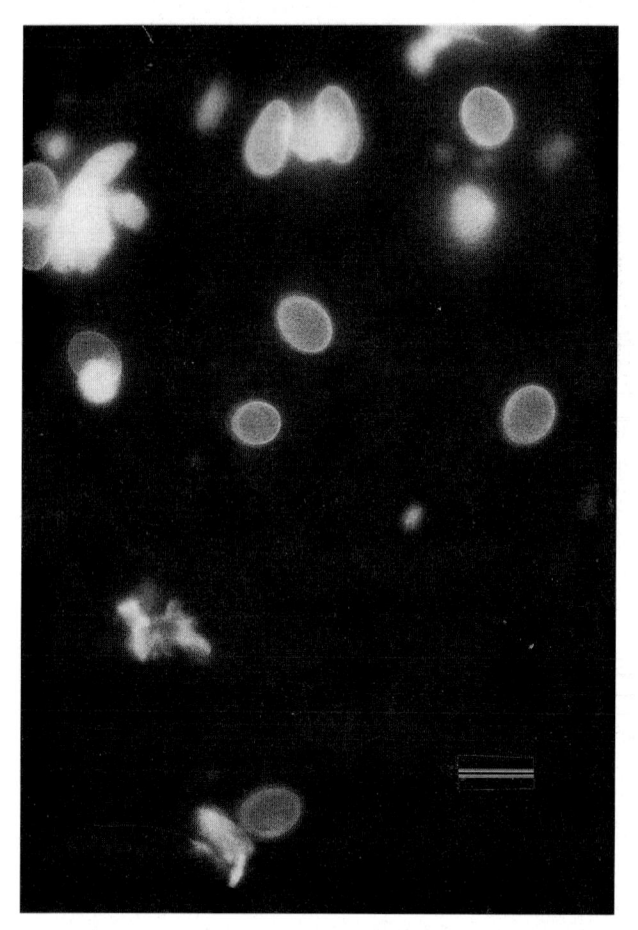

Fig. 3. Reaction of rabbit anticyst serum with intact, unfixed *Giardia* cysts from human feces. Intact, unfixed, purified (Douglas et al., 1987) cysts from a patient with acute giardiasis were reacted with the rabbit antiserum or preimmune serum [diluted 1:100 in 0.02 M PBS with 1% bovine serum (BSA) and 1% Tween-20] for 2 h, washed by centrifugation, and reacted with FITC-conjugated protein A (1:2000). The cysts show fluorescence with the antiserum, while the fecal debris is autofluorescent. There was no reaction with pre-immune serum.

10 or 20 mg/ml produced either an increase or decrease in the rate of encystation, again depending on the isolate. When the cultures were passaged a second time into their respective media with the same concentration of added bile, the encystation level was always less than the level attained during the first passage. Continued subculture resulted in a further decrease in the encystation rate.

The complete life cycle of *Giardia* was reproduced in a continuous series of trophozoite-cyst conversions (Schupp et al., 1988a,b). The first cycle was completed when strain MR4 trophozoites were stimulated to form cysts in vitro by the addition of 5 mg/ml bile (Fig. 4). The cysts forms in vitro were isolated from the remaining trophozoites by distilled water lysis and inoculated into parasite-free Mongolian gerbils by gavage. Cysts underwent excystation in vivo and yielded trophozoites that were then isolated at necropsy from the small bowel of the experimentally infected gerbils. These trophozoites were then placed into TYI-S-33 growth medium without added bile. When the re-established cultures were placed in TYI-S-33 media enriched with 5 mg/ml bile, cysts were again formed.

Gillin et al. (1988b, see section 2.1.) have reported in vitro and in vivo differentiation of trophozoite-cyst-trophozoite stages, using the WB strain of *Giardia* from a human and

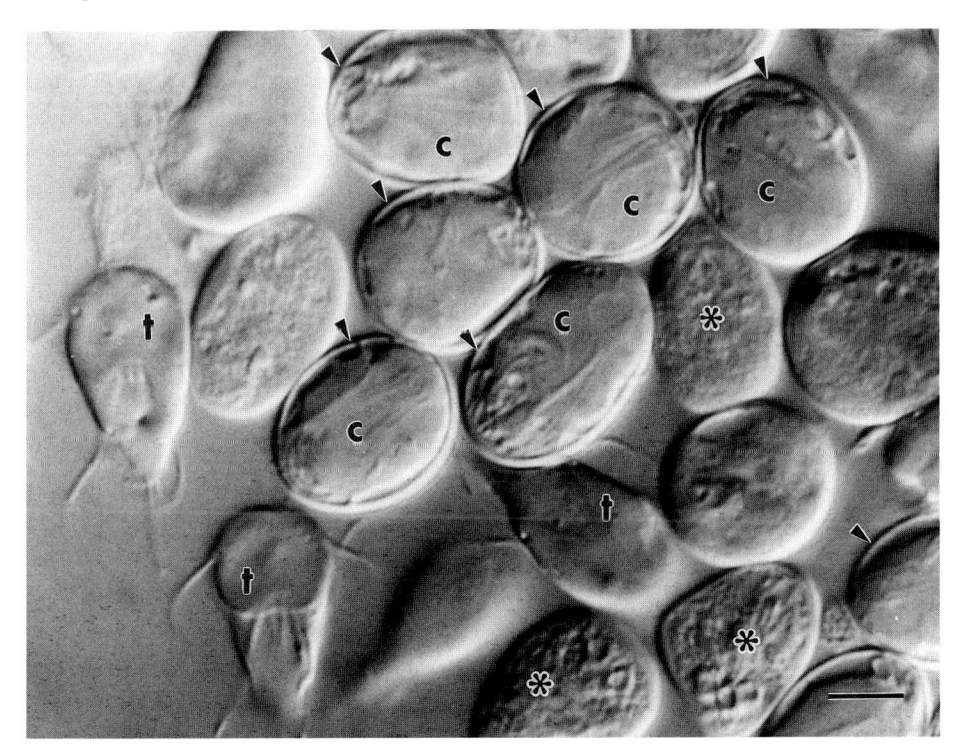

Fig. 4. A Nomarski differential interference contrast micrograph of the MR4 strain of *Giardia* induced by bile to undergo encystment. *Giardia* trophozoites (t) and cysts (c) are easily recognized with the latter being surrounded by the characteristic cyst wall. Subpopulations of cysts consistent with a nonviable morphology can also be observed (*). Magnification bar = 5 μ.

the suckling mouse model of Hill et al. (1983). With the in vitro encystation model for the MR4 strain of *Giardia*, Schupp et al. (1988) have demonstrated: (1) Morphologically distinct *Giardia* cysts were produced in TYI-S-33 media with bile supplementation. (2) In vitro formed cysts were immunostained by antisera raised in rabbits using in vivo isolated *Giardia* cysts. (3) The cysts produced in vitro were shown to be viable as measured by three different tests of viability: (a) fluorogenic dye staining, (b) excystation and (c) animal infectivity. (4) The complete life cycle of *Giardia* was reproduced in a series of trophozoite-cyst transformations that demonstrated that the MR4 isolate used was still capable of animal infectivity and further, could still be recultured and stimulated to undergo encystation in bile-supplemented media.

2.3. Giardia *trophozoites of human origin (Peruvian isolate) (Sterling et al., 1988)*

The in vitro encystation procedure was developed to provide antigen for generating monoclonal antibodies that could be utilized for immunodiagnostic screening of fecal and water samples.

Giardia cysts were produced after modifying in vitro incubation conditions for trophozoites from a human-derived, Peruvian isolate. Trophozoites were grown in modified TYI-S-33 medium without bile for 4 days. Then the cells were concentrated and incubated for 48 h in a 90:10 nitrogen to carbon dioxide atmosphere in a limited volume of similar medium (1.5 ml). The in vitro formed *Giardia* cysts were identified by SEM, but viability of these cysts could not be demonstrated either by excystation or by their ability to produce infection in an animal model.

The monoclonal antiserum that was derived from the in vitro-produced cysts was shown by indirect immunofluorescence (IIF) to be specific for the cyst wall of *Giardia* and, also, did not cross react with *Entamoeba histolytica, E. coli, E. hartmanni, Eimeria* sp., *Cryptosporidium, Candida* sp., *Rhodotorula* sp., or algae. Studies using IIF with this monoclonal (D.S.; S.L.E.) have shown that cysts from a variety of species of *Giardia* were immunostained, including those from mice, voles, muskrats, beavers, dogs, birds and humans. Additionally, immunoreactivity for this monoclonal antibody resided on the filamentous component of the cyst wall (D.S., S.L.E., unpublished observation). This provides further support for the thesis that cysts formed in vitro are similar not only in morphology but also in antigenic constitution to in vivo derived cysts.

3. Cyst morphology

Giardia cysts prepared in vitro have an oval shape and a size variation between 6 and 15 μm (usual range 8-12 μm). Morphologic markers at the light microscopic level include 2-4 nuclei associated with one pole of the cyst, cytoplasmic organelles such as linear fibrils representing flagellar axonemes or stacks of curved elements known to be either dissembled adhesive disc or the median body.

In addition, the fibrillar cyst wall (0.20-0.25 μm in width), peripheral vacuoles beneath the cytoplasmic membrane, basal bodies, and peritrophic spaces between cyst wall and cytoplasm are demonstrated by electron microscopy.

Current microscopic or serologic analysis cannot differentiate between *Giardia* isolated from different hosts (Filice, 1952). Therefore, morphological descriptions of cysts (with the exception of the cysts isolated from microtine rodents which are termed binary cysts) are essentially the same (refer to Chapter 2 on cyst morphology).

Using fluorogenic dyes that are either metabolically incorporated or excluded from the cyst (Schupp and Erlandsen, 1987a; Schupp et al., 1987b) suggests that individual cysts within populations of cysts isolated from the mouse model for giardiasis can be divided further into subpopulations of viable and nonviable cysts. The basis for distinguishing viable cysts is the incorporation of fluorescein diacetate (see below) and also morphology characterized by the presence of a clearly delineated cyst wall, a space between cyst wall and the cytoplasm (peritrophic space) and a cytoplasmic appearance by light microscopy that is glassy or hyaline. In contrast, the nonviable MR4 cysts stain with propidium iodide and do not have a clearly delineated cyst wall, but possess a granular appearing cytoplasm that permits better visualization of the intracytoplasmic organelles.

3.1. Light and electron microscopic comparisons of in vivo and in vitro produced cysts

Utilizing the above criteria for cyst morphology it was demonstrated by Schupp et al. (1988) and Gillin et al. (1986, 1987, 1988a,b) that in vitro-produced cysts possessed the morphology described for *Giardia* cysts formed in vivo (see Fig. 3). In addition, morphologic subpopulations that correspond to the viable and nonviable phenotype were observed by differential interference contrast microscopy in cysts produced in vitro (Fig. 4). Although the characteristic morphology identical to that described previously for viable and nonviable *Giardia muris* cysts (Schupp et al., 1987b) can be demonstrated within in vitro cysts derived from MR4 cultures, further correlation using a fluorescence-activated cell sorter to investigate the association between viability as measured by morphology or dye exclusion and the ability of cysts to produce an animal infection, have not yet been performed.

Ultrastructural comparison of the cyst wall from cysts isolated from feces and in vitro-derived cysts can be seen using low voltage scanning electron microscopy (Fig. 4). In all cysts examined, the external surface of the cyst wall was composed of a woven interlacing network of filaments ranging from 7-20 nm in diameter. In a previous study using transmission electron microscopy (Schupp et al., 1988a), the appearance of the cyst wall of in vitro and in vivo derived *Giardia* cysts revealed a strikingly similar fibrillar nature. In addition to this similar ultrastructure, immunogold labeling of thin sections using antisera produced against human cysts (a gift from Dr Judith Sauch) revealed specific immunolabeling of the fibrillar component of the cyst wall of in vitro-derived cysts (Fig. 5) and also labeling of vacuoles within trophozoites from those cultures stimulated to undergo encystation. This pattern of immunolabeled intracellular vacuoles

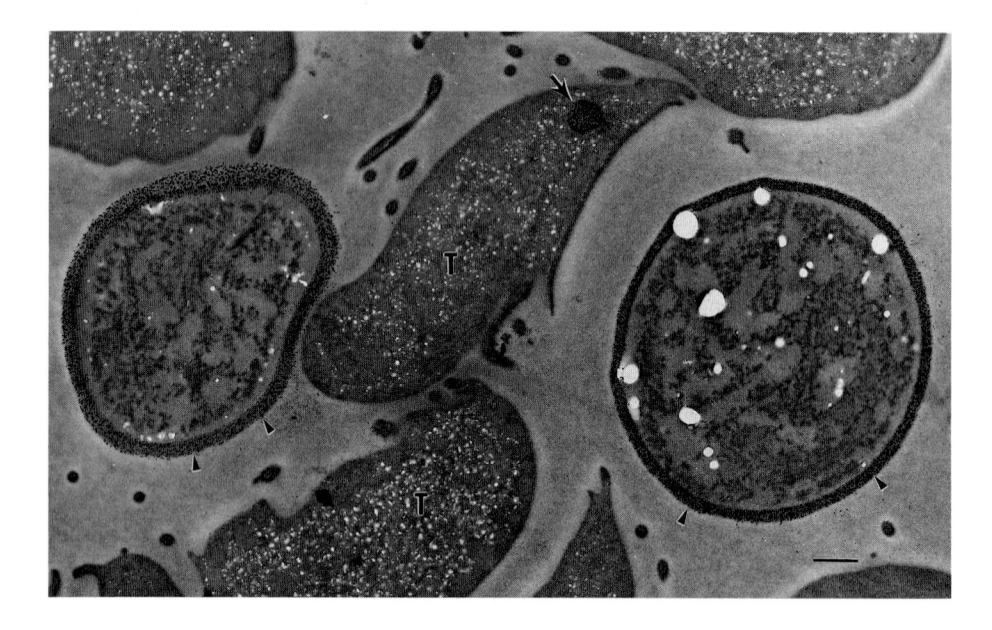

Fig. 5. Post-embedment immunogold (15 nm) labeling of thin sections from MR4 cultures undergoing encystation after induction using bile supplemented TYI-S-33. Dense immunogold labeling for cyst wall antigen is seen over the filamentous component of the wall of two *Giardia* cysts (arrowheads) and also in a cytoplasmic vacuole (arrow) within a trophozoite (T). Cyst morphology is consistent with nonviability and may reflect the prolonged exposure to culture conditions (48 h) or poor infiltration by the LR White embedment. Bar = 1μm.

raises questions as to the mode of synthesis, time required for encystation and the mechanism of secretion for the fibrillar component of the cyst wall. The immunostaining corroborates the ultrastructural similarities in the cyst wall between in vitro- and in vivo-derived cysts and indicates that the composition of the in vitro-derived cyst wall may be similar in antigenicity to those formed in vivo.

4. Viability of in vitro-produced cysts

The *Giardia* cyst is the infective form of this zooflagellate, and information regarding its viability and resistance to disinfecting agents has been of interest to water quality control engineers, clinicians, other public health workers, and environmental groups. Techniques used to determine cyst viability have been based on light microscopic staining methods (including the use of fluorogenic dyes), cyst morphology and physiological indicators of *Giardia* function such as excystation and animal infectivity.

4.1. Fluorogenic dyes

Fluorogenic dye staining is based on the hydrolysis by intracellular enzymes of the fluorogenic substrate fluorescein diacetate (FDA). FDA is a colorless, molecule which diffuses into, and is concentrated by, cells with intact bilayer lipid membranes. The nonpolar fluorescein molecule that results from the enzymatic cleavage of the acetate groups remains within cells that are viable and can be visualized under fluorescent excitation of 450-490 nm wavelength. This assay of viability has been correlated with infectivity of animals and cyst morphology in the mouse model for giardiasis (Schupp et al., 1987c).

Propidium iodide (PI) is a large planar molecule that will not traverse an intact lipid bilayer. When a cell membrane is compromised, this molecule will enter and intercalate into nucleic acids; it thus serves as a marker for nonviable cysts.

Using the FDA/PI method, in vitro-derived *Giardia* cysts can have a viability as high as 50%. Unfortunately, the percentages obtained with this procedure have been variable, whereas, with in vivo-derived cysts isolated from animals models for giardiasis, the percentage of viable cysts was more constant. Numerous factors could be responsible for the variation in the results obtained with this procedure. Total cell number at the onset of induction of encystation affect the availability of essential components of medium that are involved in cyst wall formation or the buildup of byproducts of metabolism. In addition, older or more dense cultures induced to undergo encystation would have a larger fraction of senescent trophozoites, which would release proteases and hydrolases from cellular lysis. Additionally, previous studies have shown that storage at 37°C for 24 h of *Giardia* cysts isolated from feces greatly reduced their viability as judged by excystation. Such cysts never survived longer than 4 days at 37°C (Bingham and Meyer, 1979; Bingham et al., 1979).

4.2. Excystation

The excystation procedure was performed using a modification of the technique of Bingham and Meyer (1979). Seven tubes were inoculated with 7.5 × 10⁵ strain MR4 cysts that had been produced in vitro. Contaminating trophozoites were removed from the cysts by lysis in distilled water. Signs of excystation, including motile trophozoites and excysting forms, were observed in 2/7 tubes (Schupp et al., 1988a). Although the excystation rate was low (<1%), cultures were established and maintained in bile-supplemented TYI-S-33 medium.

4.3. Animal models

The viability of in vitro derived cysts from MR4 cultures was investigated by determining animal infectivity using both the Mongolian gerbil model (Belosevic et al., 1983) and the newborn mouse model (Hill et al., 1983) for giardiasis. In both models, 35% of the animals inoculated with 2×10^5 strain MR4 cysts were shown to have trophozoites in the small intestine at necropsy. Furthermore, scanning electron microscopic examination of the villous epithelial cells in the gerbil revealed mucosal lesions that were morphologically similar to the ventral adhesive disc of the trophozoites.

These results demonstrate that cysts formed in vitro are viable by three separate criteria of *Giardia* cysts with normal functions.

5. Biochemical evidence for in vitro cyst wall formation

5.1. Identification of Giardia cyst wall-specific components with Western blots

Cellular differentiation is generally characterized by synthesis of stage-specific structural or functional components. As a tool for analysis of cyst-specific antigens, polyspecific antibodies were raised in rabbits (Gillin et al., 1986, 1987). Cysts (from feces of a patient with chronic symptomatic giardiasis) to be used as antigens were highly purified by removing fecal debris and bacteria by passage over a Sephadex G-50 column (Douglas et al., 1987), incubation with antibiotics and washing. The purified cysts were injected without adjuvant intravenously into rabbits in order to minimize release of trophozoite antigens by cyst breakage.

The antiserum proved specific for cysts. It did not react with cultured trophozoites by indirect immunofluorescence (IIF, Fig. 2), ELISA, or Western blots (Gillin et al., 1986, 1987). It did react with unfixed cysts from human feces by IIF, suggesting that at least some of the antigenic determinants are exposed on the outer surface of the cyst wall (Gillin et al., 1987a) (Fig. 3).

The antiserum reacted in Western blots with cysts purified from human feces and also with in vitro-derived cysts of strain WB (Gillin et al., 1987, 1988). Reactivity with in vitro-produced cysts of strain WB establishes that the antigens are specific to *Giardia* and not of fecal origin. Moreover, the antiserum was prepared against cysts from a patient from the San Diego area, whereas strain WB was isolated from a patient infected in Afghanistan (Smith et al., 1982b), suggesting that antigens are conserved among isolates of differing geographic origin.

The cyst-specific antigens have been analyzed by Western blots of strain WB trophozoites induced to encyst in vitro (Gillin et al., 1987a; Reiner et al., 1989). As above, no reaction was observed with trophozoites. The major antigens recognized by this serum were four discrete bands between 66 and 103 kDa and a set of polydisperse bands of lower weight (21 to 39 kDa). All the antigens were sensitive to proteolytic digestion demonstrating proteinaceous components in the cyst wall.

The next question addressed was whether all the cyst antigens appear in parallel, i.e., whether they are co-ordinately or independently regulated. SDS-PAGE and Western blots of cultures harvested over time showed that the antigens of lower weight (21 to 39 kDa) appeared earlier and seemed to be under less stringent regulation because they were also

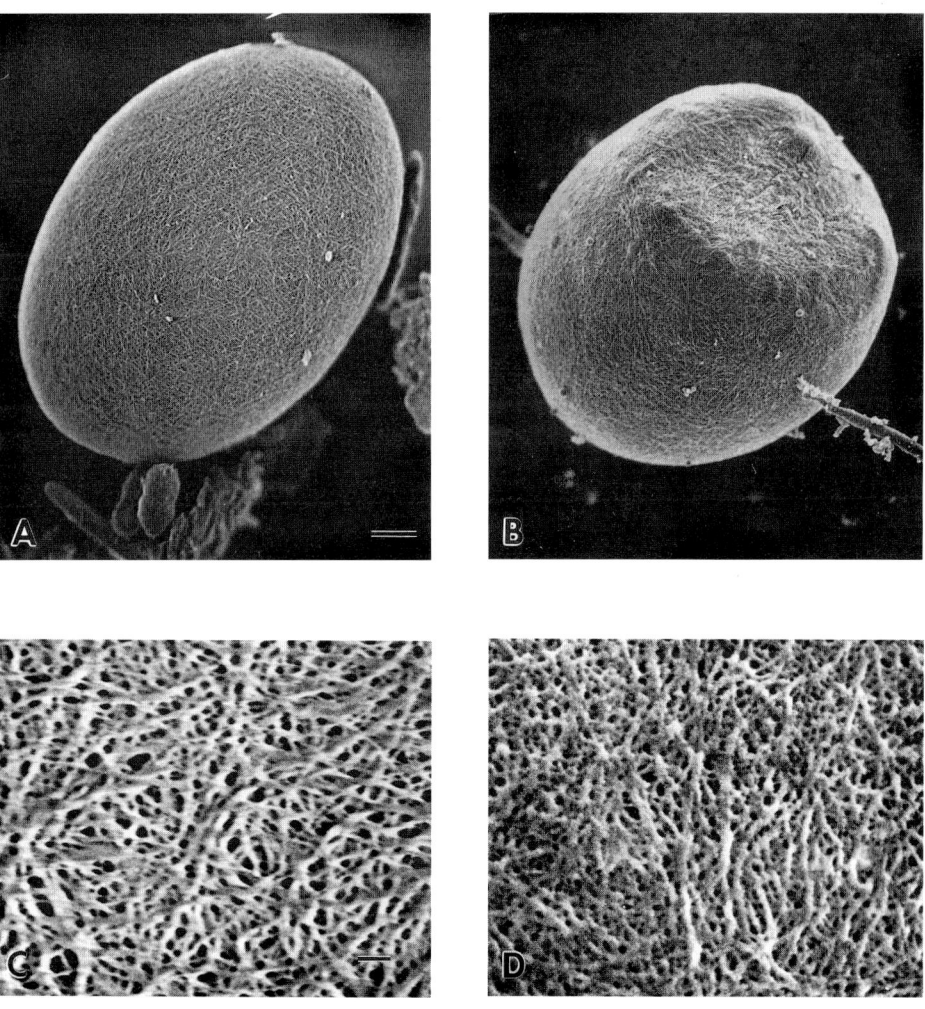

Fig. 6. Low voltage scanning electron micrographs of the filamentous cyst wall of the MR4 strain of *Giardia*, recovered after natural in vivo encystment in the gerbil (panels A and C) or by induction with bile using axenic cultures of the MR4 strain (panels B and D). Cysts forms either in vitro or in vivo both possessed an anastomotic filamentous cyst wall. Bar = 1 μ for panels A and D. Bar = 0.1 μ for panels C and D.

observed under suboptimal conditions of encystation. The antigen pattern exhibited by the total culture at 48 h (Fig. 7) was the same as that exhibited by isolated, water-resistant cysts of strain WB (Reiner et al., in press).

Because the first antiserum was prepared by injection of cysts purified from feces, it would recognize only those antigens of strain WB which are shared with the fecal cyst strain and are present in mature cysts (although, as shown, they are expressed earlier). In order to identify other encystation-specific antigens, especially those which may not be exposed on the surface of mature cysts, additional antiserum was prepared in rabbits

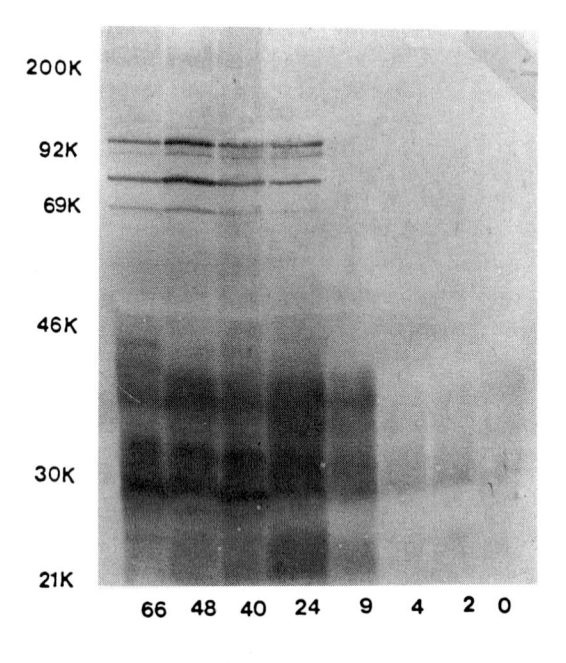

Fig. 7. Time of appearance of cyst specific antigens during in vitro encystation of *Giardia* strain WB. Trophozoites were incubated at 37°C in TYI-S-33 without bovine bile with 8 mM Na glycocholate, 0.5 mM myristic acid and 0.1 M oleic acid, initial pH 7.8. At the times indicated, the parasites were harvested, and 6×10^6 parasites/lane subjected to SDS-PAGE and immunoblotting with the rabbit anticyst serum (1:200) as described (Gillin et al., 1987).

by subcutaneous injection of cysts derived from strain WB in vitro. Western blots with this serum reveal a complex pattern of additional, cyst-specific bands which appear at characteristic times of encystation. Some of these antigens are glycosylated (Reiner et al., in press). Thus, differentiation of the motile, flagellated, parasitic trophozoite into the cyst stage, which is highly adapted to survival outside the host, entails the regulated synthesis of a large number of new antigenic components (Gillin et al., 1987, 1988; Reiner et al., in press).

Antibodies with reactivity against cysts have been reported by others. Sauch (1985) raised antibodies in rabbits against Percoll-purified cysts from human feces. This antiserum was useful for detecting and identifying *Giardia* cysts in water samples. Rosoff and Stibbs (1986a,b) demonstrated a 65 kDa, highly glycosylated antigen (GSA 65) in both trophozoites and cysts by Western blots. Although it is not stage-specific, IIF studies with dried, acetone-fixed cysts suggested that GSA 65 is present in the cyst wall. This antigen was prominent in stools of patients with giardiasis.

5.2. Isotope incorporation

The cyst wall of *Giardia* is important because it is probably responsible for the resistance of this stage to hypotonic lysis and to disinfection. The chemical composition of the cyst wall is not currently known.

Ward et al. (1985) reported that chitin, a polymer of *N*-acetylglucosamine (Glc-NAC) is a component of the cyst wall on the basis of lectin binding, which was prevented by pre-treatment of cysts with purified chitinase, but not by trypsin. Arroyo-Begovich and Carabez-Trejo (1982) had previously demonstrated chitin in the *Entamoeba* cyst wall. Data of Gillin et al. (1987) and Das and Gillin (1987 a,b; unpublished data) are consistent with the activity of chitin synthetase (CS). They observed polymerization of ^{3}H- or ^{14}C-Glc-NAc from UDP Glc-NAC (the substrate for CS) by extracts of encysting WB strain *Giardia* or *E. invadens*. The high molecular weight product was digested to characteristic dimers by purified endochitinase, but was not digested by proteases. After further enzymatic digestion of the isolated dimers (chitobiose), only labelled Glc-NAC was recovered. Thus chitin synthetase is a developmentally regulated enzyme in human origin *Giardia* and *E. invadens*.

5.3. Carbohydrate analysis of cyst wall components

Identification of the carbohydrate composition of the *Giardia* cyst wall has been based largely on two different experimental approaches and has yielded conflicting information as to the type of carbohydrate moieties present (see Chapter 2 for discussion of the cyst wall). In addition to the proteins described above (Section 1), Ward et al. (1985) proposed chitin to be a constituent of the cyst walls of *Giardia muris* and human-source *Giardia*. This conclusion was based on histochemical staining using plant lectins (wheat germ agglutinin and succinylated wheat germ agglutinin) with putative specificity for *N*-acetylglucosamine and sialic acid, which was abolished after treatment of the cysts with chitinase. Further support for the presence of chitin in the *Giardia* cyst wall was provided by Gillin et al. (1987). In these studies on in vitro encystment, the enzyme chitin synthetase was detected in extracts of encysting trophozoites by incorporation and recovery of isotopically labeled *N*-acetylglucosamine.

Using gas chromatography and mass spectrometry, Jarroll et al. (1989) reported that the amino sugar galactosamine was detected in both *Giardia muris* and human-source *Giardia* cysts (ca 47 nmoles/10^6 cells). A similar biochemical analysis was performed on *Giardia* cysts produced in vitro using the MR4 strain, and 37 nmoles of galactosamine per 10^6 cells was detected. Galactosamine was hypothesized to be stage-specific for cysts because it was not detected in trophozoites either by the biochemical techniques mentioned above or by lectin staining for galactosamine. The inability to detect glucosamine within cyst wall hydrolysates led to their conclusion that the *Giardia* cyst wall is not composed of chitin but instead contains galactosamine, perhaps as N-acetylgalactosamine. Detection of β-N-acetylgalactosaminidase in *Giardia* cysts suggests that this hydrolase might participate in excystation.

The use of histochemical and biochemical approaches to the identification of cyst wall carbohydrates has yielded dramatically different results. Further biochemical analysis of the *Giardia* cyst wall will be required to clarify these findings. It seems likely that the use of *Giardia* cysts formed in vitro may provide a model system for characterizing both the protein and the carbohydrate composition of the cyst wall.

6. Summary

Giardia encystation in vitro offers significant research opportunities on an important aspect of the life cycle of this intestinal pathogen. Prior to the development of in vitro encystation, cyst isolation required rigorous purification methods to remove fecal debris and contaminating microorganisms. Additionally, naturally infected humans and experimentally infected animal models provided potentially heterogenous sources of cysts that could hinder biochemical or biologic analysis of a population of cysts. Further development of in vitro encystation techniques will offer unique opportunities to study wall assembly, either morphologically with immunogold labeling at the electron microscopic level or biochemically, with the aid of radiolabeled precursor molecules.

Development of in vitro techniques utilizing different *Giardia* species has opened a new era in *Giardia* research because the life cycle of this protozoan can now be completed outside the host. Collectively, these techniques should aid in elucidating the biochemical composition of the *Giardia* cyst wall as well as the nature of the molecular signal that initiates the production and subsequent assembly of cyst wall components, and results in the formation of viable *Giardia* cysts.

References

Arroyo-Begovich, A. and Carabez-Trejo, A. (1982) Location of chitin in the cyst wall of *Entamoeba invadens* with colloidal gold tracers. J. Parasitol. 68, 253-258.

Belosevic, M., Faubert, G.M., MacLean, J.D., Law, C. and Croll, N.A. (1983) *Giardia lamblia* infections in Mongolian gerbils: an animal model. J. Infect. Dis. 147, 222-226.

Bingham, A.K., Jarroll, E.L., Meyer, E.A. and Radulescu, S. (1979) *Giardia* sp: physical factors of excystation in vitro and excystation vs eosin exclusion as determinants of viability. Exp. Parasitol. 47, 284-291.

Bingham, A.K. and Meyer, E.A. (1979) *Giardia* excystation can be induced in vitro in acidic solutions. Nature (London) 227, 301-302.

Das, S. and Gillin, F.D. (1987a) Cell fractionation of chitin synthetase from encysting *Giardia lamblia* and *Entamoeba invadens*. Am. Soc. Cell. Biol. Abstr. No. 932.

Das, S. and Gillin, F.D. (1987b) Chitin synthetase in encysting *Giardia lamblia* and *Entamoeba invadens*. Molecular Parasitology Symposium. Am. Soc. Biol. Abstract No. 1295.

Douglas, H., Reiner, D.S. and Gillin, F.D. (1987) A new method for purification of *G. lamblia* cysts. Trans. R. Soc. Trop. Med. Hyg. 81, 315-316.

Erlandsen, S.L. and Bemrick, W.J. (1987) Waterborne giardiasis: sources of *Giardia* cysts and evidence pertaining to their implication in human infection. In: P.M. Wallis and B.R. Hammond (Eds.), Advances in *Giardia* Research. University of Calgary Press (in press).

Filice, F.P. (1952) Studies on the cytology and life history of a *Giardia* from the laboratory rat. Univ. Calf. Publ. Zool. 57, 53-146.

Fordtran, J.S. and Locklear, T.W. (1966) Ionic constituents and osmolality of gastric and small-intestinal fluids after eating. Am. J. Digest. Dis. 11, 503-521.

Gillin, F.D., Gault, M.J., Reiner, D.S., Douglas, H., Wunderlich, A. and Sauch, J.F. (1986) In vitro encystation of *Giardia lamblia*. Am. Soc. Trop. Med. Hyg. Abstract No. 37.

Gillin, F.D., Reiner, D.S., Gault, M.J., Douglas, H., Das, S., Wunderlich, A. and Sauch, J. (1987) Encystation and expression of cyst antigens by *Giardia lamblia* in vitro. Science 235, 1040-1043.

Gillin, F.D., Reiner, D.S. and Boucher, S.E. (1988a) Small intestinal factors promote encystation of *Giardia lamblia* in vitro. Infect. Immun. 56, 705-707.

Gillin, F.D. (1988b) Excystation and Encystation Workshop Summary. In: P.M. Wallis and B.R. Hammond (Eds.), Advances in *Giardia* Research. University of Calgary Press, p. 273.

Hill, D.R., Guerrant, R.L., Pearson, R.D. and Hewlett, E.L. (1983) *Giardia lamblia* infection of suckling mice. J. Infect. Dis. 147, 217-221.

Hofmann, A.F. (1984) Chemistry and enterohepatic circulation of bile acids. Hepatology 4, 4S-14S.

Hofmann, A.F. and Roda, A. (1984) Physicochemical properties of bile acids and their relationship to biological properties: an overview of the problem. J. Lipid Res. 25, 1477-1489.

Jarroll, E.L., Manning, P., Lindmark, D.G., Coggins, J.R. and Erlandsen, S.L. (1989) *Giardia* cyst wall-specific carbohydrate: evidence for the presence of galactosamine Mol. Biochem. Parasitol. 32, 121–132.

Lavier, G. (1942) Les modalites de l'enkystement chez les flagelles du genre *Giardia*. Comptes Rendus Soc. Biol. Paris 136, 67-70.

Perroncito, E. (1887) Incapsulamento del Megastoma intestinale. G. Accad. Med. Torino 35, 349-351.

Reiner, D.S., Wang, C.-S. and Gillin, F.D. (1986) Human milk kills *Giardia lamblia* by generating toxic lipolytic products. J. Infect. Dis. 154, 825-831.

Reiner, D.S., Douglas, H. and Gillin, F.D. (1989) Identification and localization of cyst-specific antigens of *Giardia lamblia*. Infect. Immun. 57, 963–968.

Roberts-Thomson, I.C., Stevens, D.P., Mahmoud, A.A.F. and Warren, K.S. (1976) Giardiasis in the mouse: an animal model. Gastroenterology 71, 57-61.

Rosoff, J.D. and Stibbs, H.H. (1986a) Isolation and identification of a *Giardia lamblia* - specific stool antigen (GSA 65) useful in coprodiagnosis of giardiasis. J. Clin. Microbiol. 23, 905-910.

Rosoff, J.D. and Stibbs, H.H. (1986b) Physical and chemical characterization of a *Giardia lamblia*-specific antigen useful in the coprodiagnosis of giardiasis. J. Clin. Microbiol. 24, 1079-1083.

Sauch, J.F. (1985) Use of immunofluorescence and phase-contrast microscopy for detection and identification of *Giardia* cysts in water samples. Appl. Env. Microbiol. 50, 1434-1438.

Schupp, D.G. and Erlandsen, S.L. (1987a) A new method to determine *Giardia* cyst viability: correlation of fluorescein diacetate and propidium iodide staining with animal infectivity. Appl. Env. Microbiol. 53, 704-707.

Schupp, D.G., Januschka, M.M. and Erlandsen, S.L. (1988b) Assessing *Giardia* cyst viability with fluorogenic dyes: comparisons to animal infectivity and cyst morphology by light and electron microscopy. In: P.M. Wallis and B.R. Hammond (Eds.), Advances in *Giardia* Research. University of Calgary Press, pp. 265–269.

Schupp, D.G., Januschka, M.M. and Erlandsen, S.L. (1988a) Morphology of *Giardia* encystation in vitro. In: P.M. Wallis and B.R. Hammond (Eds.), Advances in *Giardia* Research. University of Calgary Press pp. 29–32.

Schupp, D.G., Januschka, M.M., Sherlock, L.F., Stibbs, H.H., Meyer, E.A., Bemrick, W.J. and Erlandsen, S.L. (1988b) Production of viable *Giardia* cysts in vitro: determination by fluorogenic dye staining, excystation, and animal infectivity in the mouse and Mongolian gerbil. Gastroenterology 95, 1-10.

Smith, P.D., Gillin, F.D., Brown, W.R. and Nash, T.E. (1982a) IgG antibody to *Giardia lamblia* detected by enzyme-linked immunosorbent assay. Gastroenterology 80, 1476-1480.

Smith, P.D., Gillin, F.D., Spira, W.M. and Nash, T.E. (1982b) Chronic giardiasis: studies on drug sensitivity toxin production, and host immune response. Gastroenterology 83, 797-803.

Sterling, C., Kutob, R.M., Gizinski, M.J., Verastegui, M. and Stetzenbach, L.G. (1988) In: P.M. Wallis and B.R. Hammond (Eds.), Advances in *Giardia* Research. University of Calgary Press pp. 219–222.

Ward, H.D., Alroy, J., Lev, B.I., Keusch, G.T. and Pereira, M.E.A. (1985) Identification of chitin as a structural component of *Giardia* cysts. Infect. Immun. 49, 629-634.

Giardiasis (E.A. Meyer, ed.)
© 1990 Elsevier Science Publishers B.V. (Biomedical Division)

9

Pathology and pathogenesis of the intestinal mucosal damage in giardiasis

ANNE FERGUSON, J. GILLON and G. MUNRO

Western General Hospital, University of Edinburgh, Edinburgh, U.K.

1. Introduction	156
2. Pathological changes in the mucosa of the small intestine in human giardiasis	156
2.1. Distribution of parasites in the intestine	156
2.2. Attachment of trophozoites to the mucosa and penetration of the epithelium	157
2.3. Histological changes in patients without immunodeficiency	157
2.3.1. General mucosal appearances	157
2.3.2. Intra-epithelial lymphocyte counts	158
2.3.3. Lamina propria plasma cells	158
2.4. Histological changes in immune-deficient patients with giardiasis	158
2.5. *Giardia* infection in patients with AIDS	159
3. Small intestinal abnormalities in experimental murine giardiasis	159
3.1. Time course of infection and distribution of trophozoites	160
3.2. Effects of primary infection on the small intestinal mucosa	161
3.2.1. Mucosal architecture	161
3.2.2. Intra-epithelial lymphocyte counts	161
3.2.3. Lamina propria plasma cells	161
3.3. Effects of chronic, endemic infection on the intestinal mucosa	163
4. Host response in *Giardia* enteropathy and manipulation of immune status	164
4.1. Spectrum of host-parasite relationships	164
4.2. Attempts to alter plateau parasite load	164
4.3. Modulation of host-immune status	166
4.4. Intestinal morphology in steroid-treated, *Giardia*-infected mice	166
4.5. Intestinal morphology in athymic, *Giardia*-infected mice	168
5. Parasite- and host-related factors in the pathogenesis of the mucosal lesion	169
References	171

1. Introduction

Clinical effects of human infection with *Giardia* range from the asymptomatic carrier state to a severe malabsorption syndrome. Similarly, histopathological changes in the affected mucosa may be minimal, or there may be significant enteropathy with enterocyte damage, villus atrophy and crypt hyperplasia. Reasons for this extreme variation in host susceptibility are poorly understood. Our working hypothesis is that host factors such as nutritional status, systemic immune responses and mucosal immunity contribute significantly to the tissue damage in giardiasis, almost independently of the local effects produced directly by the parasites and their secreted products. In this chapter we first describe the patterns of change in small intestinal structure that have been reported in human giardiasis, bearing in mind that the data on pathological changes in human infection is patchy and many of the clinical studies in the literature concern unusual presentations or highly selected groups of patients. Subsequently we review information obtained using the mouse model of the disease, in which more extensive investigation is possible. The chapter concludes with an analysis of the likely relative roles of host and parasite factors in producing tissue damage.

2. Pathological changes in the mucosa of the small intestine in human giardiasis

2.1. Distribution of parasites in the intestine

In humans, the small intestine is accessible only by means of invasive techniques involving intubation. There is therefore practically no information on the distribution of the parasite along the length of intestine in man. As discussed elsewhere in this book, trophozoites are readily detected in the duodenum and proximal jejunum of infected patients. However, Wright et al. (1977) found evidence of vitamin B_{12} malabsorption in 20 of 40 patients with giardiasis. The degree of B_{12} malabsorption seemed to correlate with the severity of histological change in the jejunal mucosa, and absorption returned to normal in the majority of treated patients. This is perhaps circumstantial evidence of the presence of parasites, and associated enteropathy, in the ileum in some patients.

Another important point that has not been studied in man is whether the distribution of the parasites along the intestine alters in abnormal circumstances – for instance, in disorders of intestinal motility. It is clear that, when conditions are favorable, the parasite may be found in various extraintestinal sites such as the gallbladder (Goldstein et al., 1978) and urinary tract (Meyers et al., 1977).

2.2. Attachment of trophozoites to the mucosa and penetration of the epithelium

Present evidence suggests that trophozoites do not normally penetrate the intestinal epithelium in humans. Brandborg et al. (1967) found evidence of mucosal invasion in patients who had diarrhea and large numbers of trophozoites in the lumen, but not in asymptomatic subjects. Similarly, Lupascu et al. (1970) found the organism within the mucosa of spontaneously infected mice when overwhelming infection was present. However, Owen et al. (1979), in a careful ultrastructural study using the murine model of the infection, found mucosal invasion only in areas where necrosis or mechanical trauma was present, casting doubt on the significance of reports of invasion in human studies performed on peroral suction or forceps biopsy specimens, which are bound to be traumatized.

The parasite is normally adherent to the epithelial cell surface by means of its ventral adhesive disk, the edges of which are embedded in the fuzzy coat over the microvilli, which themselves appear normal (Morecki and Parker, 1967).

2.3. Histological changes in patients without immunodeficiency

The earlier published reports of the pathological changes in the small intestine in patients with giardiasis were often based on small numbers of patients, but these reports were valuable in helping to establish that the infection could cause a clinical syndrome accompanied by pathological damage to the mucosa and that the abnormalities reverted to normal after treatment.

2.3.1. General mucosal appearances

Zamchek et al. (1963) described three patients with diarrhea caused by giardiasis in whom the jejunal morphology ranged from normal to subtotal villus atrophy. Both acute (polymorphonuclear leukocytes and eosinophils) and chronic inflammatory cells were noted in the lamina propria, and the number of epithelial mitoses was increased. These changes reverted to normal after treatment. Yardley et al. (1964) found that the presence of eosinophils and polymorphs within the epithelium was associated with epithelial cell damage. Morecki and Parker (1967) and Brandborg et al. (1967) reported that patients with symptomatic giardiasis could have normal jejunal histology with no inflammatory infiltrate. In a careful and detailed study, Hoskins et al. (1967) reported a spectrum of morphological change from normal to almost complete villus atrophy. Crypt mitoses were increased in proportion to the degree of villus damage. In one patient with severe mucosal damage, the changes had returned almost to normal 2 days after completion of a course of treatment with atabrine.

More recent studies (Wright et al., 1977; Duncombe et al., 1978; Gillon, 1985) have confirmed a range of histological change from normal to subtotal villus atrophy, with greater density of the inflammatory infiltrate in the lamina propria when villus atrophy was present. There is a correlation between the degree of villus abnormality and the severity of malabsorption (Hoskins et al., 1967; Wright et al., 1977; Duncombe et al., 1978). Wright and Tomkins (1978) also showed that patients with giardiasis had reduced mucosal surface area measurements compared with controls; the degree of abnormality correlated with indices of malabsorption and improved after treatment.

2.3.2. Intra-epithelial lymphocyte counts
The presence of acute inflammatory cells in the epithelial layer was reported by Yardley et al. (1964) and Hoskins et al. (1967), but the numbers of intra-epithelial lymphocytes (IEL) were not remarked upon in either study. IEL counts performed both in adults (Wright and Tomkins, 1977; Gillon, 1985) and children (Ferguson et al., 1976) showed high IEL counts at the time of infection, falling after treatment. Studies of IEL counts in murine giardiasis are reviewed later in this chapter.

2.3.3. Lamina propria plasma cells
Direct immunofluorescence on jejunal biopsy specimens has been used by several workers to enumerate the lamina propria plasma cells of different immunoglobulin classes, but no clear pattern has emerged. During active infection, Popovic et al. (1974) showed that IgA cell numbers were reduced while IgM cells were increased in number; Thompson et al. (1977) found raised numbers of both IgA and IgM cells; Blenkinsopp et al. (1978) found increases in IgA, IgM, and IgG cells; and Ridley and Ridley (1976) described raised IgM cell numbers but normal numbers of IgG and IgA cells. When plasma cells of all five immunoglobulin classes were studied (Gillon et al., 1982b), IgA and IgM cell numbers were similar to those in controls during infection, but IgA cell numbers rose significantly when patients were rebiopsied following successful treatment with metronidazole. Giardiasis patients had significantly raised numbers of IgE and IgD cells in the lamina propria at the time of infection, and the numbers of IgE cells returned to normal after treatment. No attempt was made to determine whether these cells were plasma cells, mast cells, or a mixture. Taken together, these studies suggest that *Giardia* infestation initially provokes IgM and IgE synthesis, perhaps with relative suppression of local IgA production.

2.4. Histological changes in immune-deficient patients with giardiasis

Studies of patients presenting de novo with symptomatic giardiasis have usually revealed no underlying abnormality of serum immunoglobulins (Jones and Brown, 1974; Wright et al., 1977). Nevertheless, a high incidence of giardiasis has been shown to occur in patients with immunodeficiency syndromes, especially common variable hypogammaglobulinemia (Ament et al., 1973). Giardiasis was the commonest cause of diarrhea in these patients and was associated with abnormalities of mucosal architecture ranging from mild to severe villus atrophy. No plasma cells were seen in the lamina propria, but immunofluorescence studies were not performed. The authors did not comment on other lymphoid cells. Ament and Rubin (1972) reported that two of seven patients with giardiasis had nodular lymphoid hyperplasia, two had severe villus atrophy, and three had mixed lesions. The severity of villus damage seemed to correlate with the degree of malabsorption, and successful treatment of giardiasis led to symptomatic cure and improvement in all abnormalities of mucosal architecture except nodular lymphoid hyperplasia.

Although no direct comparisons have been reported, it seems likely from the above studies that giardiasis produces a more severe degree of villus damage in hypogammaglobulinemic patients than in otherwise normal individuals. Ament and Rubin (1972) found bacterial colonization of the jejunum in five of eight patients with giardiasis and suggested that this might contribute to the enteropathy.

2.5. Giardia infection in patients with AIDS

Shortly after the clinical features of acquired immunodeficiency syndrome AIDS were defined and the infectious etiology confirmed, studies of jejunal biopsies showed histological abnormalities in many affected patients (Kotler et al., 1984). Giardiasis is not uncommon in homosexual men (Quinn et al., 1983), so theoretically this organism might be an important pathogen in immunodeficient AIDS patients. However, clinical experience does not bear this out. *Giardia* infection was found in none of 10 homosexual AIDS patients without diarrhea and in only 3 of 22 patients with diarrhea (Smith et al., 1988). In Africa, giardiasis and amebiasis are notably absent as important infections in immunocompromised AIDS patients (Professor A. Bailey, personal communication).

3. Small intestinal abnormalities in experimental murine giardiasis

An experimental model of murine giardiasis, first described by Roberts-Thomson et al. (1976), has proved very useful for studies of host-parasite relationships. This system offers the advantage that changes in the host intestine can be studied in sequence and with precise knowledge of parasite numbers and distribution. We have studied various features of small intestinal pathology in primary *Giardia* infection of mice and also in mice with endemic giardiasis (Gillon et al., 1982a; MacDonald and Ferguson, 1978; Munro, 1985). We used techniques based on those that are applied clinically in the examination of small intestinal biopsies – measurements of mucosal architecture, quantitation of brush border disaccharidases, and enumeration of IEL and plasma cells. For study of a primary *Giardia muris* infection, animals were usually infected by oral inoculation of 1000 to 2000 cysts (initially obtained from Dr. Roberts-Thomson, Melbourne). The effects of endemic giardiasis were established by study of strains of mice that were found to be infected when we screened a number of strains maintained under conventional conditions in one of the animal houses in Glasgow.

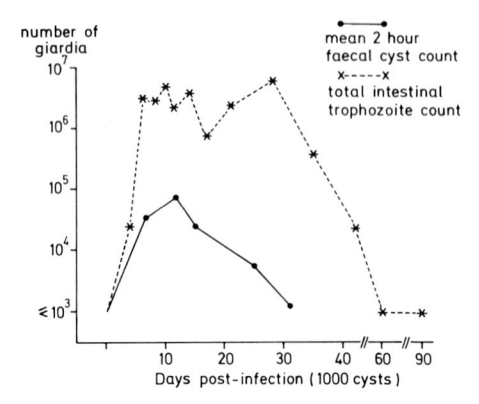

Fig. 1. Time course of a primary *Giardia muris* infection of CBA mice, as monitored by fecal cyst excretion and total intestinal trophozoite count.

3.1. Time course of infection and distribution of trophozoites

The magnitude and time course of *Giardia* infection can be monitored by performing serial cyst counts, and total small intestinal trophozoite load can be measured by a vibration technique (Gillon et al., 1982a). Results for mice of the CBA strain are shown in Fig. 1. Both cyst excretion and trophozoite count peak at 2 weeks, cysts being undetectable in the majority of animals after 4 weeks. However, small numbers of trophozoites could be found in 50% of the animals studied at 3 or more months postinfection. The existence of a latent infection, undetectable by fecal cyst counts, was confirmed by using systemic corticosteroids (Nair et al., 1981); in a majority of previously infected mice, residual trophozoites proliferate rapidly (Fig. 2). The nature of the constraining influence in normal animals is still unknown.

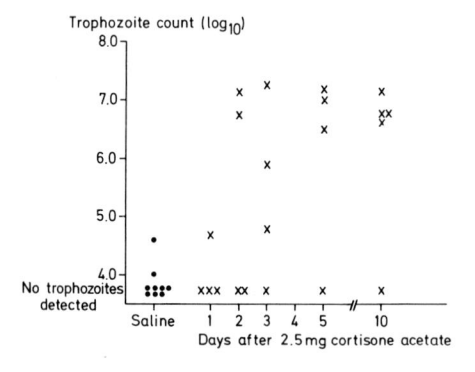

Fig. 2. Recrudescence of *Giardia muris* infection in CBA mice, eight months after a primary infection. Each mouse was given 2.5 mg cortisone acetate subcutaneously; animals were killed at intervals thereafter. Although in a minority no trophozoites were subsequently detected, substantial counts of trophozoites, comparable to those in a primary infection, were observed from day 2.

Trophozoite counts can also be used to study the distribution of parasites along the small intestine (Gillon et al., 1982a). In CBA mice the highest trophozoite density was in the proximal small intestine, though early in infection substantial numbers (several thousand trophozoites per centimeter length of intestine) were present in the ileum and only as infection progressed were the parasites clearly localized to the jejunum. This predilection for the mid small bowel suggests that the organism requires a high concentration of nutrients at a relatively stable pH.

3.2. Effects of primary infection on the small intestinal mucosa

3.2.1. Mucosal architecture
In their original description of the animal model of giardiasis, Roberts-Thomson et al. (1976) reported that in CF-1 mice the ratio of villus length to crypt length was significantly reduced in the upper jejunum at the time of maximum trophozoite numbers. In our more detailed study of CBA mice, animals were killed at intervals from 1-10 weeks postinfection. Mice received intraperitoneal colchicine at a measured time interval before they were killed to allow subsequent measurement of crypt cell production rate (MacDonald and Ferguson, 1977). Very similar results have been obtained recently in BALB/c mice (Munro and Ferguson, submitted).

In the jejunum, significant shortening of the villi was found only at 1 week postinfection, with crypt hyperplasia from 1-4 weeks. At 2 weeks postinfection, lactase, sucrase, and maltase levels in the jejunum were significantly lower than in control animals. An unexpected finding was that late after infection (weeks 8 and 10) there was expansion in villus size in the jejunum with increased brush border enzyme content; reciprocal changes occurred in the ileum, diminution in villi and crypts with reduced disaccharidases, presumably adaptive to the expanded mass of the gut proximally.

3.2.2. Intra-epithelial lymphocyte counts
Counts of jejunal and ileal IEL were performed in the mice used in the morphology experiment described above. In the jejunum, the counts were significantly higher than control from week 3 and remained so thereafter. In the ileum a significant fall occurred at 3 weeks, and raised counts were obtained from 6 weeks onwards. The sustained rise in IEL count, which persists after trophozoites have largely been eliminated, suggests that the occasional isolated finding of a high IEL count in the jejunal biopsy of a patient investigated for diarrhea may indicate recent, self-cured protozoal infection.

3.2.3. Lamina propria plasma cells
Studies of plasma cells were performed in *Giardia*-infected BALB/c mice (Munr, 1985). Specimens of jejunum were taken, fixed in mercuric buffered formalin, paraffin embedded and immunostained by using a PAP schedule and a range of isotype-specific antisera. Mice were studied on days 11, 25 and 32 of infection, and IEL counts were also performed. Results are shown in Fig. 3. By day 11 of infection, the total plasma cell

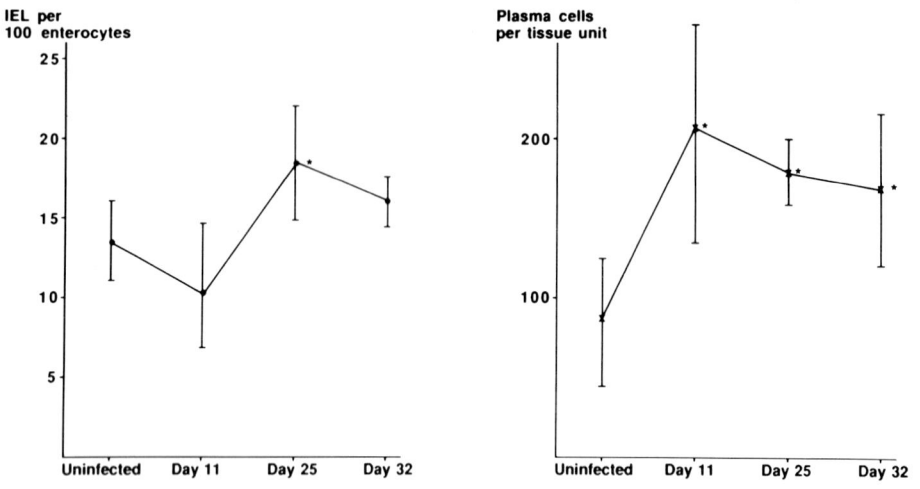

Fig. 3. Counts of IEL (per 100 enterocytes) and plasma cells (per 100 μm muscularis mucosae tissue unit) in BALB/c mice uninfected and at three stages of a primary *Giardia muris* infection. *P < 0.05 when compared with uninfected.

count had risen, when compared with uninfected controls, and remained high on days 25 and 32. The rise in IEL count occurred later, on day 25.

There were no significant changes in the relative proportions of k and ? plasma cells in the four groups of mice, but the patterns of isotype-specific plasma cell distribution were influenced by infection (Table 1). In uninfected mice the majority of cells contained IgA, with small numbers of IgE and IgG cells. IgM and IgA cell counts were higher than controls from day 11 until the end of the study, whereas for IgG cells there was

TABLE 1

Immunoglobulin isotype-specific staining of plasma cells in the intestinal mucosa of uninfected BALB/c mice, and of mice on days 11, 25 and 32 of a primary *G. muris* infection.

Immunoglobulin	Uninfected	*Giardia muris* infection		
		Day 11	Day 25	Day 32
Ig:		*	*	
	0.6±1.0	5.7±4.6	3.5±2.5	5.8±5.6
IgG		*		
	3.2±2.3	14.3±9.2	5.7±2.1	6.7±4.8
IgA		**	**	
	52±30	142.2±44	125.2±29	87.8±53
IgE			*	†
	5.2±5.3	11.2±7.2	19±9.6	16.3±11

* $P < 0.05$ when compared with uninfected;
** $P < 0.01$ when compared with uninfected;
† $0.05 < P < 0.10$ when compared with uninfected.

a sharp, transient rise on day 11. The observed rise in IgE-containing cells was later, on day 25, and sustained.

3.3. Effects of chronic, endemic infection on the intestinal mucosa

Some years ago, we found that some mouse strains in a busy, conventional animal house were infected with *Giardia* and *Hexamita*. Histological assessment, quantitation of IEL, microdissection and measurement of individual villi and crypts, and epithelial cell kinetic studies (using a stathmokinetic technique with colchicine injection) were used to compare the intestines of these mice and also of accidentally infected and fostered mice derived from generally uninfected strains (MacDonald and Ferguson, 1978). The histology of the small intestine from infected mice appeared normal, apart from an increase in numbers of IEL. Mean IEL counts per 100 epithelial cells were 11.6 and 13.6 in two groups of uninfected mice and 17.6 and 21.8 in two groups of infected mice. Tissue measurements showed no effects of infection on villus length, but chronically infected mice had significantly longer crypts than did uninfected mice. Cell production rate per crypt per hour ranged from 6.2 to 8.2 in uninfected animals, and from 11.8 to 17.1 in *Giardia*-infected mice (Fig. 4).

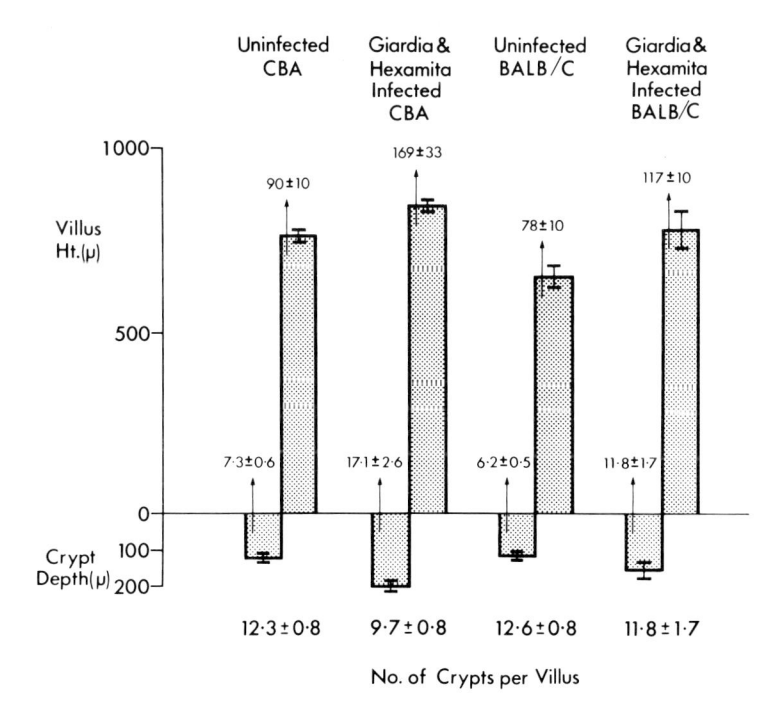

Fig. 4. Measurements of villus and crypt lengths, and crypt cell production rate (by a stathmokinetic technique) in CBA and BALB/c mice, uninfected, and from animals, derived from the same colonies, chronically infected with *Giardia* and *Hexamita*. Chronic protozoal infection led to hyperplasia of the crypts of Lieberkuhn.

4. Host response in Giardia enteropathy and manipulation of immune status

4.1. Spectrum of host-parasite relationships

Our working hypothesis is that the changes in the gut mucosa in *Giardia* infection are partly due to direct effect of the parasite and partly due to antigen-specific host-immune response (e.g. immune complexes and delayed-type hypersensitivity ([DTH]) (Gillon et al., 1982a), with a variable contribution by other host factors such as diet, gut motility and nutritional status (Ferguson et al., 1980). An antigen nonspecific 'innocent bystander' effect of DTH may be the pathogenesis of many of the features of enteropathy in this and other diseases, with the changes in epithelial cell kinetics, intra-epithelial lymphocyte infiltration and enterocyte integrity being caused by lymphokines secreted by activated T-cells in the lamina propria (Ferguson, 1987). In order to analyze these various factors experimentally, only one should be changed and all others remain the same.

A further point to consider is that the extent of parasite- and host-related phenomena will vary during the different phases of infection. This variation is related to the following characteristics of an infection: (i) the duration of the prepatent phase, (ii) the slope of the exponential growth phase, (iii) the magnitude of parasite load achieved during the plateau phase, (iv) the time of onset and slope of the elimination phase, and (v) the constraints on reproduction of residual trophozoites at the end of the expulsion phase.

An important aspect, which can be monitored but which is proving extremely difficult to manipulate, is the total parasite load in the plateau phase. This can be assessed either as trophozoite count or by fecal cyst excretion. In most situations in which host response is altered by interfering with immune capacity, not only is there a prolonged time course, but also the parasite burden is substantially greater than in control mice – often tenfold higher. This is clearly shown for infection in athymic mice (Fig. 5) and in steroid-treated mice (Fig. 6). Thus, when seeking to define the 'thymus dependent' components of the enteropathy by comparing gut histology in athymic and control animals, any contribution by the parasite is likely to be substantially greater in immune-deficient mice.

4.2. Attempts to alter plateau parasite load

We have unsuccessfully pursued a number of avenues, in immunologically intact animals, to produce very high levels of plateau infection. For example, we found differences between male and female BALB/c mice in the time course of infection. The pre-patent and logarithmic growth phase were identical, but in female mice parasite expulsion occurred during the third week, whereas in male mice expulsion was delayed to the fifth week. However, the magnitude of parasite infection during the short and prolonged plateau phase in the two sexes was similar. Another approach was based on the idea that a decrease in intestinal motility would allow larger numbers of parasites to reside in the small bowel. Daily treatment of animals with 0.4 mg loperamide, achieved a 45

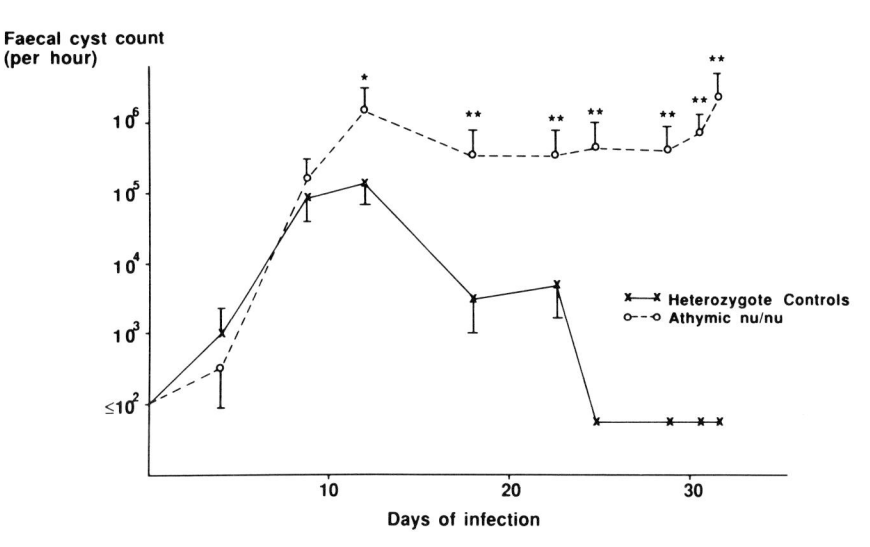

Fig. 5. Course of *Giardia muris* infection in heterozygote (*nu/+*) and athymic (*nu/nu*) mice on a BALB/c background; $^*P < 0.05$ when compared with heterozygotes; $^{**}P < 0.01$ (mean ± 1 SD).

percent reduction in wet fecal output per day and delayed transit of dye through the gut. However, cyst excretion was similar to that of untreated infected animals; studies of intestinal architecture, crypt cell production rate and IEL count were identical in loperamide-treated and control animals.

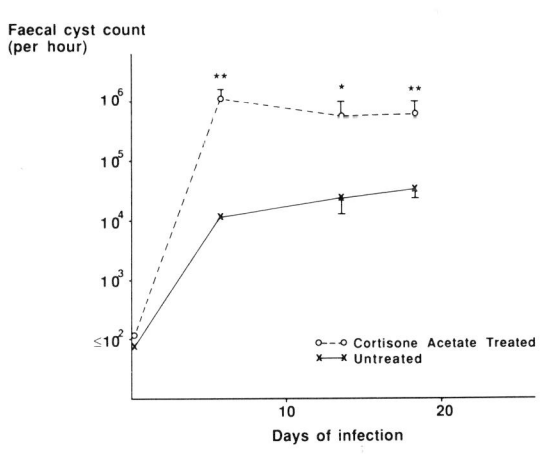

Fig. 6. Development of primary *Giardia muris* infection in untreated BALB/c mice and in mice treated weekly with 2.5 mg cortisone acetate subcutaneously. $^*P < 0.05$ when compared with untreated; $^{**}P < 0.01$ (mean ± 1 SD).

4.3. Modulation of host-immune status

There have been a number of studies of giardiasis in mice with genetically or experimentally altered parasite resistance. Previous work with *nu/nu* athymic mice has already been mentioned. Infection is greatly prolonged in mice lacking T-cells (Roberts-Thomson and Mitchell, 1978; Munro and Ferguson, unpublished data). It has recently been shown that clearance of *Giardia muris* infection requires helper/inducer rather than suppressor/cytotoxic T lymphocytes (Heyworth et al., 1987). Whether the helper T-cells act via specific cellular immunity or via their helper effect on immunoglobulin production remains a matter of dispute. Treatment of mice with cyclosporin A, producing pharmacological inhibition of T helper cells, has also been found to increase cyst output and delay the elimination phase of primary infection (Belosevic et al., 1986).

In order to study the protective role of antibody, Snider et al. (1985) treated mice from birth with rabbit anti-IgM antisera. This produced immunoglobulin deficiency. When these mice were infected with *Giardia muris*, they had high trophozoite counts and prolonged cyst excretion, very similar to the findings in athymic animals. Further evidence to support a role of antibodies rather than antigen-specific T-cells in immunity is the absence of evidence of DTH in parasite resistant mice (Anders et al., 1982). On the other hand, mice deficient in natural killer cells have entirely normal clearance of *Giardia muris* (Heyworth et al., 1986).

To confuse the issue further, a relationship exists between the capacity of mice to mount inflammatory responses and the ability of the same strains to control a *Giardia* infection (Belosevic and Faubert, 1986). We reasoned that the non-specific inflammatory effects associated with a DTH reaction in the gut might confer parasite resistance and tested this by studying the course of *Giardia muris* infection in mice with graft-versus-host reaction (GvHR). However, although there were greater changes in gut architecture and in IEL counts in mice with concurrent *Giardia* infection and GvHR than in either experimental group alone or in controls, there was no evidence that an on-going DTH reaction in the gut conferred any resistance to the parasites as measured by cyst or trophozoitic counts (Ferguson and Munro, 1988). Finally, mice deficient in mast cells develop chronic giardiasis (Erlich et al., 1983). The most likely explanation would be that the mast cell is an important component of a DTH, but since DTH appears to have been excluded as an important component of parasite resistance in primary infection, other explanations will have to be sought.

Regrettably, the pathology of the intestine in immunomodulated, infected mice has not been reported in the studies described above. Our own work on the enteropathy in athymic mice and in steroid-treated mice is in the public domain only as a thesis (Munro, 1985), but some salient points are summarized below.

4.4. Intestinal morphology in steroid-treated Giardia-*infected mice*

Mice, previously infected with *Giardia muris* and then given corticosteroids, develop

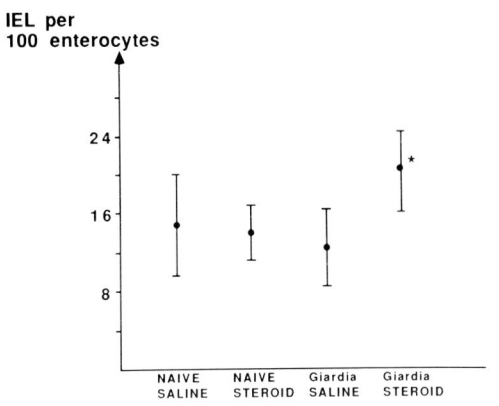

Fig. 7. Effects on IEL count of steroid administration (2 mg hydrocortisone sodium sc for 5 days) to BALB/c mice previously infected with *Giardia muris*. Steroids alone, or saline treatment after *Giardia* infection, had no significant effect on IEL count, whereas there was a significant ($P < 0.01$) increase in IEL count as a result of the recrudescence of infection associated with steroid administration.

recrudescent infection with the trophozoite count rising from undetectable to a level some tenfold higher than the trophozoite count in the plateau phase of a primary infection in the same strain. Groups of adult female BALB/c mice were infected at 6 weeks of age and left for 6 weeks, by which time fecal cyst counts were negative. Some of these mice then received daily subcutaneous injections of saline and others received 2 mg hydrocortisone sodium succinate daily for 5 days. Uninfected mice of the same age were also treated with saline and hydrocortisone as controls. Recrudescence of infection, evidenced by a high fecal cyst excretion and the presence of many trophozoites in smears of jejunal contents, occurred only in the previously infected and then steroid-treated mice. Studies of jejunal mucosal architecture showed no effect of this recrudescent parasite infection on villi, crypts or disaccharidase activity when the mice were compared to saline-treated, previously infected mice. However, the recrudescent infection resulted in a significant increase in IEL count in jejunum and ileum (Fig. 7).

We interpret these findings as follows. The recently infected mice presumably have secretory antibodies to *Giardia*. These antibodies cannot prevent parasite duplication, but neutralize, in some way, the toxic effect of a high parasite load on enterocytes. The normal villus architecture and enterocyte integrity (as assessed by brush border enzyme content) are in striking contrast to these parameters in the second week of a primary infection (Gillon et al., 1982a), when the number of trophozoites in the gut is similar or lower. This component of host immunity is different from the factor that constrains parasite reproduction after the elimination phase, perhaps luminal phagocytes. Neither of these host factors, IgA antibodies or mucosal phagocytes, appear to be enteropathic. The rise in IEL in steroid-treated recrudescent infection is a marker of the mucosal DTH reaction in animals with low grade T-cell sensitization, which can be expressed in the presence of a large antigenic load in the lumen of the gut. In keeping with our GvHR experiments, this does not confer resistance or interfere with trophozoite duplication. The fact that a high trophozoite load can be sustained in steroid-treated animals without any significant enteropathy, may be an experimental parallel of the situation in the healthy human carrier with normal small bowel mucosa.

4.5. Intestinal morphology in athymic, Giardia-*infected mice*

Some years ago, we suggested, on the basis of experiments with *Nippostrongylus brasiliensis*, that many of the components of tissue damage in an intestinal parasite infection were due, not to the presence of the parasite itself, but to the host immune response, probably the T-cell-mediated component (Ferguson and Jarret, 1975). Similar experiments with *Trichinella spiralis* supported this concept (Manson-Smith et al., 1979). In their paper on the thymus dependence of host resistance to *Giardia* infection in the mouse, Roberts-Thomson and Mitchell (1978) reported measurements of villus and crypt lengths. They found that there was a relative reduction in villus length in *Giardia* infection of immunologically normal mice and that gut architecture was almost normal in athymic, infected animals.

We have recently completed a series of experiments, to examine further the enteropathy of *Giardia muris* infection in adult female *nu/nu* mice and adult female heterozygote (*nu/+*) littermates on a BALB/c background. Some of the *nu/nu* mice were reconstituted with T cells at four weeks after infection. We found, as anticipated, the *Giardia muris* infection proceeded in heterozygote mice with a time course of fecal cyst excretion similar to that of our previous experience with BALB/c mice, the infection resolving by day 25. In contrast, in infected *nu/nu* mice, from day 9 there was a significantly increased fecal cyst output, and this remained high for the duration of the experiment, 98 days.

The intestinal mucosa of mice with a primary infection was studied on days 3, 10, 17 and 24. Heterozygotes showed significant reduction in villus height on day 17; this returned to control levels by day 24. Crypt length was increased at all times from day 3, crypt cell production rate increased by day 10 and remained elevated to day 24, and brush border disaccharidases were all significantly reduced from day 3 to day 24 in heterozygotes. Contrary to our predictions based on work with helminth infections, a rather similar enteropathy was observed in *nu/nu* mice. Villus height did not show any significant variation, but there was significant crypt lengthening by day 10 and maintained to day 24, with increased crypt cell production rate of similar magnitude to that found in *nu/+* mice. Disaccharidase deficiency was similar to that in heterozygotes. In fact, the only difference between heterozygote and *nu/nu* mouse enteropathy was the absence of any change in IEL numbers with infection of *nu/nu* mice; numbers of IEL in uninfected *nu/nu* mice were also significantly lower than in age- and sex-matched uninfected heterozygotes (Fig. 8). We had previously documented the absence of a rise in IELs in infected *nu/nu* mice from retrospective studies of the tissue sections used by Dr Roberts-Thomson in his initial study (Gillon and Ferguson, 1984).

The results of this experiment refute our previous suggestion that the enteropathy in giardiasis is substantially due to the host T cell response. However, it must be

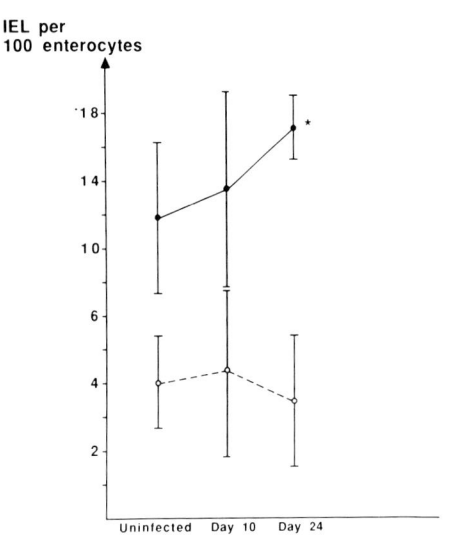

Fig. 8. Effects of *Giardia muris* infection on IEL counts in immunologically normal *nu/+* heterozygotes (solid line), and in athymic *nu/nu* mice (dashed line). *$P < 0.05$ when compared with uninfected *nu/+* mice. (Mean ± 1 SD, 6 mice per group).

borne in mind, as mentioned above, that the parasite contribution to enteropathy will be substantially greater in *nu/nu* mice than in *nu/+* controls, because the magnitude of infection is tenfold higher in the *nu/nu* animals. Clearly, a great deal of work remains to be done on the interplay between parasite and host in producing the enteropathy.

5. Parasite- and host-related factors in the pathogenesis of the mucosal lesion

Despite the recent findings in *nu/nu* mice, it remains probable that some components of the enteropathy are parasite-related and that local hypersensitivity reactions also produce tissue injury as an unavoidable side effect of the antiparasite immune response. We envisage several phases of infection with different host-parasite interactions, and thus different and overlapping explanations for the observed enteropathy and immunity in the prepatent and early parasite proliferative phase; early plateau, when trophozoite-related damage is likely; late plateau, with parasites still in situ and T cell immunity developing; expulsion phase, when animals are immune but their antigenic load is lower than in the plateau phase; and finally post-infection, when there may or may not be a few residual trophozoites. Early in infection, some features of the pathology are related to the size of the parasite load; on the other hand, later in infection there are characteristics of the enteropathy, crypt hyperplasia and IEL infiltrate, indicative of T cell-mediated hypersensitivity. Our recent work shows that humoral components of the mucosal immune response may also contribute to the local tissue damage, as well as conferring resistance.

Damage to enterocytes, as monitored by brush border disaccharidases, and, in some experiments, villus shortening, is maximal in the second week of a primary infection, and correlates well with the trophozoite count (Ferguson et al., 1980). We had previously attributed these enteropathic effects to the presence of a very heavy parasite load, perhaps with high concentrations of toxins or local interference with tissue nutrition. However, IgG plasma cell counts also increase transiently at this stage, and the presence of an enhanced mucosal IgG response creates a situation in which transient immune-complex-mediated hypersensitivity is possible. The relevant antigens could be derived from the parasites or could be those of commensal gut flora or foods.

A distinct pattern of small intestinal mucosal damage has been observed in association with gut mucosal DTH reactions. Experimental models used have included allograft rejection, GvHR, enteral challenge after immunization with protein antigen, and helminth infections. The features described in some or all of these situations are hyperplasia of the crypts of Lieberkuhn, with or without shortening of the villi; an increase in the proportion of goblet cells; brush border enzyme deficiency; increased count of IEL; an increased mitotic index of IEL; expansion in the population of mucosal mast cells; and expression of class II antigens by crypt enterocytes (reviewed by Ferguson, 1987). The precise role of IEL in the intestine remains unknown, but direct cytotoxicity by IEL against *Giardia muris* trophozoites has been reported (Kanwar et al., 1986). The roles of specific DTH or other T cell-mediated reactions in protection are still uncertain and, on current evidence, are less likely than secretory antibody as the mechanism of parasite elimination in a primary infection. Effects of DTH on the gut require both antigen-reactive T cells and antigen; these effects are probably enhanced when the epithelium is damaged and thus more permeable than normal.

High counts of IgM and IgA cells in early and late infection are typical of a developing mucosal immune response to any enteric pathogen. In mouse and rat giardiasis models, serum (Owen, 1980; Andre et al., 1983) and secretory (Andrews and Hewlett, 1983; Loftness et al., 1984; Anders et al., 1982) IgA antibodies to trophozoite antigens have been described, in some experiments associated with immunity. Locally produced IgG might also contribute to immunity. In mice, IgG and IgA promote adherence to and phagocytosis of trophozoites by neutrophils and macrophages (Kaplan et al., 1985). However, the ability of antibody to influence trophozoites in the gut lumen will be limited by differential access of immunoglobulins, complement and accessory effector cells to the pathogen, although the hyperpermeable mucosa in giardiasis may allow plasma proteins and blood cells to leak into the gut lumen.

The number of IgE-containing plasma cells also increases in murine giardiasis, although later in the infection time course than the other immunoglobulin classes. In human giardiasis, Kraft (1979) described increased counts of IgE-containing cells in jejunal biopsies, although this was not reflected in serum IgE levels, perhaps due to its binding to receptors on mucosal mast cells and eosinophils. There is some evidence that IgE is associated with immunity in that the SJL/J mouse strain supports a chronic *Giardia* infection and is a low IgE producer (Mitchell et al., 1982). In unpublished experiments, we have found an increase in mucosal mast cell count in mice with *Giardia* infection. Thus there is potential for enteropathic and protective roles of anaphylactic reactions in addition to the other types of humoral immunity discussed above.

References

Ament, M.E. and Rubin, C.E. (1972) Relation of giardiasis to abnormal intestinal structure and function in gastrointestinal immunodeficiency syndromes. Gastroenterology 62, 216-226.

Ament, M.E., Ochs, H.D. and David, S.D. (1973) Structure and function of the gastrointestinal tract in primary immunodeficiency syndromes: a study of 39 patients. Medicine (Baltimore) 52, 227-248.

Anders, R.F., Roberts-Thomson, I.C. and Mitchell, G.F. (1982) Giardiasis in mice: analysis of humoral and cellular immune responses to *Giardia muris*. Parasite Immunol. 4, 47-57.

Andre, E., Gillon, J., Andre, C., Lafont, S. and Jourdan, G. (1983) Pesticide containing diets augment anti-sheep red blood cell non-reaginic antibody responses in mice, but may prolong murine infection with *Giardia muris*. Environ. Res. 32, 145-150.

Andrews, J.S. and Hewlett, E.L. (1983) Protection against infection with *Giardia muris* by milk containing antibodies to *Giardia*. J. Infect. Dis. 143, 242-246.

Belosevic, M. and Faubert, G.M. (1986) Comparative studies of inflammatory responses in susceptible and resistant mice infected with *Giardia muris*. Clin. Exp. Immunol. 65, 622-630.

Belosevic, M., Faubert, G.M. and MacLean, J.D. (1986) The effects of cyclosporin A on the course of infection with *Giardia muris* in mice. Am. J. Trop. Med. Hyg. 35, 496-500.

Blenkinsopp, W.K., Gibson, J.A. and Haffenden, G.P. (1978) Giardiasis and severe jejunal abnormality. Lancet 1, 994.

Brandborg, L.L., Tankersley, C.B., Gottlieb, S., Barancik, M. and Sartor, V.E. (1967) Histological demonstration of mucosal invasion by *Giardia lamblia* in man. Gastroenterology 52, 143-150.

Duncombe, V.M., Bolin, T.D., Davis, A.E., Cummins, A.G. and Crouch, R.L. (1978) Histopathology in giardiasis: a correlation with diarrhoea. Aust. N.Z. J. Med. 8, 392-396.

Erlich, J.H., Anders, R.F., Roberts-Thomson, I.C., Schrader, J.W. and Mitchell, G.F. (1983) An examination of differences in serum antibody specificities and hypersensitivity reaction as contributing factors to chronic infection with the intestinal protozoan parasite, *Giardia muris*, in mice. Aust. J. Exp. Biol. Med. Sci. 61, 599-615.

Ferguson, A. (1987) Models of immunologically driven small intestinal damage. In: M.N. Marsh (Ed.), Immunopathology of the Small Intestine. John Wiley, Chichester, pp. 225-252.

Ferguson, A., Gillon, J. and Al Thamery, D. (1980) Intestinal abnormalities in murine giardiasis. Trans. R. Soc. Trop. Med. Hyg. 74, 445-448.

Ferguson, A. and Jarrett, E.E.E. (1975) Hypersensitivity reactions in the small intestine. I. Thymus dependence of experimental 'partial villous atrophy.' Gut 16, 114-117.

Ferguson, A., Logan, R.F.A. and MacDonald, T.T. (1980) Increased mucosal damage during parasite infection in mice fed an elemental diet. Gut 21, 37-43.

Ferguson, A., McClure, J.P. and Townley, R.R.W. (1976) Intraepithelial lymphocyte counts in small intestinal biopsies from children with diarrhoea. Acta Paediatr. Scand. 65, 541-546.

Ferguson, A. and Munro, G.H. (1988) *Giardia muris* infection in mice with concurrent graft-versus-host reaction. Parasite Immunol. 10, 589–592.

Gillon, J. (1985) Clinical studies in adults presenting with giardiasis to a gastro-intestinal unit. Scott. Med. J. 30, 89-95.

Gillon, J., Al Thamery, D. and Ferguson, A. (1982) Features of small intestinal pathology (epithelial cell kinetics, intraepithelial lymphocytes, disaccharidases) in a primary *Giardia muris* infection. Gut 23, 498-506.

Gillon, J., Andre, C., Descos, L., Minaire, Y. and Fargier, N.L. (1982b) Changes in mucosal immunoglobulin containing cells in patients with giardiasis before and after treatment. J. Infect. 5, 67-72.

Gillon, J. and Ferguson, A. (1984) Changes in the small intestinal mucosa in giardiasis. In: S.L. Erlandsen and E.A. Meyer (Eds.), *Giardia* and Giardiasis. Plenum Press, New York, pp. 163-183.

Goldstein, F., Thornton, J.J. and Szydlowski, T. (1978) Biliary tract dysfunction in giardiasis. Am. J. Dig. Dis. 23, 559-560.

Heyworth, M.F., Carlson, J.R. and Ermak, T.H. (1987) Clearance of *Giardia muris* infection requires helper/inducer T lymphocytes. J. Exp. Med. 165, 1743-1748.

Heyworth, M.F., Kung, J.E. and Eriksson, E.C. (1986) Clearance of *Giardia muris* infection in mice deficient in natural killer cells. Infect. Immun. 54, 903-904.

Hoskins, L.C., Winawer, S.J., Broitman, S.A., Gottlieb, L.S. and Zamcheck, N. (1967) Clinical giardiasis and intestinal malabsorption. Gastroenterology 53, 265-279.

Jones, E.G. and Brown, W.R. (1974) Serum and intestinal immunoglobulins in patients with giardiasis. Am. J. Digest. Dis. 19, 791-796.

Kanwar, S.S., Ganguly, N.K., Walia, B.N.S. and Mahajan, R.C. (1986) Direct and antibody dependent cell mediated cytotoxicity against *Giardia lamblia* by splenic and intestinal lymphoid cells in mice. Gut 27, 73-77.

Kaplan, B.S., Uni, S., Aikawa, M. and Mamhoud, A. (1985) Effector mechanism of host resistance in murine giardiasis: specific IgG and IgA cell mediated immunity. J. Immunol. 134, 1975-1981.

Kotler, D.P., Gaetz, H.P., Lange, M., Klein, E.B. and Holt, P.R. (1984) Enteropathy associated with the acquired immunodeficiency syndrome. Ann. Intern. Med. 101, 421-428.

Kraft, S.C. (1979) The intestinal immune response in giardiasis. Gastroenterology 76, 877-879.

Loftness, T.J., Erlandsen, S.L., Wilson, I.D. and Meyer, E.A. (1984) Occurrence of specific IgA in bile after inoculation of *Giardia lamblia* trophozoites into rat duodenum. Gastroenterology 87, 1022-1029.

Lupascu, G.H., Radulescu, S. and Cernat, M.J. (1970) The presence of *Lamblia muris* in the tissues and organs of mice spontaneously infected. J. Parasitol. 56, 444-445.

MacDonald, T.T. and Ferguson, A. (1977) Hypersensitivity reactions in the small intestine. 3. The effects of allograft rejection and of graft-versus-host disease on epithelial cell kinetics. Cell Tissue Kinet. 10, 301-312.

MacDonald, T.T. and Ferguson, A. (1978) Small intestinal epithelial cell kinetics and protozoal infection in mice. Gastroenterology 74, 496-500.

Manson-Smith, D.F., Bruce, R.G. and Parrott, D.M.V. (1979) Villous atrophy and expulsion of intestinal *Trichinella spiralis* are mediated by T-cells. Cell. Immunol. 47, 285-292.

Meyers, J.D., Kuharic, H.A. and Holmes, K.K. (1977) *Giardia lamblia* infection in homosexual men. Br. J. Vener. 53, 54-55.

Mitchell, G.F., Anders, R.F., Brown, G.V., Handman, E., Roberts-Thomson, I.C., Chapman, C.B., Forsyth, K.P., Kahl, L.P. and Cruise, K.M. (1982) Analysis of infection characteristics and anti-parasite immune responses in resistant compared with susceptible hosts. Immunol. Rev. 61, 137-188.

Morecki, R. and Parker, J.G. (1967) Ultrastructural studies of the human *Giardia lamblia* and subjacent jejunal mucosa in a subject with steatorrhoea. Gastroenterology 52, 151-164.

Munro, G.H. (1985) Murine giardiasis: intestinal mucosal immune responses. Ph.D. thesis, University of Edinburgh.

Nair, K.V., Gillon, J. and Ferguson, A. (1981) Corticosteroid treatment increases parasite numbers in murine giardiasis. Gut 22, 475-480.

Owen, R.L. (1980) The immune response in clinical and experimental giardiasis. Trans. R. Soc. Trop. Med. Hyg. 74, 443-445.

Owen, R.L., Nemanic, P.D. and Stevens, D.P. (1979) Ultrastructural observations of giardiasis in a murine model. Gastroenterology 76, 757-769.

Popovic, O., Pendic, B., Paljm, A., Andrejevic, M. and Trpkovic, D. (1974) Giardiasis, local immune defense and responses. Eur. J. Clin. Invest. 4, 380.

Quinn, T.C., Stamm, W.E., Goodell, S.E., Mkrtichian, E., Benedetti, J., Corey, L., Schuffler, M.D. and Holmes,

K.K. (1983) The polymicrobial origin of intestinal infections in homosexual men. N.Engl.G.Med. 309, 516–582.

Radulescu, S., Lupascu, G., Ciplea, A.G. and Cernat, M.J. (1971) Presence of the flagellate *Giardia muris* in tissues and organs of spontaneously infected mice. Arch. Roum. Pathol. Exp. Microbiol. 30, 405-411.

Rendtorff, R.C. (1954) The experimental transmission of human intestinal protozoal parasites. II. *Giardia lamblia* cysts given in capsules. Am. J. Hyg. 59, 209-220.

Rey, J., Schmitz, J., Rey, F. and Jos, J. (1971) Cellular differentiation and enzymatic defects. Lancet 2, 218.

Ridley, M.J. and Ridley, D.S. (1976) Serum antibodies and jejunal histology in giardiasis associated with malabsorption. J. Clin. Pathol. 29, 30-34.

Roberts-Thomson, I.C. and Mitchell, G.F. (1978) Giardiasis in mice: I. Prolonged infections in certain mouse strains and hypothymic (nude) mice. Gastroenterology 75, 42-46.

Roberts-Thomson, I.C., Stevens, D.P., Mahmoud, A.A.F. and Warren, K.S. (1976) Giardiasis in the mouse: an animal model. Gastroenterology 71, 57-61.

Smith, P.D., Lane, H.C., Gill, V.J., Manischewitz, J.F., Quinnan, G.V., Fauci, A.S. and Masur, H. (1988) Intestinal infections in patients with the acquired immunodeficiency syndrome (AIDS). Ann. Intern. Med. 108, 328-333.

Snider, D.P., Gordon, J., McDermott, M.R. and Underdown, B.J. (1985) Chronic *Giardia muris* infection in anti-IgM-treated mice. I. Analysis of immunoglobulin and parasite-specific antibody in normal and immunoglobulin-deficient animals. J. Immunol. 6, 4153-4162.

Thompson, A., Rowland, R., Hecker, R., Gibson, G.E. and Reid, D.P. (1977) Immunoglobulin-bearing cells in giardiasis. J. Clin. Pathol. 30, 292-294.

Wright, S.G. and Tomkins, A.M. (1977) Quantification of the lymphocyte infiltrate in jejunal epithelium in giardiasis. Clin. Exp. Immunol. 29, 408-412.

Wright, S.G. and Tomkins, A.M. (1978) Quantitative histology in giardiasis. J. Clin. Pathol. 31, 712-716.

Wright, S.G., Tomkins, A.M. and Ridley, D.S. (1977) Giardiasis: clinical and therapeutic aspects. Gut 18, 343-350.

Yardley, J.H., Takano, J. and Hendrix, T.R. (1964) Epithelial and other mucosal lesions of the jejunum in giardiasis: jejunal biopsy studies. Bull. Johns Hopkins Hosp. 115, 389-406.

Zamcheck, N., Hoskins, L.C., Winawer, S.J., Broitman, S.A. and Gottlieb, L.S. (1963) Histology and ultrastructure of the parasite and the intestinal mucosa in human giardiasis: effects of atabrine therapy. Gastroenterology 44, 860 (Abstract).

Giardiasis (E.A. Meyer, ed.)
© 1990 Elsevier Science Publishers B.V. (Biomedical Division)

10

Clinical symptoms and diagnosis by traditional methods

MARTIN S. WOLFE

Tropical Medicine Unit, Office of Medical Services, Department of State, Washington, D.C. 20520, U.S.A.

1. Clinical symptoms	175
1.1. Incubation and prepatent periods	176
1.2. Acute stage	176
1.3. Subacute and chronic stages	177
1.4. Asymptomatic cyst-passing stage	179
1.5. Giardiasis in the nutritionally deprived	179
1.6. Post-*Giardia* lactose intolerance	180
1.7. Differential diagnosis	180
1.7.1. Identification of parasites	180
1.7.2. Stool examinations	181
1.7.3. Examination of intestinal fluid	181
1.7.4. Small bowel biopsy	182
1.7.5. Radiologic findings	183
1.7.6. Other tests	183
1.7.7. Empiric treatment	183
References	183

1. Clinical symptoms

In this chapter, the range of symptomatology observed in *Giardia* infections will be described. A point to be emphasized in considering the clinical features of giardiasis is that those individuals who are infected present a spectrum of symptomatology the precise aspects of which depend to a significant degree on the duration of the infection. The role of host factors in *Giardia* symptomatology is discussed in this chapter, and in Chapters 13 and 14. Although, in the last decade, we have increased our understanding of many aspects of this disease, we still do not clearly understand the mechanism(s) of its pathogenesis. Further, we do not yet know why the result of *Giardia* infection is, in some cases, acutely ill individuals, and, in other cases, asymptomatic infections.

1.1 Incubation and prepatent periods

Based on his experiments with human volunteers, Rendtorff in 1954 determined that the prepatent period, as established by the first detection of stool parasites, averaged 9.1 days. On the other hand, the most reliable data on the incubation period in giardiasis comes from investigations of travellers returned from the Soviet Union. The mean time period from entrance into the Soviet Union until the onset of illness in American travellers has been 12 to 15 days, with a range of 1 to 75 days (Walzer et al., 1971; Brodsky et al., 1974). In returned Finnish travellers from the Soviet Union, Jokipii and Jokipii (1977) found a median incubation time of 8 days and a median prepatent period of 14 days. Much of the present knowledge of the incubation period of giardiasis comes from cases contracted in Leningrad, prior to recognition of cryptosporidiosis. In recent years, cryptosporidiosis has been recognized as the cause of a short incubation period (3-12 days) diarrheal illness contracted in Leningrad. It now seems that those cases of disease with short incubation periods may represent cryptosporidiosis and that the incubation period for giardiasis may more typically be in the range of 12 of 19 days. (Jokipii et al., 1985).

1.2. Acute stage

A variety of symptoms may signal the onset of giardiasis; these include nausea, anorexia, an uneasiness in the upper intestine, malaise, and perhaps low-grade fever and chills. There is then usually the sudden onset of explosive, watery, foul smelling diarrhea, associated with increased foul flatulence and abdominal distention. Foul belching and upper to midepigastric cramps may occur. Mucus occurs only rarely in the stool, and when blood is present it is invariably secondary to anal irritation from the diarrhea. Some of the best available data on the symptomatology of acute infections comes from investigations of individuals recently returned from the Soviet Union. Table 1 shows the frequency of symptoms in a series of 32 of these cases with proven giardiasis (Walzer et al., 1971). Frequency of similar primarily acute stage symptoms, in acute waterborne outbreaks in the United States, are given by Moore et al. (1969) from Aspen, Colorado; Shaw et al. (1977) from Rome, New York; Dykes et al. (1980) from Camas, Washington; and Lopez et al. (1980) from Berlin, New Hampshire. Jokipii and Jokipii (1983) analyzed the clinical features of 201 Finnish cases with acute giardiasis.

If the acute stage lasts only a few days, as it occasionally does, giardiasis may not be recognized as the cause. The initial acute symptoms of giardiasis may mimic those of acute viral enteritis, *Campylobacter* infection, bacillary dysentery, bacterial or other food poisoning, acute intestinal amebiasis, or 'traveller's diarrhea' caused by toxigenic *Escherichia coli*. Giardiasis, however, can be suspected over these other acute diarrheas

TABLE 1

Clinical features of 32 patients with proven giardiasis recently returned from the Soviet Union[a] compared with 105 State Department cases with undetermined duration of proven infection.

Symptom	State Dept. % (N=105)	USSR % (N=32)
Flatulence	46.7	56.5
Foul stool	44.8	52.2
Cramps	32.4	59.4
Distention	31.4	–
Anorexia	20.0	56.2
Nausea	20.0	59.4
Weight loss	18.1	–
Belching	15.2	30.4
Heartburn	14.3	–
Headache	11.4	–
Constipation	11.4	–
Vomiting	4.8	34.4
Fever	3.8	17.4
Chills	2.9	–
Diarrhea	62.9[b]	71.9
Blood in stool	0	0
Mucus in stool	3.8	4.4
Fatigue	28.6	87.5

[a] From Walzer et al. (1971) Giardiasis in travelers. J. Infect. Dis. 124; 235-237.
[b] 52.4% had soft or mushy stools; 10.5% had watery stools.

by its longer incubation period and the more characteristic symptoms of foul-smelling soft or loose stools, foul-smelling flatus and belching, marked abdominal distention, and the virtual absence in the stool of blood, mucus, and cellular exudate.

Commonly, the acute infection resolves spontaneously, and cysts may disappear from the feces. Some patients become asymptomatic cyst-passers for a period and have no further clinical manifestations. Others may have periodic brief recurrences of acute symptoms. In occasional patients, the acute stage may last for months, leading to malabsorption, steatorrhea, debility, and weight loss. This last situation appears to be more common in young children than adults and perhaps helps explain why giardiasis had formerly been considered primarily a disease of childhood.

1.3. Subacute and chronic stages

Most commonly, the acute stage is followed by the development of this infection into the subacute or chronic stage. In returnees from residence or lengthy travel abroad, the acute stage is often not recognized or recalled; these individuals frequently present with persistent or recurrent mild to moderate symptoms. A series of 105 cases with uncertain duration of infection was seen by the author in 1974 at the Department of State; from one-third to one-half presented with flatulence, mushy foul stools, primarily upper intestinal

TABLE 2

Characteristics of the stools of 105 State Department cases with proven giardiasis

	No.	%
Type of stool		
Formed	35	33.3
Mushy	55	52.4
Watery	11	10.5
Unknown	4	3.8
Presence of		
Blood	0	0
Pus	0	0
Mucus	4	3.8
Frequency		
Normal	65	61.9
Increased	22	21.0
Very frequent	13	12.4

cramps, and abdominal distention. Other symptoms included anorexia, nausea, weight loss, belching, heartburn, headache, and constipation. Vomiting, fever and chills rarely occurred. These symptoms are shown in Table 1 and are compared to the symptoms of the 32 acute cases. Type of stool passed, frequency of bowel movements, and virtual absence of blood, pus, and mucus in the stool of these 105 State Department cases from 1974 is shown in Table 2. Of these 105 cases, 39% were judged by our criteria to have mild symptoms (cramps, constipation, flatulence, foul stool, mushy stool); 41% were judged to have moderate symptoms (above mild symptoms and/or belching, nausea, anorexia, vomiting, distention, heartburn, weight loss, fatigue, chills, fever, headache); and 6.7% were considered to have incapacitating severe symptoms (above symptoms plus frequent watery diarrhea, marked weight loss, and marked fatigue). No symptoms were present in 13% of this group. Thus, 80% of these cases were considered to have mild to moderate subacute or chronic symptoms. Black et al. (1977) compared clinical findings in *Giardia*-positive and *Giardia*-negative children infected in two day-care centers, and found *Giardia* infection to be significantly associated with diarrhea lasting more than ten days, and flatulence. In a series of cases from India, the *Giardia*-positive children had significantly increased diarrhea, abdominal discomfort, failure to thrive, and general weakness, whereas there was relatively little difference between *Giardia*-positive and -negative children in appetite, abdominal distention, pallor, and weight loss (Gupta and Mehta, 1973).

Symptoms of the typical patient with non-acute infection include recurrent brief, or less commonly persistent, episodes of loose foul stools; these may be yellowish, frothy, and float in the toilet water, accompanied by increased distention and foul flatus. Between exacerbations, stools are usually mushy, but normal stools or constipation may also occur. Abdominal discomfort is often caused by marked distention, with complaints such as 'feeling blown up', 'having a gas bubble I can't get rid of', or 'my belt has to be loosened'. Cramps are not common in established infections and when present they are usually in the mid to upper epigastrium. Sulfuric belching with a rotten egg taste, called the 'purple burps' by some, and substernal burning, are not uncommon. Anorexia, nausea, and a gurgling or bubbling or uneasiness in the epigastrium are frequent complaints, but vomiting is unusual in this stage. There may be tenderness to paltation in the right, and less commonly in the mid and left upper quadrants. Urticaria is occasionally associated with giardiasis. Such constitutional complaints as weight loss, lassitude or fatigue, headaches, and myalgias may occur. Some question whether these constitutional symptoms, considerably remote from the bowel, are caused by *Giardia*, but personal experience indicates that these symptoms usually disappear following effective treatment of this parasite. In rare cases symptoms may persist for years, but in the great majority of cases spontaneous disappearance of parasites and symptoms occurs after variable periods of time. If eosinophilia occurs, it is usually related to another concomitant cause.

The presence of *Giardia* infection rarely has been associated with cholecystitis (Soto and Dreiling, 1977) and pancreatitis (Kosyarska, 1977). Uncommon manifestations suggesting immunologic reactions, including arthritis (Shaw and Stevens, 1987) and retinal arteritis and iridocyclitis (Knox and King, 1982) have responded to specific anti-giardiasis treatment. Various types of malabsorption have been confirmed (Hoskins et al., 1967; Wright et al., 1977; Hartong et al., 1979), including steatorrhea, disaccharidase (particularly lactose and xylase) deficiency, Vitamin B_{12} malabsorption, hypocarotenemia, low serum folate, and protein-losing enteropathy.

1.4. Asymptomatic cyst-passing state

In our series of Department of State cases, 13% of adults and 17% of children were passing cysts asymptomatically when diagnosed. Powell (1956) in Ireland reported 8 of 28 *Giardia*-positive children to be asymptomatic. Keystone et al. (1978) in Canada found between 20 and 39% of infected children in two day-care nurseries and their household contacts to have symptomatic giardiasis. In day-care center outbreaks of giardiasis, 50% or more of infected young children may be asymptomatic. When studied by jejunal biopsy, however, Barbicri et al. (1970), found eleven symptom-free children in Brazil to have changes in the jejunal mucosa and a mild degree of malabsorption of lipiodol and D-xylose. The duration of the asymptomatic cyst-passing state has not been determined.

1.5. Giardiasis in the nutritionally deprived

This subject has been well summarized in a review article by Solomons (1982). He stated that giardiasis might contribute to an impaired protein-energy status, but that the magnitude of the contribution is not major. He believed it likely that giardiasis in some individuals increases their requirements for total energy, vitamins, and their inability to utilize fat as a form of energy. No systematic epidemiologic data were found to support the nutriture of an individual in promoting the development of *Giardia* infection. Evidence, however, was given which suggests that the relationship between malnutrition and giardiasis is synergistic. Solomons also felt that if assumptions about causality are accepted, three factors common to human protein-energy malnutrition: immune deficiency, decreased gastric acid secretion, and bacterial or fungal overgrowth of the intestine could all promote a more favorable environment for *Giardia* to infect the human host.

1.6. Post-Giardia *lactose intolerance*

Lactose intolerance, which is common during active infection, may persist following apparent eradication of giardiasis with specific treatment, particularly in patients from ethnic groups with a predisposition to lactase deficiency. This must be considered before administering further anti-*Giardia* treatment, in individuals with negative post-treatment specimens who have persistent soft stools and excessive gas and distention.

1.7. Differential diagnosis

Acute diarrhea caused by *Giardia* must be differentiated from other acute viral, bacterial, and protozoal agents (see section 2, acute stage). Giardiasis should be suspected in the absence of blood or mucus in the stool, and in the presence of upper abdominal cramps and distention and the foul odor of feces and gas.

Chronic diarrhea from giardiasis must be differentiated from amebiasis and other pathogenic intestinal parasites such as *Dientamoeba fragilis, Cryptosporidium, Isospora belli, Strongyloides stercoralis*, and from inflammatory bowel disease and irritable colon. When giardiasis symptoms include upper intestinal discomfort, heartburn, belching, and intestinal rumbling, the disease must be differentiated from duodenal ulcer, hiatal hernia, and gallbladder and pancreatic disease.

Chronic diarrhea with malabsorption and weight loss from giardiasis must be differentiated from celiac disease in children, and from sprue, tropical enteritis, and other less common malabsorption disorders in adults. Intestinal biopsy may be required to make the correct diagnosis.

Eosinophilia and intestinal symptoms occurring together are rarely due to giardiasis, but are much more likely caused by infecting hookworm, *S. stercoralis, D. fragilis* or *I. belli*.

1.7.1. Identification of parasites
Traditionally, *Giardia* infection is diagnosed by finding cysts or trophozoites in feces, or by finding trophozoites in duodenojejunal aspirate or biopsy. Detection of the organism in feces may be difficult, as the number of cysts passed can vary considerably from day to day and in some individuals there is an extreme paucity of parasites. In some cases, aspiration and biopsy may also be negative, likely due to the patchy nature of the loci of infection.

1.7.2. Stool examinations

An experienced technician, utilizing appropriate collection and laboratory procedures, should confirm the majority of (perhaps up to 70%), but not all *Giardia* infections by stool examinations, which should be the initial diagnostic procedure of choice. When formed stools are being passed, which is the more usual situation after the initial acute diarrheal stage, the hardy cyst form is often present and examination of unpreserved stools may be adequate to make the diagnosis. Stools are often loose or watery in the acute stage, as well as intermittently in more established infections, and may contain only the more labile trophozoites. It is then very important to either immediately examine a wet smear of a just-passed stool specimen, or to preserve stool for later examination in vials of 10% formalin, merthiolate-iodine-formalin (MIF), or polyvinyl alcohol (PVA). Commercial kits containing these preservatives are now available. Purging does not appear to aid in the diagnosis, and routine stool culture methods are not presently available.

Timing of stool collection is also important. A single negative stool specimen cannot rule out infection and at least 3 stool specimens should be examined by appropriate methods by a well-trained parasitology technician before moving on to other diagnostic procedures. Examination of stools on alternate days has given us an increased positive yield over specimens collected on 3 consecutive days, likely being related to the intermittent passage of parasites due to periods of their active multiplication. Indeed, some of those infected may be low excretors and it has been suggested that examination of 2 or 3 stools a week for 4 or 5 weeks might be required to find *Giardia* cysts in these individuals (Danciger and Lopez, 1975). It has also been shown that symptoms may be present before parasites become detectable in the stool and repeated examinations on a weekly basis may be necessary until the infection becomes patent (Jokipii and Jokipii, 1977). These prolonged periods of examinations however, are often impractical, tedious, and expensive for the patient.

If parasites are numerous in a particular case, direct smear examination in drops of saline or Lugol's iodine may be sufficient. If this is negative, a formol-ether concentration procedure should be performed. Zinc-sulfate flotation may occasionally reveal an infection when the other methods have not.

Many antibiotics, antacids, kaolin products, paregoric, most enema preparations, and oily laxatives may cause a temporary masking of or disappearance from the stool of parasites. Examination of stool and intestinal contents should therefore be deferred for approximately five to ten days after use of these products.

1.7.3. Examination of intestinal fluid

Where parasites cannot be found following a reasonable number of stool examinations in suspected cases, examination of duodenal or upper jejunal fluid may allow for their recovery. Fluid can be obtained with a duodenal tube or endoscopically, or with the Enterotest (HEDECO, Mountain View, CA 94043). The latter is a rubber-lined weighted gelatin capsule containing a nylon line. It comes in a 140 cm adult size, and 90 cm pediatric size in a smaller gelatin capsule. With the patient fasting, the free end of the string is taped to the side of the mouth and the capsule is swallowed with water. Water is drunk after the first and second hours but no other food or drink should be taken. The line occasionally does not pass through the pylorus, but in most cases the line extends to its full length in 4 h and can then be removed. Some workers prefer to leave the line in place for 6 to 8 h or overnight, reporting results to be somewhat better. The distal half or so of the line is usually saturated with bile-stained mucus, which is scraped off onto slides by gloved fingers. A few drops of saline are mixed with the scraped-off material and microscopic examination is performed. *Giardia* trophozoites, as well as other parasites of the duodenum and bile ducts, may be found by this method (Beal et al., 1970; Rosenthal and Liebman, 1980). The Enterotest has been shown by some workers to be simpler than, and as effective as, duodenal intubation (Bezjak, 1972).

However, by using a tube or endoscope, larger quantities of fluid may be obtained, sampling can be made at various levels of the duodenum and jejunum, and a biopsy can be taken at the same time. Centrifugation of duodenal fluid adds little to the diagnostic sensitivity. Intestinal fluid should be examined immediately. There are mixed reports on the value of intestinal fluid examination; some workers report it to be more reliable diagnostically than stool examinations (Kamath and Murugasu, 1974), while others have shown that stools can be positive when duodenal fluid and biopsies are negative (Naik et al., 1978; Madanogopalan et al., 1975). Personal experience has shown that after a series of negative stool examinations, we are rarely able to confirm an infection in intestinal fluid however obtained, possibly due to the patchy nature of loci of infection (which may be lower down in the small bowel), or to the extreme paucity of parasites in a hyperreactive individual with marked symptoms. The examination of intestinal fluid should therefore supplement but not substitute for stool examinations.

1.7.4. Small bowel biopsy
Occasionally, in patients in whom infection cannot be confirmed after multiple examinations of stool and intestinal fluid, diagnosis may be made via small intestinal biopsy (Kamath and Murugasu, 1974). Biopsy is best made at the area of the duodenojejunal junction, or preferably from multiple duodenal and jejunal sites. The intestinal juice remaining in the capsule should first be examined for parasites, along with touch impression smears of the mucosal surface. These are air-dried for one hour, fixed in methanol for 30 min, washed in tap water, and then Giemsa-stained for 10 min (Ament, 1972). With Giemsa stain, *Giardia* are purple and epithelial cells are pink. Biopsy samples should also be serially sectioned and stained and carefully screened since trophozoites may appear in only a few of the sections. *Giardia* in extraluminal sites may be difficult to recognize with conventional hematoxylin and eosin staining, and special staining with a modification of Masson's trichrome stain after fixation in Bouin's solution was found to be preferable by Brandborg et al. (1967). It is rare, however, for *Giardia* to be recognized as a mucosal invader and parasites are much more likely to be seen attached to the microvillus border, particularly in the crypts.

1.7.5. Radiologic findings
Although small intestinal radiography is often normal in *Giardia* infections, a wide variety of abnormalities may occur. These are usually seen in the duodenum or jejunum, associated with diffuse or focal mucosal inflammation. Findings include altered motility, thickened mucosal folds, increased secretions, and a suggestive pattern of edema and segmentation. Although not specific for giardiasis, these findings can suggest the infection in a clinically suspect case. Barium examination of the small bowel may show these particular diagnostic features in about 20% of *Giardia*-infected patients (Marshak and Lindner, 1976). Barium examination should ideally be preceded by examination of stool, intestinal fluid, or mucosal biopsy, since it is virtually impossible to recognize intestinal parasites for one week or longer after barium use.

1.7.6. Other tests
The hemogram is usually normal and eosinophilia is rare. Malabsorption of fat, glucose, lactose, xylose, carotene, folic acid and vitamin B12 is present in some patients. Serologic tests to detect circulating antibodies in serum have been developed and are described in Chapter 11. Unfortunately, these have proved to be of limited usefulness in a clinical setting. No serodiagnostic procedure yet available has proven capable of distinguishing symptomatic and asymptomatic infection.

A number of reports are available describing methods for the immunologic detection of *Giardia* antigen in stool specimens; commercial diagnostic kits have been introduced, and remain to be thoroughly evaluated. These are described in detail in Chapter 11.

1.7.7. Empiric treatment
Varying rates of success have been attributed by different workers for the above diagnostic methods. At least in part, this is related to the expertise and care used in the various techniques. Most workers agree that the initial and simplest diagnostic technique is repeated stool examinations. If this fails to confirm infection, the Enterotest, intestinal intubation or endoscopy, or intestinal biopsy can be used. It is evident, however, that no method or combination of methods presently available is capable of diagnosing all *Giardia* infections, and in patients with a strong clinical and epidemiological basis for having giardiasis, marked improvement and apparent cure may occur after empiric treatment with quinacrine or metronidazole.

References

Ament, M.E. (1972) Diagnosis and treatment of giardiasis. J. Pediatr. 80, 633-637.
Barbieri, D., DeBrito, T., Hoshino, O., Nascimento, O.B., Martins-Campos, J.V., Quarentei, G. and Marcondes, E. (1970) Giardiasis in childhood. Arch. Dis. Child. 45, 466-472.
Beal, C.B., Viens, P., Grant, R.G.L. and Hughes, J.M. (1970) A new technique for sampling duodenal contents. Demonstration of upper small bowel pathogens. Am. J. Trop. Med. Hyg. 19, 349-352.

Bezjak, B. (1972) Evaluation of a new technique for sampling duodenal contents in parasitologic diagnosis. Am. J. Digest. Dis. 17, 848-850.

Black, R.E., Dykes, A.C., Sinclair, M.S. and Wells, J.G. (1977) Giardiasis in day care centers: evidence of person-to-person transmission. Pediatrics 60, 486-491.

Brandborg, L.I., Tankersley, C.B., Gottlieb, S., Barancik, M. and Sartor, V.E. (1967) Histological demonstration of mucosal invasion by *Giardia lamblia* in man. Gastroenterology 52, 143-150.

Brodsky, R.E., Spencer, H.C. and Schulz, M. (1974) Giardiasis in American travellers to the Soviet Union. J. Infect. Dis. 130, 319-323.

Danciger, M. and Lopez, M. (1975) Numbers of *Giardia* in the feces of infected children. Am. J. Trop. Med. Hyg. 24, 237-242.

Dykes, A.C., Juranek, D.D., Lorenz, R.A., Sinclair, S., Jakubowski, W. and Davies, R. (1980) Municipal waterborne giardiasis: an epidemiologic investigation. Beavers implicated as a possible reservoir. Ann. Intern. Med. 92, 165-170.

Gupta, R.K. and Mehta, S. (1973) Giardiasis in children: a study of pancreatic functions. Indian J. Med. Res. 61, 743-748.

Hartong, W.A., Gourley, W.K. and Arvanitakis, C. (1979) Giardiasis: clinical spectrum and functional-structure abnormalities of the small intestinal mucosa. Gastroenterology 77, 61-69.

Hoskins, L.C., Winawer, S.J., Broitman, S.A., Gottlieb, L.S. and Zamcheck, N. (1967) Clinical giardiasis and intestinal malabsorption. Gastroenterology 53, 265-279.

Jokipii, A.M.M. and Jokipii, L. (1977) Prepatency of giardiasis. Lancet 1, 1095-1097.

Jokipii, L. and Jokipii, A.M.M. (1983) Traveller's giardiasis: an analysis of clinical features. Travel Traffic Med. Int. 1, 75-80.

Jokipii, A.M.M., Hemila, M. and Jokipii, L. (1985) Prospective study of acquisition of *Cryptosporidium, Giardia lamblia*, and gastrointestinal illness. Lancet 2, 487-489.

Kamath, K.R. and Murugasu, R. (1974) A comparative study of four methods for detecting *Giardia lamblia* in children with diarrheal disease and malabsorption. Gastroenterology 66, 16-21.

Keystone, J.S., Krajden, S. and Warren, M.R. (1978) Person-to-person transmission of *Giardia lamblia* in day-care nurseries. Can. Med. Assoc. J. 119, 241-248.

Knox, D. and King, J. (1982) Retinal arteritis, iridocyclitis, and giardiasis. Ophthalmology 89, 1303-1308.

Kosyarska, J. (1977) Lambliasis as a cause of acute pancreatitis. Wiad. Lek. 30, 875-877.

Lopez, C.E., Dykes, A.C., Juranek, D.D., Sinclair, S.P., Conn, J.M., Christie, R.W., Lippy, E.C., Schultz, M.G. and Mires, M.H. (1980) Waterborne giardiasis: a community-wide outbreak of disease and a high rate of asymptomatic infection. Am. J. Epidemiol. 112, 495-507.

Madanogopalan, N., Rao, V.P., Somasundaram, A. and Lakshmipathi, T. (1975) A correlative study of duodenal aspirates and feces examination in giardiasis, before and after treatment with metronidazole. Current Med. Res. Opinion 3, 99-103.

Marshak, R.H. and Lindner, A.E. (1976) Radiology of the Small Intestine, 2nd ed., W.B. Saunders Co., Philadelphia, pp. 123-124.

Moore, G.T., Cross, W.M., McGuire, D., Mollohan, C.S., Gleason, M.S., Healy, G.R. and Newton, L.H. (1969) Epidemic giardiasis at a ski resort. N. Engl. J. Med. 281, 402-407.

Naik, S.R., Rau, N.R. and Vinayak, V.K. (1978) A comparative evaluation of examination of three stool samples, jejunal aspirate and jejunal mucosal impression smears in the diagnosis of giardiasis. Ann. Trop. Med. Parasitol. 72, 491-492.

Powell, E.D. (1956) Giardiasis. Irish J. Med. Sci. 34, 509-517.

Rendtorff, R.C. (1954) The experimental transmission of human intestinal protozoan parasites II. *Giardia lamblia* given in capsules. Am. J. Hyg. 59, 209-220.

Rosenthal, P. and Liebman, W.M. (1980) Comparative study of stool examinations, duodenal aspiration, and pediatric Entero-Test for giardiasis in children. J. Pediatr. 96, 278-279.

Shaw, P.K., Brodsky, R.E., Lyman, D.O., Wood, B.T., Hibler, C.P., Healy, G.R., MacLeod, K.I.E., Stahl, W. and Schultz, M.G. (1977) A community-wide outbreak of giardiasis with evidence of transmission by a municipal water supply. Ann. Intern. Med. 87, 426-432.

Shaw, R.A. and Stevens, M.B. (1987) The reactive arthritis of giardiasis. A case report. J. Am. Med. Assoc. 258, 2734-2735.

Solomons, N.W. (1982) Giardiasis: nutritional implications. Rev. Infect. Dis. 4, 859-869.

Soto, J.M. and Dreiling, D.A. (1977) *Giardia lamblia*. A case presentation of chronic cholecystitis and duodenitis. Am. J. Gastroenterol. 67, 265-269.

Walzer, P.D., Wolfe, M.S. and Schultz, M.G. (1971) Giardiasis in travelers. J. Infect. Dis. 124, 235-237.

Wright, S.G., Tomkins, A.M. and Ridley, D.S. (1977) Giardiasis: clinical and therapeutic aspects. Gut 18, 343-350.

Giardiasis (E.A. Meyer, ed.)
© 1990 Elsevier Science Publishers B.V. (Biomedical Division)

11

Detection of *Giardia* by immunologic methods

PAUL G. ENGELKIRK and LARRY K. PICKERING

Program in Medical Technology/Cytogenetics, School of Allied Health Sciences, and Program in Infectious Diseases and Clinical Microbiology and Department of Pediatrics, Medical School, University of Texas Health Science Center at Houston, U.S.A.

1. Introduction	187
2. Serodiagnosis of giardiasis and detection of anti-*Giardia* antibodies in clinical specimens other than serum	188
2.1. Anti-*Giardia* antibodies in serum	188
2.2. Anti-*Giardia* antibodies in saliva	190
2.3. Anti-*Giardia* antibodies in human milk	190
2.4. Anti-*Giardia* antibodies in intestinal secretions	190
2.5. Summary	191
3. Detection of *Giardia* antigen in clinical specimens	191
3.1. Immunofluorescence	191
3.2. Counterimmunoelectrophoresis	193
3.3. Enzyme-linked immunosorbent assays	194
3.4. Immunologic detection of *Giardia* in tissue sections	196
4. Summary	196
References	196

1. Introduction

Traditionally, *Giardia* infection has been diagnosed by microscopic examination of stool specimens, using procedures which lack sensitivity and are cumbersome to perform (Chapter 10; Pickering and Engelkirk, 1988). Examination of duodenal material obtained via aspiration of contents, string test or biopsy may increase sensitivity, but these are invasive techniques. Fortunately, methods have been developed for in vitro culturing of *Giardia* trophozoites (Chapter 6) and concentration of *Giardia* cysts from stool specimens (Chapter 6). These technologic advances make it possible to collect sufficient *Giardia* antigen for the immunization of laboratory animals and production of anti-*Giardia* antiserum for use in immunologic methods for detection of *Giardia*. Additional impetus for the development of such techniques arose from a need for rapid and sensitive methods for screening water samples for the presence of *Giardia* cysts. Immunologic techniques for detection of *Giardia* are reviewed in this chapter.

2. Serodiagnosis of giardiasis and detection of anti-Giardia antibodies in clinical specimens other than serum

2.1. Anti-Giardia antibodies in serum

The pre-1984 literature pertaining to detection of anti-*Giardia* antibodies in serum was reviewed by Visvesvara and Healy (1984). Thus, neither the historic aspects nor a chronologic record of this particular diagnostic approach will be presented here. A variety of methodologies have been employed for detection of anti-*Giardia* antibodies in serum, including immunodiffusion (Vinayak et al., 1978; Jokipii and Jokipii, 1982), hemagglutination (Ganguly et al., 1981), immunofluorescence (Ridley and Ridley, 1976; Radulescu et al., 1976; Wright et al., 1977; Lopez-Brea et al., 1979; Visvesvara and Healy, 1979; Visvesvara et al., 1980; Baveja et al., 1981; Ganguly et al., 1981; Winiecka, 1984), and enzyme-linked immunosorbent assay (ELISA) (Smith et al., 1981; Haralabidis, 1984; Miotti, 1985; Goka et al., 1986) techniques. Table 1 contains a brief synopsis of representative reports.

All investigations reviewed by Visvesvara and Healy (1984) utilized methods for

TABLE 1

Procedures for detection of anti-*Giardia* antibodies in serum

Type of procedure	Reference	Antigen used	Antibody class(es) detected	% Sensitivity	Specificity
Immuno-diffusion	Vinayak et al. (1978)	Sonicated cysts	All	91	100
Immuno-fluorescence	Visvesvara et al. (1980)	Trophozoites	All	97	–
Hemagglutination	Ganguly et al. (1981)	Trophozoites	All	73	–
ELISA	Smith et al.. (1981)	Trophozoites	IgG	81	–
ELISA	Goka et al. (1986)	Trophozoites	IgM	96	96

detection of either total human globulin or IgG. The problems associated with attempts to diagnose any disease by testing a single serum sample for IgG antibodies are well known, but several specific examples of potential difficulties are discussed below.

Using an indirect human globulin immunofluorescence procedure, Visvesvara et al. (1980) demonstrated that serum titers of anti-*Giardia* antibodies did not decrease by more than a single dilution for periods of up to 2.5 months following treatment. Smith et al. (1981) reported that only 80% of patients with symptomatic giardiasis developed a detectable IgG response by ELISA, and that IgG antibodies were detectable between two weeks and 15 months following therapy. When McNally et al. (1988) used an immunofluorescence antibody (IFA) technique to test sera of patients with microscopically proven giardiasis, only 42% of the patients had positive results. The authors concluded that the IFA technique was of limited utility in detecting giardiasis in a clinical setting.

When immunofluorescence and ELISA procedures were compared by Wittner et al. (1983), they found the procedures to be equally sensitive, but the immunofluorescence procedure was more specific. The authors concluded that although serologic procedures might be reliable in the diagnosis of symptomatic patients, they were unreliable in asymptomatic patients due to nonspecific antibody titers caused by intestinal parasites other than *Giardia*. Jokipii et al. (1988) concluded that their ELISA procedure, which employed *Giardia* cysts as antigen, was unsuitable for diagnosis of patients with giardiasis because the anti-*Giardia* antibody titers in the patient population studied were indistinguishable from titers in healthy controls.

Haralabidis (1984) demonstrated that sera from patients with microscopically-proven *Giardia* infection reacted by ELISA with a variety of protozoan and helminth parasite antigens, including *Toxoplasma gondii* (15% of sera tested) and *Sarcocystis* spp. (12% of sera tested). These results could indicate either cross-reactivity between anti-*Giardia* antibodies and non-*Giardia* parasite antigens (thus, a lack of specificity), or coinfection with these particular organisms. None of the 92 sera reacted with *Entamoeba histolytica* antigen. Jokipii et al. (1988) concluded that sera from most people contains antibodies which cross-react with *Giardia* cysts, and that these antibodies may be induced by immunogens other than *Giardia*.

It was not until 1986 that a method was published for detection of IgM anti-*Giardia* antibodies (Goka et al., 1986). In place of methods which detected and quantitated long-lived IgG antibodies that may remain at a high titer for many months after the patient had been cured, this procedure detected and quantitated relatively short-lived IgM antibodies. Thus, results of such a procedure might prove to be more clinically relevant, in that they would be more likely to indicate the cause of a patient's *present* symptoms. Goka et al. (1986) concluded that serum IgG responses were not helpful in distinguishing active from past *Giardia* infection.

Nash et al. (1987) reported specific anti-*Giardia* serum IgM responses in 100% of human volunteers experimentally infected with human-source *Giardia*. Such responses were observed within two weeks of infection in 70% of acute episodes, but were low in chronically infected and rechallenged individuals. Thus, as noted by Nash et al. (1987), the IgM ELISA procedure of Goka et al. (1986) may have limited diagnostic usefulness in chronic or repeated infections.

Taylor and Wenman (1987) reported that convalescent sera of most patients with giardiasis contain antibodies directed against a specific 31 000 dalton *G. duodenalis* antigen. Perhaps serologic assays using this purified antigen would prove to be more sensitive and specific than assays employing a mixture of antigens, such as crude trophozoite or cyst preparations.

2.2. Anti-Giardia *antibodies in saliva*

Investigators from Russia published results of a unique approach to the immunodiagnosis of giardiasis (Osipova et al., 1984). They used an immunofluorescence procedure to detect *Giardia*-specific antibodies in *saliva*, and compared these results to serum titers. Diagnostic titers were obtained in saliva from 95% of 40 patients with giardiasis, compared to diagnostic titers in 80% of serum specimens from the same patients. These results suggest that saliva may be a more suitable specimen than serum for detection of anti-*Giardia* antibodies in patients with giardiasis. Antibody titers in saliva of 80 control patients were all below 1:4. Unfortunately, only an English abstract of this paper was available for review. Additional information would certainly be of interest, such as details of the immunofluorescence procedure, which immunoglobulin class(es) were detected, and assay reproducibility.

2.3. Anti-Giardia *antibodies in human milk*

Using ELISA techniques for detection of IgG and secretory IgA (s-IgA), Miotti et al. (1985) investigated and compared levels of anti-*Giardia* antibodies in serum and human milk samples from two populations of lactating women in Mexico and Texas. Serum IgG and human milk s-IgA anti-*Giardia* antibodies were present in both populations. However, a higher percentage of Mexican women yielded positive serum and human milk results than Texan women, and antibody concentrations were higher in the Mexican population. The authors speculated that in areas endemic for giardiasis, infants may acquire anti-*Giardia* antibodies from their mothers both transplacentally and via human milk, and that the passive transmission of such antibodies might protect the infants from *Giardia* infection.

2.4. Anti-Giardia *antibodies in intestinal secretions*

Nash et al. (1987) described humoral and intestinal fluid IgA antibody responses to *Giardia* in experimentally infected human volunteers. Humoral IgA responses were detected at the same time as intestinal IgA responses, but only 50% of the patients demonstrated significant rises in *Giardia*-specific intestinal IgA antibodies. It was apparent that the presence of such intestinal antibodies neither prevented the establishment of, nor altered the course of, *Giardia* infection in these patients.

2.5. Summary

The ideal serodiagnostic procedure for giardiasis would be 100% sensitive, yielding positive results whenever a patient is truly harboring *Giardia*. The assay should be 100% specific, being positive only when a *Giardia* infection is present. Unfortunately, no serodiagnostic procedure for *Giardia* infection fulfills these criteria. There is variability in the humoral response to *Giardia* infection. Some patients with symptomatic infections fail to develop sufficiently high antibody concentrations for results to be called positive. In some patients, concentrations of anti-*Giardia* IgG antibodies remain elevated long after the infection has been eradicated. The assay having the greatest clinical utility appears to be the one that detects IgM (Goka et al., 1986). An assay which will detect IgA anti-*Giardia* antibodies in saliva (Osipova et al., 1985) might prove to be of value, as might one that employs a potent *Giardia*-specific antigen to which all patients with *Giardia* infection respond immunologically (Taylor and Wenman, 1987). No serodiagnostic procedure has been reported that is capable of distinguishing asymptomatic from symptomatic infection. Despite these shortcomings, serologic assays have proven to be of value in epidemiologic investigations of giardiasis (Miotti et al., 1986).

3. Detection of Giardia antigen in clinical specimens

The previously mentioned disadvantages of an antibody detection procedure for immunodiagnosis of giardiasis (variability of patient immune response, prolonged elevation of titers after successful treatment, cross-reactions) provided the impetus for development of techniques for detection of *Giardia* antigen by immunologic methods. Reported methodologies for antigen detection include immunodiffusion (Goka et al., 1984), immunoelectrophoresis (Goka et al., 1984), immunofluorescence (Riggs et al., 1983), immunoperoxidase (Fleck et al., 1985), counterimmunoelectrophoresis (Craft and Nelson, 1982; Goka et al., 1984; Vinayak et al., 1985; Rosoff and Stibbs, 1986a), and enzyme-linked immunosorbent assays (Ungar et al., 1984; Goka et al., 1984; Green et al., 1985; Janoff et al., 1988; Knisley et al., 1988). Table 2 contains a brief synopsis of selected antigen detection procedures. Technical difficulties associated with detection of parasite antigen in stool specimens, including the presence of proteolytic and cross-reacting substances, have been reviewed by Green (1986), and will not be presented here.

3.1. Immunofluorescence

Riggs et al. (1983) described an immunofluorescence procedure for detection of *Giardia*

TABLE 2
Giardia antigen detection procedures

Type of procedure	Authors and reference	Antiserum source/ immunogen used	% Sensitivity	Specificity
CIE	Craft and Nelson (1982)	Rabbit/*Giardia* cysts from human fecal specimens	98	97
CIE	Vinayak et al. (1985)	Rabbit/*Giardia* trophozoites from human feces and culture	94	95
CIE	Rosoff and Stibbs (1986a)	Rabbit/GSA 65 from IEP precipitin bands (formed by reacting *Giardia*-positive stool eluates with rabbit anti-*G. lamblia* cyst serum)	90	90
CIE	Janoff et al. (1989)	Rabbit/*Giardia* cysts from human fecal specimens	88	97
ELISA	Ungar et al. (1984)	Rabbit and goat/*Giardia* trophozoites from culture	92	98
ELISA	Green et al. (1985)	Rabbit/*Giardia* trophozoites from culture and cysts from human fecal specimens	98	100
ELISA	Nash et al. (1987)	Rabbit and goat/*Giardia* trophozoites from culture	95	100
ELISA	Janoff et al. (1989)	Rabbit/*Giardia* trophozoites from culture	94	95
ELISA	Knisley et al. (1988)	Rabbit and goat/*Giardia* trophozoites from culture	92 rabbit 87 goat	87 91

antigen in human fecal smears. Stool smears were treated first with guinea pig anti-*Giardia* serum, and then with fluorescein-labeled goat anti-guinea pig gamma globulin. Since the guinea pigs were inoculated with intact cysts obtained from human fecal specimens, the antiserum was probably 'polyclonal', containing a mixture of antibodies with different specificities. Although the guinea pig anti-serum cross-reacted with cysts of *Chilomastix mesnili*, the authors felt that the two organisms could easily be differentiated by their distinctive morphologies. Cross-reactions with other intestinal protozoa were not observed. The report provided no data regarding the actual value of this technique in the diagnosis of patients with giardiasis, or the sensitivity or specificity of the procedure in comparison to other diagnostic techniques.

Immunofluorescence has also been used to detect and identify *Giardia* cysts in environmental water samples (Sauch, 1985). Following filtration of large volumes of water, membrane filters were treated with rabbit anti-*Giardia* cyst antiserum and fluorescein-conjugated goat anti-rabbit IgG, and then examined using fluorescence microscopy.

An indirect immunofluorescence procedure for detection of *Giardia* cysts in either stool or water samples is commercially available (MERIFLUOR-*Giardia* [R], Meridian Diagnostics, Cincinnati, OH). The assay employs a murine monoclonal antibody directed against a *Giardia* cyst wall component, and a fluorescein-conjugated anti-murine immunoglobulin reagent. The company claims a sensitivity and specificity of 97 and 100%, respectively. Published evaluations of the product were not available.

3.2. Counterimmunoelectrophoresis

During the late 1970s and early 1980s, counterimmunoelectrophoresis (CIE) became popular in clinical microbiology laboratories as a method for detecting bacterial antigens in cerebrospinal fluid, blood, and urine specimens. Today most CIE techniques have been replaced by less time-consuming, more rapid, and more sensitive latex agglutination and coagglutination procedures. In 1982, a CIE procedure for detection of *Giardia* antigen in feces and duodenal aspirates was reported to have a sensitivity of 98% (Craft and Nelson, 1982). In addition to being sensitive, the procedure was reported to be specific, rapid, and relatively simple to perform. Fecal specimens were diluted with distilled water and added to the 'antigen well' of a CIE agarose gel plate. Rabbit anti-*Giardia* serum was added to the 'antibody well'. Since rabbits were inoculated with whole cysts obtained from human fecal specimens, the antiserum was undoubtedly polyclonal. In most cases, a 'positive' result produced a typical double-band pattern. The authors attributed one band to rabbit IgM anti-*Giardia* antibodies and the other to rabbit IgG anti-*Giardia* antibodies, which apparently migrate at different rates in the electric field. Although there was mention of some fecal specimens having been preserved, the specific fixative(s) used were not stated.

Results obtained using a similar CIE technique were published a few years later (Vinayak et al., 1985), with a reported sensitivity of 94% and specificity of 95%. Rabbits were also used to produce the anti-*Giardia* antiserum, but in this study sonicated, axenically cultured trophozoites were used as antigen rather than cysts obtained from human fecal specimens. The polyclonal antiserum undoubtedly contained a mixture of antibodies directed against a variety of trophozoite immunogens. A typical positive CIE result was a single thick precipitin band located between the antigen and antibody wells. The lack of a second band, such as had been reported by Craft and Nelson (1982), was most likely the result of differences in methodology. Fresh frozen stool specimens were used in this study. There was no mention of how the procedure might work on formalin- or PVA-preserved specimens.

Rosoff and Stibbs (1986a, b) described the isolation and characterization of a 65 000 dalton, *Giardia*-specific antigen (GSA 65) which has proven to be of value for detection of *Giardia* antigen using immuno- and counterimmuno-electrophoresis procedures. The antigen was shown to be present in both trophozoites and cysts, although it appeared to be more plentiful in the latter. In cysts, this GSA 65 antigen is apparently located within or adjacent to the wall. Using a monospecific anti-GSA antiserum produced in rabbits, antigen was detected by CIE in 36 of 40 (90%) *Giardia* cyst-positive stool eluates.

These samples produced well-defined double precipitin lines (doublets), resembling those previously described by Craft and Nelson (1982).

Rosoff and Stibbs (1986a) believe GSA 65 to be the predominant immunologically detectable *Giardia* antigen in stools of patients with giardiasis, and that detection of GSA 65 in stool specimens would indicate an active giardial infection. Thus, for the following reasons, this particular antigen appears to be ideal for design of sensitive and specific immunodiagnostic assays for giardiasis: (1) it remains stable during prolonged storage at 4 and $-20°C$ in both 10% formalin and distilled water, (2) it is present in high concentrations in stool specimens of patients with giardiasis, and (3) it does not appear to cross-react with other intestinal protozoa (Rosoff and Stibbs, 1986b). Therefore, this antigen would seem to be a logical 'target' for commercial companies having an interest in developing such assays. It would be of interest to determine whether GSA 65 could be detected using either swab specimens or dried fecal specimens on paper discs.

Although the 65 000 dalton antigen is apparently common in stool specimens of patients with *Giardia* infection, it may not be the most immunogenic antigen in such patients. Taylor and Wenman (1987) reported that the convalescent serum of 11 of 16 patients with giardiasis contained antibodies directed against a 31 000 dalton antigen.

3.3. Enzyme-linked immunosorbent assays

In 1984, an ELISA technique for detection of *Giardia* antigen was published. Ungar et al. (1984) used an indirect double antibody 'sandwich' method to detect the presence of *Giardia* antigen in fecal specimens. *Giardia* antigen in specimens was 'captured' using goat anti-*Giardia* trophozoite antibodies which were attached to the walls of microtiter tray wells. Since sonicated, axenically cultured trophozoites were used to inoculate the goat, the resultant antiserum was probably polyclonal, containing a mixture of antibodies directed against a variety of trophozoite antigens. Following incubation and addition of rabbit anti-*Giardia* serum to the wells, alkaline phosphatase-labeled goat anti-rabbit IgG was added. Color was developed by adding *p*-nitrophenyl phosphate substrate to the wells. From the addition of clinical specimens through the spectrophotometric readings, the procedure took in excess of 4 h to perform.

The ELISA procedure of Ungar et al. (1984) had a sensitivity of 92% and a specificity of 98%. Although the procedure reportedly worked well on fresh, refrigerated, or frozen specimens, results were neither accurate nor reproducible when formalin- or PVA-preserved specimens were tested. It was suggested that both rectal swabs (Culturette [R] specimens), and specimens which had been smeared onto filter paper and allowed to dry, yielded results comparable to those obtained using fresh, refrigerated, or frozen specimens. The ability to use dried, filter paper specimens should be studied more extensively, since collection, storage, and shipment of such specimens would be practical during epidemiologic investigations of giardiasis. An antigen detection procedure permitting the use of preserved or dried specimens is of far greater value in a field setting than one requiring fresh, refrigerated, or frozen samples.

Green et al. (1985) reported results of a simplified ELISA procedure, having a sensitivity of 98% and a specificity of 100%. In their assay, *Giardia* antigen was 'captured' by affinity-purified rabbit anti-*Giardia* immunoglobulin attached to the walls of microtiter tray wells. Rabbits were inoculated either with whole or sonicated axenically cultured trophozoites, or with sonicated cysts obtained from human feces. Thus, all antisera used in this study were undoubtedly polyclonal. A conjugate consisting of horseradish peroxidase and affinity-purified rabbit anti-*Giardia* immunoglobulin was then added to the wells. Following incubation, color was developed by the addition of a substrate solution consisting of orthophenylene diamine and hydrogen peroxide.

For their ELISA procedure, Green et al. (1985) used filtered, phosphate-buffered saline suspensions of fecal samples, which remained frozen until time of testing. No information was provided on the value of the assay for specimens stored or preserved in other ways. Thus, the usefulness of this technique in a field setting or in conjunction with an epidemiologic investigation is unknown. The elimination of certain control reactions in the Green et al. (1985) technique was criticized by Yolken and Ungar (1985).

The ELISA procedure of Ungar et al. (1984) was used to detect *Giardia* antigen in experimentally-infected human volunteers (Nash et al., 1987). The authors concluded that the ELISA procedure was at least as sensitive as microscopic examination, and that the ELISA-positive/microscopic-negative results represented true antigen-positive specimens, rather than false-positive results. Stool specimens from infected volunteers were ELISA-positive for *Giardia* antigen before organisms were detected by microscopy.

Janoff et al. (1989) blindly evaluated CIE, ELISA, and microscopic procedures for detection of *Giardia*, and found results to be similar. The authors believe that the 'false-positive' ELISA results obtained for day-care center (DCC) toddlers actually represented greater sensitivity of the ELISA procedure, when compared to the 'gold standard' microscopic procedures. The 'false-positive' rate by ELISA was 24% in recurrently exposed DCC toddlers, but only 3% among healthy adults.

Knisley et al. (1989) demonstrated that a variety of environmental manipulations of *Giardia* antigen-positive stool specimens, such as repeated freezing and thawing, prolonged storage, and stool filtration, did not alter ELISA antigen detection results. Formalin, on the other hand, interfered with the assay results. These authors also demonstrated that nine protozoal and 21 bacterial enteropathogens did not interfere with the assay.

An ELISA employing anti-GSA 65 antibodies for detection of *Giardia* antigen in stool specimens is commercially available (ProSpecT/*Giardia*®, Alexon Biomedical, Inc., Rolling Meadow, IL). Clinical evaluation results available from the company indicate a sensitivity of 96% and a specificity of 100% for the ELISA, compared to a sensitivity and specificity of 74 and 100%, respectively, for a standard microscopic examination for parasites. Thirty-percent more true positives were detected using the ELISA than with the microscopic examinations.

A commercial ELISA for detection of *Giardia* antigen is currently being developed (GIARD*EIA* [R], Antibodies Incorporated, Davis, CA). Preliminary evaluation of the product revealed a sensitivity of 95% and a specificity of 90% (Abstract C329, Annual Meeting of the American Society for Microbiology, Atlanta, GA, 1987).

3.4. Immunologic detection of Giardia *antigen in tissue sections*

Rabbit antiserum to cultured *Giardia* trophozoites has been used in a peroxidase-antiperoxidase technique for detection of *Giardia* organisms and their degradation products in jejunal biopsy specimens (Fleck et al., 1985). Such a procedure might prove useful in diagnosis of *Giardia* infection, and also could prove to be of value in determining the frequency and extent with which *Giardia* trophozoites invade the lamina propria.

4. Summary

The presence of anti-*Giardia* antibodies may indicate either past or present infection with *Giardia*, whereas the presence of *Giardia* antigen in stool specimens indicates current infection. The specificity of 'second generation' antigen detection assays is being improved by incorporation of monoclonal antibodies directed against *Giardia*-specific antigens, such as the 31 or 65 kilodalton antigens previously described (Taylor and Wenman, 1987; Rosoff and Stibbs, 1986a, b). To preserve sensitivity, the monoclonal antibodies should react with antigenic determinants that are present in all *Giardia* strains, and preferably present in large quantities. It is uncertain whether antigenic differences among *Giardia* strains (Smith et al., 1982; Ungar and Nash, 1987) will affect the sensitivity of *Giardia* antigen detection procedures.

Emphasis should also be placed on modifying these procedures for use in the field and/or with specimens that have been collected and preserved in the field. Further evaluations should be performed on specimens which have been smeared and dried onto filter paper discs, eliminating the need for refrigerating, freezing, or preserving specimens, and reducing the space required to transport large numbers of samples. As the *Giardia* problem in day-care centers and other settings continues to grow, a sizeable commercial market appears to be emerging for rapid and reliable immunodiagnostic procedures for detection of *Giardia*.

References

Baveja, U.K., Bhatia, R., Agarwal, D.S. and Warhurst, D.C. (1981) Serodiagnosis of giardiasis with or without malabsorption using indirect immunofluorescent test. J. Com. Dis. 13, 244-247.
Craft, J.C. and Nelson, J.D. (1982) Diagnosis of giardiasis by counterimmunoelectrophoresis of feces. J. Infect. Dis. 145, 499-504.
Fleck, S.L., Hames, S.E. and Warhurst, D.C. (1985) Detection of *Giardia* in human jejunum by the immunoper-

oxidase method. Specific and non-specific results. Trans. R. Soc. Trop. Med. Hyg. 79, 110-113.

Ganguly, N.K., Mahajan, R.C., Vasudev, V., Radha Krishna, V., Anand, B.S., Dilawari, J.B. and Chandanani, R.E. (1981) Comparative evaluation of indirect haemagglutination and immunofluorescence tests in sero-diagnosis of giardiasis. Indian J. Med. Res. 73 (Suppl.), 111-113.

Goka, A.K.J., Inge, P.M.G. and Farthing, M.J.G. (1984) Immunoassay of *Giardia* antigen for diagnosis of giardiasis. Gut 25, A1162.

Goka, A.K.J., Rolston, D.D.K., Mathan, V.I. and Farthing, M.J.G. (1986) Diagnosis of giardiasis by specific IgM antibody enzyme-linked immunosorbent assay. Lancet 2, 184-186.

Green, E.L. (1986) Immunological detection of parasite antigen in faeces. Parasitol. Today 2, 198-200.

Green, E.L., Miles, M.A. and Warhurst, D.C. (1985) Immunodiagnostic detection of *Giardia* antigen in faeces by a rapid visual enzyme-linked immunosorbent assay. Lancet 2, 691-693.

Haralabidis, S.TH. (1984) Immunodiagnosis of giardiasis by ELISA and studies on cross-reactivity between the anti-*Giardia lamblia* antibodies and some heterologous parasitic antigens and fractions. Ann. Trop. Med. Parasitol. 78, 295-300.

Janoff, E.N., Craft, J.C., Pickering, L.K., Novotny, T., Blaser, M.J., Knisley, C. and Reller, L.B. (1988) Diagnosis of *Giardia lamblia* infections by detection of parasaite-specific antigens. J. Clin. Microbiol., 27, 431–435.

Jokipii, A.M.M. and Jokipii, L. (1982) Serum IgG, IgA, IgM, and IgD in giardiasis: the most severely ill patients have little IgD. J. Infect. 5, 189-193.

Jokipii, L., Miettinen, A. and Jokipii, A.M.M. (1988) Antibodies to cysts of *Giardia lamblia* in primary giardiasis and in the absence of giardiasis. J. Clin. Microbiol. 26, 121-125.

Knisley, C.V., Engelkirk, P.G., Pickering, L.K., West, S. and Janoff, E.N. (1988) Rapid detection of *Giardia* antigen in stool using enzyme immunoassays. Am. J. Trop. Med. Hyg., in press.

Lopez-Brea, M., Sainz, T., Camarero, C. and Baquero, M. (1979) *Giardia lamblia* associated with bronchial asthma and serum antibodies, and chronic diarrhoea in a child with giardiasis. Trans. R. Soc. Trop. Med. Hyg. 73, 600.

McNally, P.R., Herrera, J.L., Brewer, T.G., Visvesvara, G.S. and Engelkirk, P.G. (1988) Prospective evaluation of immunofluorescent antibody testing in the diagnosis of giardiasis. Unpublished observations.

Miotti, P.G., Gilman, R.H., Pickering, L.K., Ruiz-Palacios, G., Park, H.S. and Yolken, R.H. (1985) Prevalence of serum and milk antibodies to *Giardia lamblia* in different populations of lactating women. J. Infect. Dis. 152, 1025-1031.

Miotti, P.G., Gilman, R.H., Santosham, M., Ryder, R.W. and Yolken, R.H. (1986) Age-related rate of seropositivity of antibody to *Giardia lamblia* in four diverse populations. J. Clin. Microbiol. 24, 972-975.

Nash, T.E., Herrington, D.A. and Levine, M.M. (1987) Usefulness of an enzyme-linked immunosorbent assay for detection of *Giardia* antigen in feces. J. Clin. Microbiol. 25, 1169-1171.

Osipova, S.O., Giyasov, Z.A., Dekhkan-Khodzhaeva, N.A. and Shafer, N.P. (1984) Detection of specific antibodies in saliva in lambliasis infection. Med. Parazitol. Parazit. Bolezni. 5, 57-60.

Pickering, L.K. and Engelkirk, P.G. (1988) *Giardia lamblia*. Pediatr. Clin. N. Am., 35, 565–577.

Radulescu, S., Iancu, L., Simionescu, O. and Meyer, E.A. (1976) Serum antibodies in giardiasis (letter). J. Clin. Pathol. 29, 863.

Ridley, M.J. and Ridley, D.S. (1976) Serum antibodies and jejunal histology in giardiasis associated with malabsorption. J. Clin. Pathol. 29, 30-34.

Riggs, J.L., Dupuis, K.W., Nakamura, K. and Spath, D.P. (1983) Detection of *Giardia lamblia* by immunofluorescence. Appl. Environ. Microbiol. 45, 698-700.

Rosoff, J.D. and Stibbs, H.H. (1986a) Isolation and identification of a *Giardia lamblia*-specific stool antigen (GSA 65) useful in coprodiagnosis of giardiasis. J. Clin. Microbiol. 23, 905-910.

Rosoff, J.D. and Stibbs, H.H. (1986b) Physical and chemical characterization of a *Giardia lamblia*-specific antigen useful in the coprodiagnosis of giardiasis. J. Clin. Microbiol. 24, 1079-1083.

Sauch, J.F. (1985) Use of immunofluorescence and phase-contrast microscopy for detection and identification of *Giardia* cysts in water samples. Appl. Environ. Microbiol. 50, 1434-1438.

Smith, P.D., Gillin, F.D., Brown, W.R. and Nash, T.E. (1981) IgG antibody to *Giardia lamblia* detected by enzyme-linked immunosorbent assay. Gastroenterology 80, 1476-1480.

Smith, P.D., Gillin, F.D., Kaushal, N.A. and Nash, T.E. (1982) Antigenic analysis of *Giardia lamblia* from Afghanistan, Puerto Rico, Ecuador, and Oregon. Infect. Immun. 36, 714-719.

Taylor, G.D. and Wenman, W.M. (1987) Human immune response to *Giardia lamblia* infection. J. Infect. Dis. 155, 137-140.

Ungar, B.L.P. and Nash, T.E. (1987) Cross-reactivity among different *Giardia lamblia* isolates using immunofluorescent antibody and enzyme immunoassay techniques. Am. J. Trop. Med. Hyg. 37, 283-289.

Ungar, B.L.P., Yolken, R.H., Nash, T.E. and Quinn, T.C. (1984) Enzyme-linked immunosorbent assay for the detection of *Giardia lamblia* in fecal specimens. J. Infect. Dis. 149, 90-97.

Vinayak, V.K., Jain, P. and Naik, S.R. (1978) Demonstration of antibodies in giardiasis using the immunodiffusion technique with *Giardia* cysts as antigen. Ann. Trop. Med. Parasitol. 72, 581-582.

Vinayak, V.K., Kum, K., Chandna, R., Venkateswarlu, K. and Mehta, S. (1985) Detection of *Giardia lamblia* antigen in the feces by counterimmunoelectrophoresis. Pediatr. Infect. Dis. 4, 383-386.

Visvesvara, G.S. and Healy, G.R. (1979) The possible use of an indirect immunofluorescent test using axenically grown *Giardia lamblia* antigens in diagnosing giardiasis. In: W. Jakubowski and J.C. Hoff (Eds), Waterborne Transmission of Giardiasis. Environmental Protection Agency, Washington, D.C., pp. 53-63.

Visvesvara, G.S. and Healy, G.R. (1984) Antigenicity of *Giardia lamblia* and the current status of serologic diagnosis of giardiasis. In: S.L. Erlandsen and E.A. Meyer (Eds), *Giardia* and Giardiasis: Biology, Pathogenesis, and Epidemiology. Plenum Press, New York, pp. 219-232.

Visvesvara, G.S., Smith, P.D., Healy, G.R. and Brown, W.R. (1980) An immunofluorescence test to detect serum antibodies to *Giardia lamblia*. Ann. Intern. Med. 93, 802-805.

Winiecke, J., Kasprzak, W., Kociecka, W., Plotkowiak, J. and Myjak, P. (1984) Serum antibodies to *Giardia intestinalis* detected by immunofluorescence using trophozoites as antigen. Tropenmed. Parasit. 35, 20-22.

Wittner, M., Maayan, S., Farrer, W. and Tanowitz, H.B. (1983) Diagnosis of giardiasis by two methods. Arch. Pathol. Lab. Med. 107, 524-527.

Wright, S.G., Moody, A.H., Tomkins, A.M. and Ridley, D.S. (1977) Fluorescent antibody studies in giardiasis. Abstract, Gut 18, 986.

Yolken, R.H. and Ungar, B. (1985) ELISA detection of *Giardia lamblia* (letter). Lancet 2, 1120.

Giardiasis (E.A. Meyer, ed.)
© 1990 Elsevier Science Publishers B.V. (Biomedical Division)

12

Nonspecific defenses against human *Giardia*

FRANCES D. GILLIN, SIDDHARTHA DAS and DAVID S. REINER

Department of Pathology H811F, University of California, San Diego Medical Center, San Diego, 92103, U.S.A.

1. Introduction	199
2. Killing of *Giardia* trophozoites by normal human milk	202
2.1. Antibody-independent killing by NHM	202
2.2. Evidence that bile salt-stimulated lipase is required for killing	202
2.3. Conversion of *Giardia*-cidal activity of NHM from bile salt-dependent to bile salt-independent	203
2.4. The role of bile salts in killing by NHM	204
2.4.1. Activation by cholate	204
2.4.2. Activation by conjugated bile salts	204
3. Killing of *Giardia* trophozoites by products of lipolysis	204
4. Killing of *Giardia* trophozoites by human intestinal fluid in vitro	206
4.1. The mechanisms of killing by intestinal fluid	206
4.2. Intestinal components that protect human *Giardia* from killing	209
4.2.1. Bovine serum albumin	209
4.2.2. Bile salt	209
4.2.3. Mucus	209
References	211

1. Introduction

Data from a number of investigations of outbreaks of giardiasis (e.g., Craun, 1984) and studies of travellers document that both the severity of symptoms and the duration of infection are extremely variable (Wolfe, 1984). This was also reflected in a recent well-controlled study of experimental human infections with a single *Giardia* strain (Nash et al., 1987). Moreover, the severity and duration of giardiasis bore no apparent relationship to the magnitude of the serum or secretory antibody responses (Nash et al., 1987). We have proposed (Gillin et al., 1983a) that variability in giardiasis may be due in part to trophozoite interactions with non-immune elements of the host intestinal milieu.

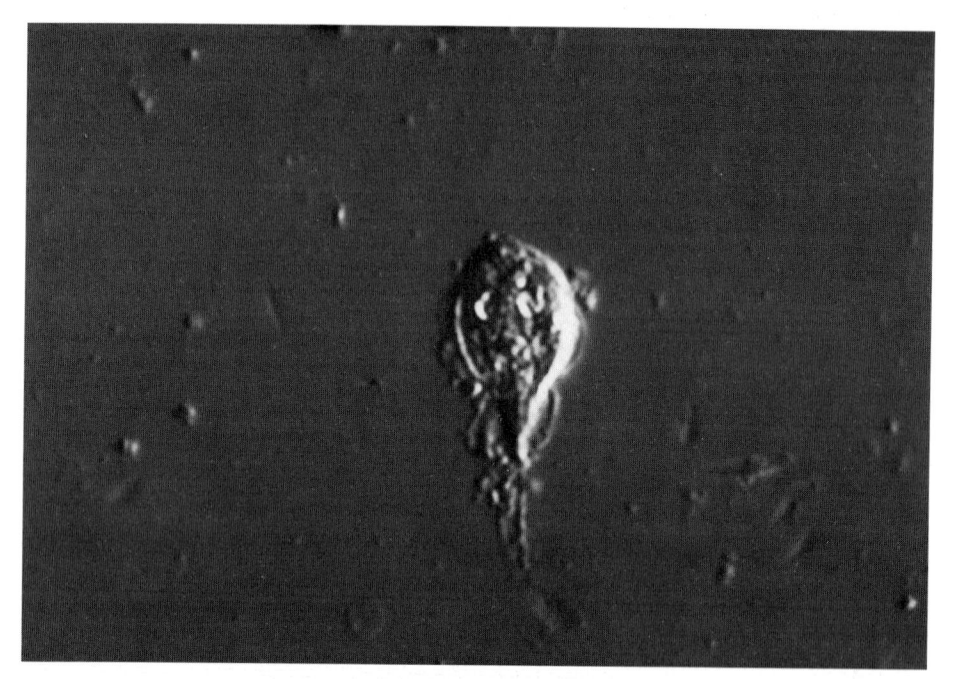

Fig. 1. A partially digested trophozoite in the fluid phase of a duodenal aspirate from a patient with chronic symptomatic giardiasis, photographed with Nomarski differential interference contrast optics (×4000).

The upper human small intestine colonized by *Giardia* is a complex and everchanging environment, which is normally inhabited by relatively few microbes (Simon and Gorbach, 1981). *Giardia* trophozoites 'swim' in the intestinal lumen where they are exposed to fluctuating pH and concentrations of bile, nutrients, digestive enzymes and their products. Trophozoites also penetrate the mucus layer and attach to the underlying epithelial cells (Morecki and Parker, 1967).

The intestinal tract has a unique system of defenses which is less well understood than circulating defenses. Secretory defenses may be produced locally, secreted into the duodenum, or ingested – as by breast-fed babies. This system has both immune (secretory antibody) and non-immune components (lysozyme, lactoferrin, lipases – see below), many of which are found in both breast milk and intestinal fluid (McNabb and Tomasi, 1981). We have frequently observed dead trophozoites and ghosts in the clear fluid phase of aspirates from patients (Fig. 1), while live, motile trophozoites tended to be associated with mucus strands (Fig. 2) (Das et al., 1988). This suggested that certain intestinal fluid factors might be toxic to the parasites, while other factors such as mucus might protect them.

The work summarized below supports this hypothesis since we (Gillin et al., 1983a, b, 1985) and others (Hernell et al., 1986; Rohrer et al., 1986) have shown that *Giardia*

Fig. 2. Live trophozoites isolated from the same patient, showing association with intestinal mucus. Photographed with Nomarski differential interference contrast optics. Inset: detail at higher magnification (×2000).

201

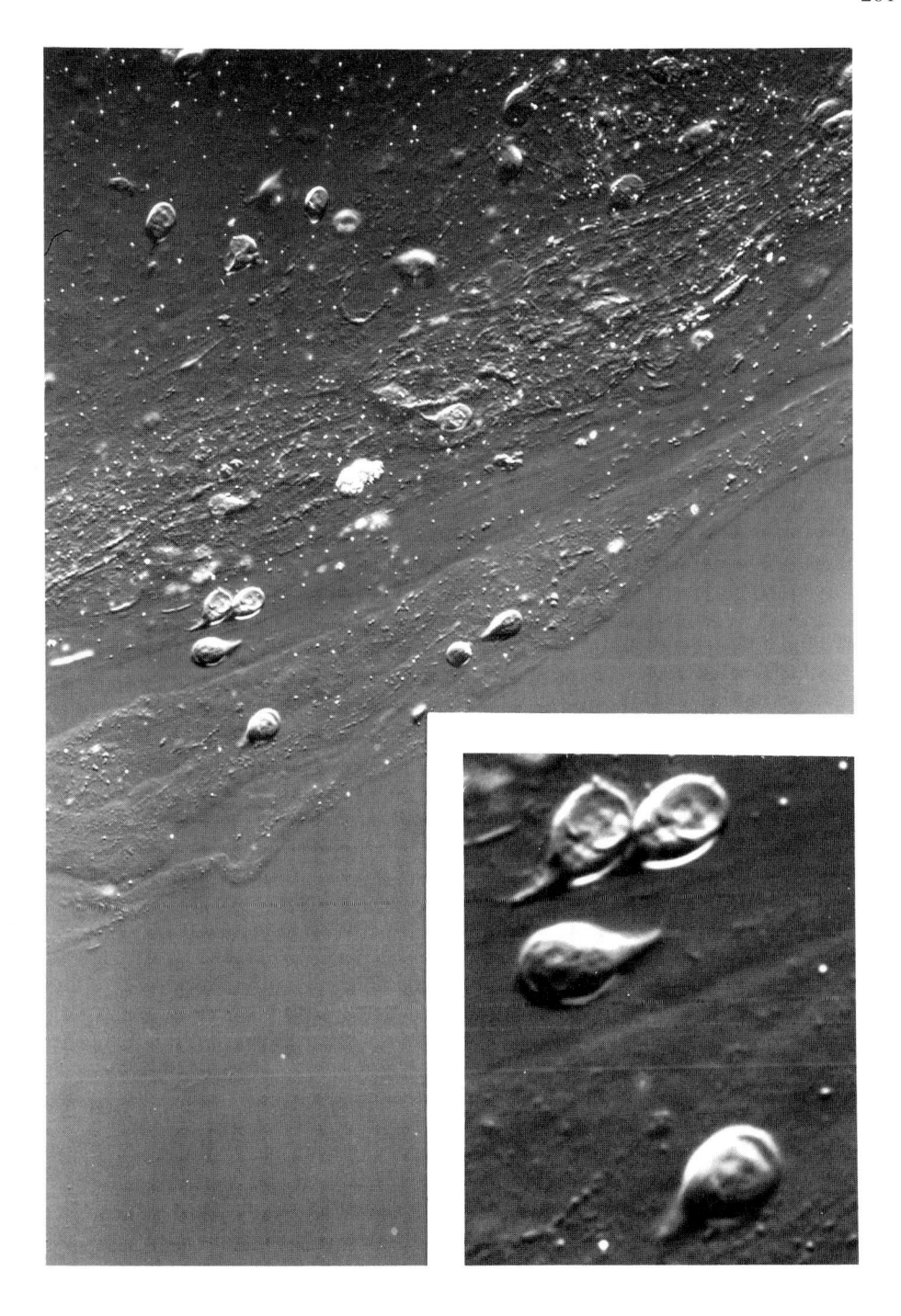

trophozoites are killed in vitro by normal human milk (NHM) and by human intestinal fluid (IF) (Das et al., 1988). Products of lipolysis such as unsaturated free fatty acids (FFA) (Reiner et al., 1984, 1986; Hernell et al., 1986; Rohrer et al., 1986), lysophospholipids or monoglycerides generated by lipases in NHM (Reiner et al., 1984, 1986) or IF (Das et al., 1988) appear to mediate killing. On the other hand, specific intestinal factors such as mucus and bile salts which bind lipolytic products protect trophozoites from killing by NHM (Zenian and Gillin, 1987; Gillin, 1987) and IF (Das et al., 1988), as well as FFA (Reiner et al., 1984, 1986). This may help explain how *Giardia* specifically colonizes the human small intestine.

2. Killing of Giardia trophozoites by normal human milk

Human breast milk is a rich source of both secretory antibodies and of non-immune secretory defense factors (McNabb and Tomasi, 1981). Prior to testing the idea that milk from women with histories of giardiasis would inhibit attachment of *Giardia*, preliminary experiments were designed to detect any effects of normal human milk (NHM, from women without histories of giardiasis) on parasite attachment and survival.

Quite unexpectedly, we found that NHM rapidly killed *Giardia* trophozoites. Killing increased with time and milk concentration (Gillin et al., 1983a). Parasites first lost motility and swelled, then lysed (Gillin et al., 1983b). All the milk samples we have tested (at 1%) to date (from 15 women) killed >95% of the parasites in less than 3 h, but unheated cow's milk and goat's milk (1-20%) did not. Thus, killing activity appeared specific to human milk.

2.1. Antibody-independent killing by NHM

The *Giardia*-cidal activity of NHM is not due to its high concentration of secretory IgA (sIgA) because full activity was retained after passage over a column of sheep anti-human sIgA coupled to Sepharose 4B (Gillin et al., 1983a). This decreased the sIgA concentration of the milk to below that detectable by an ELISA for non-specific sIgA (<0.1 μg/ml). Neither IgG nor IgM was detected in the milk by radial immunodiffusion (<5 μg/ml). Thus, the killing activity was not due to 'natural' antibodies or antibodies raised in response to previous subclinical or undiagnosed giardiasis.

2.2. Evidence that bile salt-stimulated lipase is required for killing

Several lines of evidence supported the idea that killing requires the activity of the bile salt-stimulated lipase (BSL) of human milk.

a. The *Giardia*-cidal activity of NHM is absolutely dependent on the presence of bile salts which activate BSL (Gillin et al., 1985; Hernell et al., 1986) and inhibit the other minor lipase in human milk (lipoprotein lipase, Hernell et al., 1981).

b. Heating NHM (100°C, 20 min) destroyed both BSL enzymatic and killing activities. Moreover, cow's milk and goat's milk lacked both activities (Gillin et al., 1985).

c. BSL is a carboxylesterase which is inhibited by diisopropylfluorophosphate (DIFP), a specific irreversible inhibitor of serine esterases (Hernell et al., 1981). Modification by DIFP reduced the BSL activity of an NHM sample by 90% and also greatly reduced its killing activity (Gillin et al., 1983a,b).

d. Trophozoites were killed by incubation with pure BSL in the presence of a bile salt and substrate triglycerides (Hernell et al., 1986).

2.3. Conversion of Giardia-*cidal activity of NHM from bile salt-dependent to bile salt-independent*

If BSL is responsible for the *Giardia*-cidal activity of milk, bile salts should be required and the activity should be heat-labile. In our early studies, however, we observed that NHM which had been stored at $-10°C$ or $-20°C$, killed trophozoites in the absence of bile salts and the killing was largely heat-stable (Gillin et al., 1983a,b). In contrast, in more recent studies (Gillin et al., 1985), we found that killing by *fresh* NHM (from other donors) or milk which was stored at $-70°C$, was completely cholate-dependent and heat-labile.

Bitman et al. (1983) have shown that BSL activity in milk stored at $-20°C$ can lose its cholate-dependence. In addition, free fatty acids (FFA) accumulate in human milk stored at $-20°C$, as a result of cleavage of milk triglycerides.

The following data support the idea that BSL can function at $-20°C$, producing FFA which are responsible for heat-stable, cholate independent killing activity. Fresh milk from a single donor was frozen in small volumes at $-10°C$, $-20°C$, or $-70°C$ and its activity tested periodically. No change in activity was observed after two days' storage at $-10°C$. However, after 6 days at $-10°C$, the killing activity had increased 4-fold, but was still completely cholate-dependent. The LD_{50} of milk stored for 23 days at $-10°C$ had decreased further and the killing activity was mostly cholate-independent and heat-stable (Gillin et al., 1985). The changes in killing activity were mirrored by alterations in the enzyme. The basal BSL enzyme activity (in the absence of cholate) of $-10°C$ milk had increased and no stimulation by cholate was observed (Gillin et al., 1985) but the enzyme remained heat-labile. Concomitantly, the FFA concentrations in NHM stored at $-10°C$ or $-20°C$ (measured by GLC) increased greatly compared with milk kept at $-70°C$ (Gillin et al., 1985; Reiner et al., 1986). These observations were confirmed by Hernell et al. (1986), who showed that NHM stored at $4°C$ for 5 days gained bile salt-independent killing activity. This did not occur in the presence of eserine, which inhibited both BSL and lipoprotein lipase. Moreover, when fresh cows' milk was stored at $4°C$, for seven days, enough FFA were generated by action of its lipoprotein lipase to kill trophozoites (Hernell et al., 1986).

These studies suggested that NHM (fresh or stored at $-70°C$) when activated by cholate, can kill human *Giardia* indirectly via generation of FFA by BSL. Moreover, FFA (and monoglycerides) account for the heat-stable killing activity of NHM stored above $-70°C$.

An important implication of these results is that for studies with *Giardia*, it is *crucial* to store human milk samples at (or below) $-70°C$. All studies described below use milk stored at $-70°C$, activated by 0.8 mM Na cholate, unless otherwise specified. Controls lacking milk, cholate, or both were included in all experiments.

2.4. The role of bile salts in killing by NHM

2.4.1. Activation by cholate

As stated above, *Giardia* killing by NHM was absolutely dependent upon sodium cholate, an unconjugated bile salt. We have never observed killing in the absence of cholate, even at NHM concentrations of 40%. Killing by NHM was sharply dependent on the cholate concentration. No killing was observed with 0.4 mM cholate but 100% of the parasites were killed with 0.8 mM (Gillin et al., 1985).

2.4.2. Activation by conjugated bile salts

We next focused in depth on the role of bile salts in activating NHM to kill *Giardia* trophozoites. We observed that while cholate activated NHM for killing, its glycine and taurine conjugates (1-40 mM) did not. This was puzzling because (1) all primary bile salts tested activated milk BSL to hydrolyze an exogenous substrate and (2) conjugated bile salts predominate in vivo. If, however, the milk was briefly sonicated, the conjugated bile salts (1 mM) all activated it to kill (Gillin, 1987).

These observations may be understood in light of the fact that milk lipids are organized into milk fat globules (MFG) (Patton and Jensen, 1976). During and after their release from mammary epithelial cells, MFG are completely surrounded by cellular plasma membrane. In vivo, removal of the MFG membrane is accomplished by the churning action of the stomach (Patton and Jensen, 1976). This suggested that in vitro, cholate activated NHM for killing by (1) opening the MFG membrane making milk lipids accessible to BSL and (2) activating the enzyme, whereas the conjugated bile salts could activate the enzyme, but not remove the MFG membrane. In the small intestine, conjugated bile salts can activate the BSL because the MFG membrane has already been disrupted.

3. Killing of *Giardia* trophozoites by products of lipolysis

Since we proposed that killing of trophozoites was due to FFA generated by BSL activity in bile salt-activated NHM, it was necessary to determine directly whether FFA and other products of lipolysis were toxic to *Giardia*. In a large study, (Table 1) the lipids and

TABLE 1

Sensitivity of human-source *Giardia* trophozoites to products of lipid hydrolysis

Lipid or lipolytic product	LD$_{50}$ for *Giardia* (μM)
Monolaurin, 12:0	87
Monomyristin, 14:0	39
Monopalmitin, 16:0	>1,000
Monoolein, 18:1	27
Diglycerides 12:0, 14:0, 16:0, 18:1	>10,000
Triglyceride 18:1	>15,625
Glycerol	>15,625
Free fatty acids	
4:0, 6:0, 8:0, 18:0	>4,000
10:0, 14:0, 16:0	>1,600
12:0	540
16:1 cis	10
16:1 trans	400
18:1 cis	6
18:1 trans	440
18:2	9
18:3	12
20:4	11
Lysophosphatidylcholine	
12:0	886
14:0	81
16:0	8
18:0	8
18:1	8
Phosphatidylcholine 12:0, 14:0, 16:0, 18:0, 18:1	>850
Phosphatidic acid, Na salt, 18:1	>4,000
Fatty acid esters and alcohol	
Oleic acid methyl or ethyl ester	>4,000
Oleoyl alcohol	>4,000
Linolenic acid methyl ester	1,160
Linolenic acid ethyl ester	1,369
Arachidonic acid methyl ester	73
Arachidonic acid ethyl ester	261

lipolytic products tested could be classified into 3 groups according to their LD$_{50}$ for trophozoites. Group I: *Giardia* was most sensitive to C$_{16}$ to C$_{20}$ cis-unsaturated FFA and to certain monoglycerides (LD$_{50}$ < 20 μM) or lysophospholipids. Group II: Medium chain (C$_{12}$-C$_{14}$) saturated FFA comprised an intermediate group (LD$_{50}$~100-1000 μM). Group III: Parasites were not killed (LD$_{50}$ >1 mM) by saturated FFA of chain length ≤ C$_{10}$ or ≥ C$_{16}$ or by diglycerides, triglycerides, or glycerol (Reiner et al., 1984, 1986).

Of the class I lipids, oleic acid (18:1) and linoleic acid (18:2) comprise a large proportion (approximately 38 and 14%, respectively) of the fatty acids in milk triglycerides. Triglycerides make up approximately 3.5% (Patton and Jensen, 1976) of human milk

(~40 mM or ~120 mM in total fatty acid). Thus release of 1-2% of the milk fatty acids (by BSL or during storage at −20°C) could explain the killing of human *Giardia*.

The specific activity of BSL in human milk with cholate was 20-40 μmol fatty acid released/min/ml milk (Gillin et al., 1985). Therefore, in our killing assays with 1% milk, 12 mM fatty acid could be released by BSL in 60 min. Thus, the activity of BSL is sufficient to explain killing by NHM (stored at −70°C).

FFA (which have detergent activity) have long been known to inhibit certain other microbes (Kabara, 1980). Interestingly, oleic acid, which was very toxic to *Giardia*, did not inhibit *Staphylococcus aureus*, pneumococci, or *Candida albicans*. Hernell et al. (1986), and Rohrer et al. (1986), respectively, have confirmed the *Giardia*-cidal activity of oleic acid and other unsaturated FFAs.

Analogs of FFA which are less polar or less flexible (trans-isomers) are less toxic to the parasites (Table 1, Reiner et al., 1986), supporting the idea that killing is due to the detergent and membrane-disrupting properties of toxic FFA (Badwey et al., 1984).

4. Killing of Giardia *trophozoites by human intestinal fluid in vitro*

In examining fresh intestinal fluid aspirates from patients with giardiasis, we frequently observe dead trophozoites in the clear fluid (Fig. 1). In contrast, active, healthy parasites are frequently adherent to mucus flecks or strands (Fig. 2). Moreover, the upper small intestine is the major site of lipolysis (Davenport, 1977). Therefore, we determined whether intestinal fluid from uninfected volunteers is toxic to cultured trophozoites in vitro (Das et al., 1988).

Samples of DF from all nine normal volunteers killed >90% of *Giardia* trophozoites of human origin during the two hour exposure (Table 2). The 50% killing concentrations ranged from 0.1 to 4.2% DF and the 90% killing concentrations from 0.5 to 8%.

To determine whether killing is a property of duodenal fluid only, we tested sequential samples from the duodenum to the upper jejunum. The data in Table 3 show that the *Giardia*-cidal activity of jejunal fluid is as potent as duodenal fluid from the same subject.

Since all the subjects in the preceding studies had fasted overnight before aspiration, we next asked whether the *Giardia*-cidal activity might be associated with the fasting state. The data in Table 4 show that DF aspirated after a liquid meal containing carbohydrate, protein, and fat was even more potent (decreased LD_{50} and LD_{90}) than fasting DF from the same subject. Thus, the *Giardia*-cidal activity was not an artifact of sampling from the duodenum or of fasting.

4.1. The mechanism of killing by intestinal fluid

To examine the mechanism of killing by intestinal fluid, we first measured the concentration of total bile salts and the activities of two pancreatic enzymes (trypsin and lipase) in each sample (Tables 2-4). None of these intestinal fluid components correlated directly

TABLE 2
Killing of human-source *Giardia* trophozoites by duodenal fluid in vitro

Volunteer	% Duodenal fluid		Bile salt	Enzyme activity (u/ml)	
	50% killing	90% killing	conc. (mM)	Trypsin	Lipase
1	3.6	6.2	1.7	50	250
2	0.1	5.0	0.7	41	150
3	0.5	1.0	5.5	13	625
4*	0.1	0.5	6.5	132	750
5	1.2	2.4	0.7	49	500
6*	2.2	5.7	3.8	100	500
7	4.2	5.7	1.2	60	750
8	0.4	8.0	3.5	10	125
9	0.4	5.0	2.5	6	260
Mean (SD)	1.4 (1.4)	4.4 (2.3)	2.9 (1.9)	51.2 (39.8)	401.1 (204.3)

* Samples with heat-stable killing activity.

TABLE 3
Killing of *Giardia* trophozoites of human origin by fluid from the duodenum and jejunum

Sample	% Intestinal fluid		Bile salt	Enzyme activity (u/ml)	
	50% killing	90% killing	conc., (mM)	Trypsin	Lipase
D_1	2.5	6.2	1.2	75	50
D_2	2.5	11.25	1.4	100	62
D_3	5.2	15	0.2	125	62
D_4	0.25	5.4	2.5	200	100
Mean (SD)	2.6 (1.7)	9.4 (3.9)	1.3 (0.8)	125 (46.1)	68.5 (18.8)
J_1	4.0	9.0	9.0	125	75
J_2	0.1	3.5	7.1	125	75
J_3	1.8	4.2	16.1	150	75
J_4	3.25	8.5	12.3	150	100
Mean (SD)	2.2 (1.4)	6.3 (2.4)	11.1 (3.4)	137.5 (12.5)	81.2 (10.8)

Note: D_1 to D_4 and J_1 to J_4 refer to samples collected during descent of the tube through the duodenum and upper jejunum.

with killing. Next, we asked whether *Giardia*-cidal activity was heat-labile and found that killing by seven of the nine DF samples in Table 2 was destroyed by heating (100°C, 20 min). In contrast, the remaining two samples in Table 2 and the DF samples from one subject before and after feeding retained activity after 20 min in a boiling water bath (data not shown). Thus, there are both heat-stable and heat-labile *Giardia*-cidal activities.

In other studies (not shown), potential inhibitors such as phenylmethylsulfonylfluoride (5 mM), EDTA (5 mM), or soybean trypsin inhibitor (50 µg/ml) did not affect killing by samples with either heat-labile or stable activity, suggesting that neither trypsin, chymotrypsin, nor complement is required for killing.

TABLE 4
Killing of *Giardia* of human origin by duodenal fluid aspirated before and after a meal

Duodenal fluid	% Duodenal fluid		Bile salt (mM)	Enzyme activity (u/ml)	
	50% killing	90% killing		Trypsin	Lipase
A. *Before meal*					
(–) 30 min	0.1	1.0	1.0	30	25
(–) 15 min	0.5	5.0	3.1	60	75
B. *After meal*					
15 min	0.05	0.1	4.3	50	50
30 min	0.02	0.1	1.6	30	50
45 min	0.025	0.1	2.4	50	50
60 min	0.05	1.0	3.0	35	75
75 min	0.065	1.0	1.1	15	25
90 min	0.1	2.4	1.0	20	50
105 min	0.01	2.5	0.67	30	25

TABLE 5
Free fatty acid concentrations of duodenal fluid samples

Duodenal fluid samples	Free fatty acids, mM					
	16:0	16:1	18:0	18:1	18:2	20:4
Heat-labile (2)	0.03	ND	0.02	0.03	0.05	0.009
Heat-stable (2)	0.86*	0.04*	0.12*	0.63*	1.95*	0.4*
Before meal						
(–) 30 min	0.12	ND	0.06	0.08	0.19	0.05
(–) 15 min	0.14	ND	0.01	0.16	0.22	0.16
After meal						
15 min	1.23	0.02	0.22	3.36	8.71	0.50
30 min	0.34	ND	0.08	1.54	4.55	0.18
60 min	7.78	0.05	1.40	14.06	30.1	0.27
105 min	1.45	0.003	0.22	3.4	7.7	0.03

Note: Killing by pre-meal and post-meal samples was heat-stable. ND not detectable. * $P < 0.02$ significantly higher FFA concentration than the samples with heat-labile killing activity.

Since it was shown earlier that killing of *Giardia* trophozoites by normal human milk is due to unsaturated FFA cleaved from milk triglycerides *during* (heat-labile killing) or before (heat-stable killing) incubation with the parasites, we compared FFA concentrations in DF samples with heat-labile and -stable killing activities. The latter have much greater FFA concentrations (Table 5), which may account for their heat-stable *Giardia*-cidal activity (Das et al., 1989).

4.2. Intestinal components that protect human Giardia from killing

4.2.1. Bovine serum albumin
Since trophozoites colonize the small intestine, we tested the hypothesis that agents which bind FFA might protect *Giardia* from killing by intestinal fluid as well as by milk and pure FFA. Bovine serum albumin (BSA) which avidly binds FFA (Badwey et al., 1984), protects *Giardia* from killing by DF (Das et al., 1988; Fig. 3), cholate activated NHM (Gillin ct al., 1983b) and oleic acid (Reiner et al., 1986). The degree of protection depended on the concentrations of both DF and BSA.

4.2.2. Bile salts
Bile salts, which are prominent components of proximal small intestinal fluid, form mixed micelles with FFA and other products of lipolysis (Hofmann and Roda, 1984). Since the ability of a given bile salt to form micelles is a function of its critical micellar concentration (CMC, the midpoint of the concentration range of micelle formation; Roda et al., 1983), we next tested the capacity of bile salts with relatively low and high CMCs to protect *Giardia* from killing by DF, milk, and oleic acid. The data in Fig. 4 show that glycodeoxycholate (CMC ~2 mM in 0.15 M NaCl; Roda et al., 1983) protects at lower concentrations (50% protection from 3% DF at 1.4 mM and from 5% DF at 3.2 mM) than does glycocholate (CMC ~8-10 mM, 50% protection at 5.8 and 6.8 mM, Fig 4).

4.2.3. Mucus
Since human intestinal mucus has been shown to bind fatty acids (Clamp and Creeth, 1984), we asked whether it would also protect trophozoites. The data in Table 6 show that human duodenal-jejunal mucus protects human-source *Giardia* trophozoites from killing by DF (Das et al., 1988), as well as NHM and oleic acid (Zenian and Gillin, 1987).

In humans, lipid is digested by a number of lipases including pancreatic triacylglycerol lipase, carboxyl ester hydrolase, phospholipases A and B and lingual lipase (Jensen et al.,

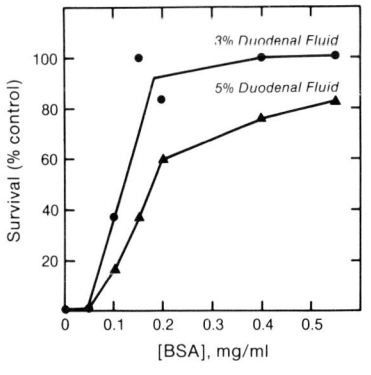

Fig. 3. Bovine serum albumin (BSA) protects human-source *Giardia* from killing by duodenal fluid. Parasites were incubated with 3% and 5% duodenal fluid for 2 h in the presence of different concentrations of BSA. After 2 h of incubation, the killing was arrested and assayed as described (Gillin et al., 1983b).

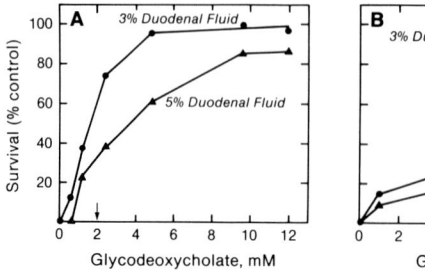

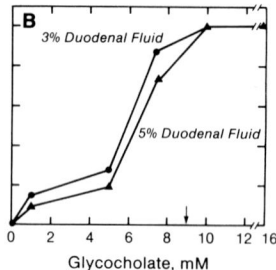

Fig. 4. Bile salts protect human-source *Giardia* from killing by duodenal fluid. Parasites were incubated with 3% and 5% duodenal fluid for 2 h in the presence of different concentrations of glycodeoxycholate (A) or glycocholate (B). After 2 h of incubation the killing was arrested by addition of complete growth medium and assayed. The arrows indicate the CMC of each bile salt.

1982). Carboxyl ester hydrolase is closely related to bile salt stimulated lipase (Blackberg et al., 1981), which is responsible for the bile salt-dependent killing of *Giardia* by human milk.

The concentrations of lipolytic products in intestinal fluid depend upon the relative rates of their production and absorption, modified by the net rates of water adsorption and excretion (Davenport, 1977). Both of these parameters might be affected by the parasite. For example, pancreatic lipase has been reported to be inhibited by *Giardia* trophozoite extracts (Smith et al., 1981) and increased water secretion in the upper intestine during diarrhea might dilute many components of the fluid, including toxic factors.

In this context, DF samples from patients with giardiasis did not appear defective in killing activity. The LD_{50} of DF from a patient with active giardiasis (of >3 years' duration) was 5.4%, and 1.8 and 2.8% for DF from two subjects with recent episodes of giardiasis (not shown). These results do not differ significantly from the range for noninfected subjects (Das et al., 1988).

Our observation that other factors in the intestinal environment protect *Giardia* from DF and from milk may help to explain parasite survival in the presence of high

TABLE 6

Intestinal mucus protects human-source *Giardia* from killing by duodenal fluid

Duodenal fluid concentration (%, v/v)	Mucus concentration (μg protein/ml)				
	0	24	49	98	196
			Survival, % control		
1.0	<0.1	68.7*	69.9*	74.1*	78.0*
3.0	<0.1	<0.1	<0.01	77.7*	82.7*
5.0	<0.1	<0.1	<0.1	78.3*	80.9*

* $P < 0.001$, significant protection.

concentrations of lipases and their products. The fact that BSA, bile salts and mucus, all bind fatty acids and other products of lipolysis strongly supports the idea that killing is due to lipolytic products.

Individual conjugated bile salts at concentrations above their CMC protect human *Giardia* from killing by human milk (Gillin, 1987) and by oleic acid (Reiner et al., 1986). Moreover, human gall bladder bile protected from killing by milk (Gillin, 1987). A contradictory report that whole bovine bile *potentiated* killing by unsaturated fatty acids was probably confounded by the presence of unconjugated bile acids in the crude bovine bile preparations (Rohrer et al., 1986). Unconjugated bile acids, which are characteristically present in the lower gut (Hofmann and Roda, 1984), are highly toxic to *Giardia* (Gillin, 1987), in contrast to the conjugated bile acids in human bile. In man, total bile salt concentrations vary from $\sim$2.5 to >20 mM (Sjovall, 1959) and could, therefore, protect these organisms from lipolytic products depending upon their local concentrations.

In vivo, *Giardia* trophozoites must penetrate the viscous mucus gel in order to attach to the underlying epithelium. Mucus fragments are also sloughed into the intestinal lumen. Our observations of active trophozoites associated with mucus strands in intestinal aspirates while ghosts tend to be in the clear fluid phase, suggest that our findings are not in vitro artifacts. We showed earlier that human intestinal mucus protects *Giardia* from killing by human milk (Zenian and Gillin, 1987) and also by oleic acid (Reiner et al., 1986).

Thus, bile salts and intestinal mucus may help explain the specific colonization of the small intestine by promoting survival of *Giardia* in the presence of toxic lipolytic products generated in intestinal fluid. Local variations in the concentrations of bile salts and mucus, as opposed to milk and pancreatic lipases and their products, may influence the variability in symptoms and duration of giardiasis.

Acknowledgements

This work was supported by grants AI 19863 and AM 35108 from the National Institutes of Health. We are grateful to Dr J. Isenberg for his generous support and helpful discussions and to Ms S. McFarlin for preparing the manuscript.

References

Badwey, J.A., Curnutte, J.T., Robinson, J.M., Berde, C.B., Karnovsky, M.J. and Karnovsky, M.L. (1984) Effects of free fatty acids on release of superoxide and on change of shape by human neutrophils. J. Biol. Chem. 259, 7870-7877.

Bitman, J., Wood, D.L., Mehta, N.R., Hamosh, P. and Hamosh, M. (1983) Lipolysis of triglycerides of human milk during storage at low temperatures: a note of caution. J. Pediatr. Gastroenterol. Nutr. 2, 521-524.

Blackberg, L., Lombardo, D., Hernell, O., Guy, O. and Olivecrona, T. (1981) Bile salt-stimulated lipase in human milk and carboxyl ester hydrolase in pancreatic juice. Are they identical enzymes? FEBS Lett. 136, 284-288.

Clamp, J.R. and Creeth, J.M. (1984) Some non-mucin components of mucus and their possible biological roles. Ciba Foundation Symposium 109, Pitman, London, pp. 121-136.

Craun, G.F. (1984) Waterborne outbreaks of giardiasis. In: S.L. Erlandsen and E.A. Meyer, (Eds.), *Giardia and Giardiasis: Biology, Pathogenesis, and Epidemiology*, pp. 243-261. Plenum Press, New York.

Das, S., Reiner, D.S., Zenian, J., Hogan, D.L., Koss, M.A., Wang, C-S. and Gillin, F.D. (1988) Killing of *Giardia lamblia* trophozoites by human intestinal fluid in vitro. J. Infect. Dis., 157, 1257–1260.

Davenport, H.W. (1977) Physiology of the Digestive Tract. Year Book Medical Publishers, Chicago.

Gillin, F.D. (1987) *Giardia lamblia*: the role of conjugated and unconjugated bile salts in killing by human milk. Exp. Parasitol. 63, 74-83.

Gillin, F.D., Reiner, D.S. and Wang, C.-S. (1983a) Human milk kills parasitic intestinal protozoa. Science 221, 1290-1292.

Gillin, F.D., Reiner, D.S. and Wang, C.-S. (1983b) Killing of *Giardia lamblia* trophozoites by normal human milk. J. Cell. Biochem. 23, 47-56.

Gillin, F.D., Reiner, D.S. and Gault, M.J. (1985) Cholate-dependent killing of *Giardia lamblia* by human milk. Infect. Immun. 47, 619-622.

Hernell, O., Ward, H., Blackberg, L. and Pereira, M.E.A. (1986) Killing of *Giardia lamblia* by human milk lipases: an effect mediated by lipolysis of milk lipids. J. Infect. Dis. 153, 715-720.

Hernell, O., Blackberg, L. and Olivecrona, T. (1981) Human milk lipases, In: E. Lebenthal (Ed.), Textbook of Gastroenterology and Nutrition in Infancy. Vol. 1, pp. 347-354. Raven Press, N.Y.

Hofmann, A.F. and Roda, A. (1984) Physicochemical properties of bile acids and their relationship to biological properties: an overview of the problem. J. Lipid Res. 25, 1477-1489.

Jensen, R.G., Clark, R.M., deJong, F.A., Hamosh, M., Liao, T.H. and Mehta, N.R. (1982) The lipolytic triad: human lingual, breast milk and pancreatic lipases: physiological implications of their characteristics in digestion of dietary fats. J. Ped. Gastroenterol. Nutr. 1, 243-255.

Kabara, J. (1980) Lipids as host-resistance factors of human milk. Nutr. Rev. 38, 65-73.

McNabb, P.C. and Tomasi, T.B. (1981) Host defense mechanisms at mucosal surfaces. Ann. Rev. Microbiol. 35, 477-496.

Morecki, R. and Parker, J.G. (1967) Ultrastructural studies of the human *Giardia lamblia* and subjacent jejunal mucosa in a subject with steatorrhea. Gastroenterology 52, 151-164.

Nash, T.E., Herrington, D.A., Losonsky, G.A. and Levine, M.M. (1987) Experimental human infections with *Giardia lamblia*. J. Infect. Dis. 156, 974-984.

Patton, S. and Jensen, R.G. (1976) Biomedical aspects of lactation with special reference to lipid metabolism and membrane functions of the mammary gland. Pergamon Press, Oxford.

Reiner, D.S., Gillin, F.D. and Zenian, A. (1984) Lethal effects of fatty acids on *Giardia lamblia* and *Entamoeba histolytica* and protection by mucus. Am. Soc. Trop. Med. Hyg., Abstract No. 144.

Reiner, D.S., Wang, C.-S. and Gillin, F.D. (1986) Human milk kills *Giardia lamblia* by generating toxic lipolytic products. J. Infect. Dis. 154, 825-831.

Roda, A., Hofmann, A.F. and Mysels, K.J. (1983) The influence of bile salt structure of self-association in aqueous solutions. J. Biol. Chem. 258, 6362-6370.

Rohrer, L., Winterhalter, K.H., Eckert, J. and Kohler, P. (1986) Killing of *Giardia lamblia* by human milk is mediated by unsaturated fatty acids. Antimicrob. Agents Chemother. 30, 254-257.

Simon, G.L. and Gorbach, S.L. (1981) Intestinal flora in health and disease. In: L.R. Johnson (Ed.), Physiology of the Gastrointestinal Tract, Vol. 2, pp. 1361-1380. Raven Press, New York.

Sjovall, J. (1959) On the concentration of bile acids in the human intestine during absorption. Acta Physiol. Scand. 46, 339-345.

Smith, P.D., Horsburgh Jr., C.R. and Brown, W.R. (1981) In vitro studies on bile acid deconjugation and lipolysis inhibition by *Giardia lamblia*. Digest. Dis. Sci. 26, 700-704.

Wolfe, M.S. (1984) Symptomatology, diagnosis, and treatment. In: S.L. Erlandsen and E.A. Meyer, (Eds.), Giardia and Giardiasis: Biology, Pathogenesis, and Epidemiology, pp. 147-162. Plenum Press, New York.

Zenian, A.J. and Gillin, F.D. (1987) Intestinal mucus protects *Giardia lamblia* from killing by human milk. J. Protozool. 34, 22-26.

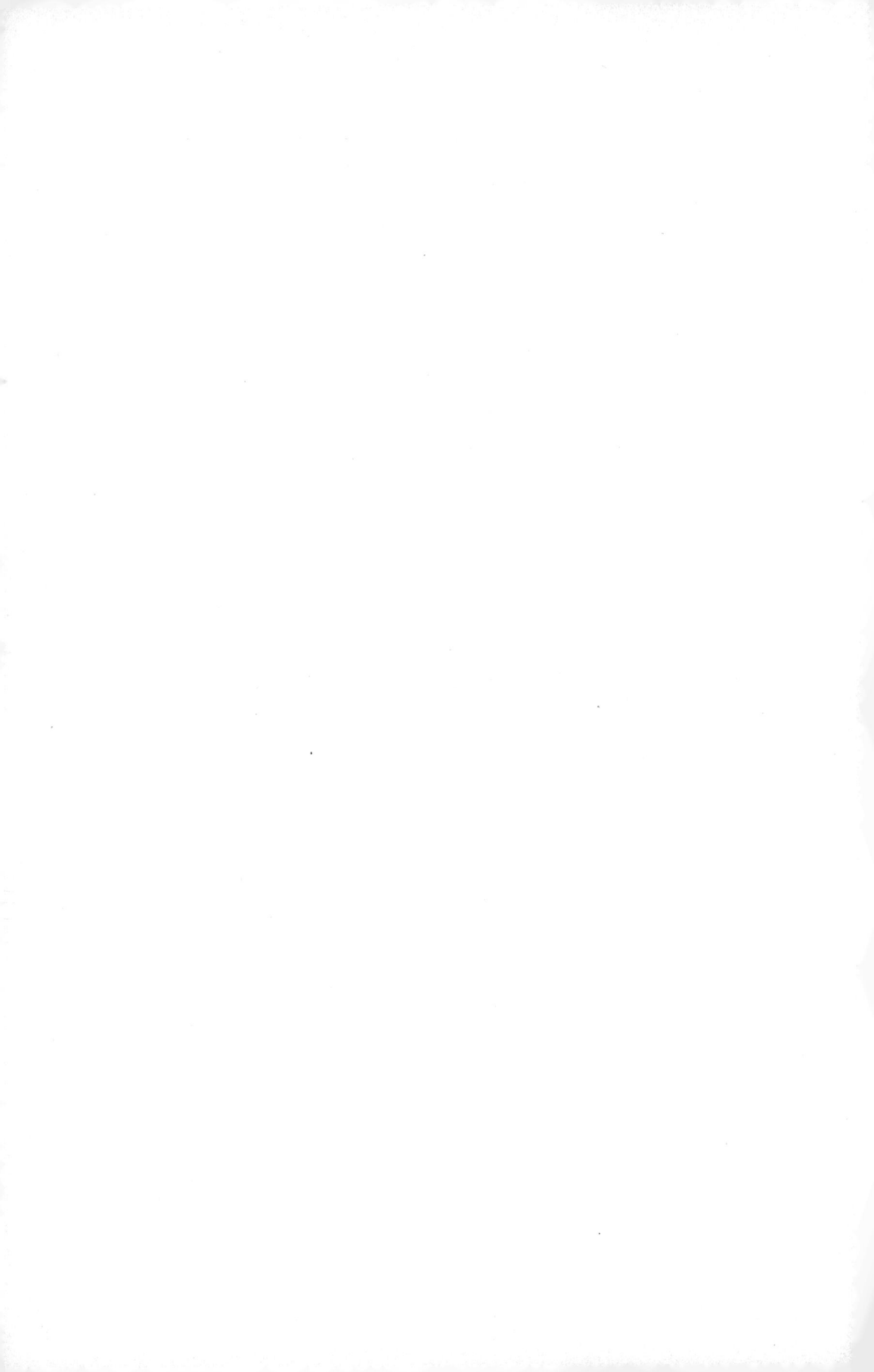

13

The role of immunity in *Giardia* infections

EDWARD N. JANOFF[1] and PHILLIP D. SMITH[2]

[1]*Infectious Disease Section, Department of Medicine, Veterans Administration Medical Center, Minneapolis, Minnesota, U.S.A. and Division of Infectious Diseases, Department of Medicine, University of Minnesota School of Medicine, Minneapolis, Minnesota, U.S.A. and* [2]*Cellular Immunology Section, Laboratory of Immunology, National Institute of Dental Research, National Institutes of Health, Bethesda, Maryland, U.S.A.*

1. Introduction	215
2. Epidemiologic perspectives	216
3. Cellular immune responses	218
4. Humoral immune responses in experimental studies	220
5. Humoral immune responses in clinical studies	221
6. *Giardia* antigens	225
7. Role of immune response in determining the course of infection	226
References	228

1. Introduction

In the classic experimental studies of Rendtorff in the 1950s, all human volunteers exposed to large doses of *Giardia* became infected, but none became ill (Rendtorff, 1954). In more natural settings, the majority of subjects in some waterborne outbreaks of giardiasis became symptomatic (Barbour et al., 1976), whereas in other outbreaks only a limited number developed symptoms (Lopez et al., 1980). Among those persons infected with *Giardia*, some experience diarrhea, malabsorption, weight loss, and abdominal pain (Wolfe, 1979; Hartong et al., 1979) but many, particularly those in developing countries, are asymptomatic (Chavalittamrong et al., 1978; Gilman et al., 1988; Islam et al., 1983; Joe et al., 1966; Zaki et al., 1986). To date, no unifying hypothesis has emerged to explain these inconsistent features of *Giardia* infections.

Convincing evidence accumulated during the past decade has confirmed that *Giardia* elicits an immune response that likely contributes to the variable human host response to the parasite. The presence of an immune response was initially suggested by epidemiologic studies that revealed a reduced incidence of symptomatic infections in persons repeatedly exposed to the parasite (Moore et al., 1969; Istre et al., 1984). Subsequent investigations in experimental animals and humans identified humoral and cellular components of host immunity to *Giardia*. Recent studies in each of these areas provide exciting new insights into the host response to this usually noninvasive parasite. Thus, the aim of this chapter is to integrate the epidemiology, immunology, and clinical features of giardiasis into a unified theory of the host response to *Giardia*.

2. Epidemiologic perspectives

Epidemiologic investigations of giardiasis in developed countries reveal that persons exposed to *Giardia* fall into two clinical categories of infection: symptomatic and asymptomatic. Regarding symptomatic giardiasis, many population studies indicate that persons episodically exposed to the parasite are far more likely to have symptoms. Such persons include travelers to certain locales (Brodsky et al., 1974; Steffen et al., 1987), backpackers (Barbour et al., 1976), expatriates (Speelman and Ljungstrom, 1986), case contacts, visitors to Colorado mountain towns (Istre et al., 1984; Moore et al., 1969), and persons exposed during waterborne outbreaks of the parasite (Lopez et al., 1980; Istre et al., 1984). In contrast, persons with recurrent or chronic exposure to the parasite are commonly asymptomatic. These persons include homosexual men (Phillips et al., 1981; William et al., 1978), toddlers in day-care centers (Black et al., 1977; Pickering et al., 1984), and long-term residents of Colorado mountain towns (Istre et al., 1984).

Similar to persons in developed countries with chronic or recurrent exposure who are commonly asymptomatic, persons infected with *Giardia* in developing countries also are usually asymptomatic (Chavalittamrong et al., 1978; Gilman et al., 1988; Islam et al., 1983; Zaki et al., 1986; Areekul and Viravan, 1986; Nacapunchai et al., 1986). Exposure to the parasite begins early in life (Zaki et al., 1986; Gilman et al., 1985; Hossain et al., 1983; Joe et al., 1966; Islam et al., 1983), high rates of carriage are present in all age groups (Zaki et al., 1986; Janoff et al., 1990), and asymptomatic reinfection occurs at a high rate (Gilman et al., 1988). In Egypt, for example, *Giardia* is detected more frequently in healthy subjects than in age-matched persons with diarrhea (Zaki et al., 1986), suggesting that high rates of exposure to and carriage of *Giardia* are associated with low rates of parasite-associated illness.

What factors explain this divergent response to *Giardia*? Symptomatic and asymptomatic infections may result from the interaction of three different aspects of the host-parasite biology of giardiasis. First, local intestinal conditions that are conducive to growth of *Giardia* may vary between individuals. As discussed in the preceding chapter, bile salts enhance the growth of *Giardia* in vitro (Keister, 1983; Farthing et al., 1985), but specific bile salts may enhance killing of *Giardia* by milk. Intestinal mucus (Gault et al., 1987; Zenian and Gillin, 1987) and possibly the presence of other intestinal organisms such as *Candida albicans* may enhance parasite growth and protect against killing. *Candida* or yeast extract is generally required for growth of *Giardia* in vitro (Meyer and Radulescu, 1984), and antibodies to *Candida* may be elevated in persons infected with *Giardia* (Haralabdis, 1984a), although an increased incidence of intestinal colonization with *Candida* is not well documented. Alternatively, some patients with giardiasis and malabsorption show bacterial colonization of the small bowel (Tomkins et al., 1978; Tandon et al., 1977), which may predispose *Giardia* to express virulence factors, similar to those proposed for *Entamoeba histolytica* (Mirelman, 1987).

Second, variability in the clinical response of the host to infection with *Giardia* may be due, in part, to differences in the pathogenicity of various strains of the parasite. Variation in the host response to different strains has been identified in both humans (Nash et al., 1987) and animals (Aggarwal and Nash, 1987). Regarding the former, none of five volunteers given trophozoites of one strain became infected or ill, whereas each of 10 volunteers given another strain of *Giardia* became infected, and 5 became ill (Nash et al., 1987). Clinically, high rates of asymptomatic infection among homosexual men (William et al., 1978) and day-care center toddlers (Black et al., 1977; Pickering et al., 1984), in contrast to low rates among other groups, may reflect strain differences. Investigating strain differences in animals, Aggarwal and Nash have shown that gerbils challenged with two distinct strains of *Giardia* clear the parasites at different rates (Aggarwal and Nash, 1987). However, both symptomatic and asymptomatic infections may follow common source exposures such as waterborne outbreaks (Lopez et al., 1980; Birkhead et al., 1989). In addition, only some household contacts may become ill with *Giardia* transmitted from asymptomatic day-care center toddlers (Polis et al., 1986; Janoff, personal observation). Moreover, some travelers, but not all, to an endemic region may become ill with giardiasis (Steffen et al., 1987). Thus, strain differences only partly explain the variable host response to the parasite.

The variable pathogenicity among strains of *Giardia* suggested by the above studies may reflect differences in certain parasite antigens. In a series of elegant experiments, Adam and his colleagues showed that cloned *Giardia* WB strain trophozoites expressed a cysteine-rich 170 kDa surface antigen (Adam et al., 1988). This antigen was absent from progeny of the clone surviving in vitro cultivation with a cytotoxic monoclonal antibody specific for the protein. This in vitro demonstration of antigenic variation, both spontaneous and in response to immunologic selection, suggests a possible mechanism by which *Giardia* survives chronically in the intestine, despite the presence of an active immune response (Smith et al., 1982b).

The third feature of the host-parasite relationship that may influence the clinical response of the host to infection with *Giardia* is the host immune response, which is described in detail below. Immunity to *Giardia* may be particularly important in recurrently exposed persons who, though often infected, are infrequently ill. For example, in Bangladesh, symptoms are reported to occur in 86% of infants newly infected with *Giardia* but in only 4% of infected mothers (Islam et al., 1983). Similarly, in

Thailand most school children and adults, who are repeatedly exposed to *Giardia*, are asymptomatic (Chavalittamrong et al., 1978; Areekul and Viravan, 1986). Thus, subjects in these and other developing countries are usually asymptomatic and have high levels of parasite-specific antibody (Hossain et al., 1983; Gilman et al., 1985; Nacapunchai et al., 1986; Miotti et al., 1986; Janoff et al., 1990). A parallel finding in healthy homosexual men is the high frequency of asymptomatic infection in association with increased levels of *Giardia*-specific antibody (Janoff et al., 1988a). In contrast, hypogammaglobulinemic subjects are commonly symptomatic when infected with *Giardia* and have no antibody to the parasite (Visvesvara et al., 1980). A closer examination of the components of the immune response to *Giardia* should provide insight into the role of immunity in the host response to this parasite.

3. Cellular immune responses

Because the cellular immune responses to *Giardia* occur at the level of the intestinal mucosa, it is important to appreciate the spectrum of mucosal inflammatory changes that may accompany giardiasis. In the mouse, trophozoites colonize the proximal small intestine (Gillon et al., 1982; Owen et al., 1979), attaching to the mucosa preferentially near the bases of villi, at the edges of Peyer's patch follicles, and less frequently on villous tips (Owen et al., 1979). Although *Giardia* may be taken up by the specialized membranous 'M' cells overlying Peyer's patches, trophozoites appear not to attach preferentially to these cells, whose function is to transport luminal antigens and microorganisms to the underlying lymphoid cells (Owen et al., 1979). Infrequently, trophozoites may invade the mucosal epithelium and penetrate the lamina propria (Brandborg et al., 1967; Morecki and Parker, 1967; Saha and Gosh, 1977), possibly coming into direct contact with lymphoid cells. However, the frequency of tissue invasion is unknown, because intestinal biopsies are not routinely performed in persons with giardiasis.

Although the mucosal histology of the proximal small intestine of persons infected with *Giardia* is frequently normal, varying degrees of histological change have been observed during giardiasis. The histological changes include infiltration of polymorphonuclear leukocytes into the epithelium and mononuclear leukocytes into the lamina propria, development of shortened villi, loss of the brush border, damage to epithelial cells, and an increase in epithelial cell mitosis (Hoskins et al., 1967; Wright and Tomkins, 1978; Duncombe et al., 1978). Rarely, infection with *Giardia* may be associated with total villous atrophy, dense mononuclear cell infiltration, and flattening of the epithelial cells, changes that resemble celiac sprue (Levinson and Nastro, 1978; Takano and Yardley, 1964; Yardley et al., 1964). These findings indicate that the parasite is capable of eliciting an inflammatory cell response, albeit of varying degree, in infected subjects.

The accumulation of inflammatory cells in the small intestinal mucosa of infected persons suggests that cellular responses may contribute to the host response to *Giardia*.

In this regard, the presence of recurrent giardiasis in some patients with high titers of antitrophozoite antibodies (Smith et al., 1982) supports the notion that circulating antibodies alone are not protective against the parasite. Indeed, investigations using an experimental animal model of giardiasis (Roberts-Thomson et al., 1976a) provide evidence that lymphoid cells, particularly T lymphocytes, contribute to host responses to the parasite. In athymic mice, which are deficient in both circulating T lymphocytes and Peyer's patch helper T lymphocytes (Heyworth et al., 1985), inoculation with *G. muris* cysts results in chronic infection with large numbers of trophozoites (Boorman et al., 1973; Stevens et al., 1978; Roberts-Thomson and Mitchell, 1978). In contrast, immunocompetent mice clear the parasite and may develop resistance to reinfection (Roberts-Thomson et al., 1976a,b), implicating a role for T lymphocytes in the pathogenesis of chronic *G. muris* infection. Strengthening this conclusion are the observations that thymus implantation or reconstitution with syngeneic lymphoid cells from thymus-intact mice causes a progressive reduction in the number of *Giardia* in the infected animals (Boorman et al., 1973; Roberts-Thomson and Mitchell, 1978). This reduction is accelerated when the reconstituted lymphoid cells are from thymus-intact mice previously infected with *Giardia* (Roberts-Thomson and Mitchell, 1978).

Based on evidence from the studies of *G. muris* infection in athymic mice, the role of T lymphocytes in the host response to *Giardia* has been investigated in normal mice. During infection with *G. muris*, the number of Peyer's patch lymphocytes may double, although the ratio of T helper to T suppressor lymphocytes (>5:1) does not change (Clark and Holberton, 1986). When these mice are depleted of T helper cells they develop chronic infection, whereas mice depleted of T suppressor cells or deficient in natural killer cells clear their infection (Heyworth et al., 1986, 1987), indicating that T helper cells may play an important role in the ability of the murine host to clear *Giardia*. Recently, T helper cells were reported to contribute, possibly as 'switch' cells, to the sequential change in Peyer's patch B cells from IgM-bearing during the first week of infection to IgA-bearing B cells during the second week of infection (Clark and Holberton, 1986). Although intriguing, the role of T helper cells in the local immune response to *G. muris* remains speculative at this time.

At the level of the intestinal mucosa, the host response to *Giardia* is initiated by the presentation of parasite antigen to T lymphocytes. Recent in vitro studies of murine, rabbit and human macrophages confirm that macrophages are capable of phagocytosing *Giardia* trophozoites (Radulescu and Meyer, 1981; Owen et al., 1981; Smith, 1985). The ability of the parasite to invade the intestinal mucosa, and the presence of macrophages in the lamina propria, would facilitate contact between the parasite and antigen-presenting cells. In addition to antigen presentation, effector cell function by monocytes-macrophages contributes to host defense mechanisms against many pathogens. In this regard, three reports indicate that human mononuclear phagocytes are capable of killing *Giardia* (Smith et al., 1982, 1984; Hill and Pearson, 1987), possibly by the products of oxidative metabolism (Hill and Pearson, 1987). Although another report has not confirmed these findings (Aggarwal and Nash, 1986), the ability of resident macrophages and local blood monocytes in the lamina propria to kill *Giardia* could provide an important mechanism of defense against invading trophozoites.

4. Humoral immune responses in experimental studies

The studies mentioned above implicate a protective role for antibody in giardiasis. Indeed, cellular mechanisms likely contribute to the regulation of the humoral response to infection with *Giardia* in mice. Several strains of mice demonstrate clear resistance to reinfection after clearing a primary *Giardia* infection (e.g., BALB/c, DBA/2, and A/J) (Roberts-Thomson and Mitchell, 1978). The protection, at least in BALB/c mice, is T-cell-dependent (Roberts-Thomson and Mitchell, 1978), and specifically L3T4 (helper/inducer) T-cell-dependent (Heyworth et al., 1987). The latter cells regulate both systemic and intestinal humoral antibody responses (Carlson et al., 1986a,b; Kawanishi et al., 1983). T-cell-deficient mice have prolonged carriage of the organism and fail to produce local antibody. Although intestinal anti-trophozoite antibodies of the IgA isotype appear to have a protective role against *G. muris* in mice (Snyder et al., 1986), the role of antibody (or its absence) in facilitating chronic giardiasis in T-cell-deficient mice is currently under investigation. Preliminary evidence indicates that *Giardia* isolated from the intestine of nude mice contain slightly less surface Ig than those isolated from immunocompetent mice (Heyworth, 1986), but the significance of this observation awaits elucidation.

Snyder and colleagues (Snyder et al., 1985) have corroborated clinical observations of giardiasis in hypogammaglobulinemic patients with a murine model in which mice treated with anti-IgM antibodies develop immunoglobulin deficiency and chronic *G. muris* infection. The inability of immune serum to transfer protection to naive mice (Roberts-Thomson and Mitchell, 1978; Andrews and Hewlett, 1981; Underdown et al., 1981) is consistent with antibody protection occurring at the level of the intestinal mucosa and/or lumen, where antibody transferred in serum likely would have little effect. Here, antibody protection could involve a direct cytotoxic effect, complement-mediated lysis, or opsonization to augment effector cell killing. Regarding a direct cytotoxic mechanism, immune serum (Hill et al., 1984), immune milk (Andrews and Hewlitt, 1981; Underdown et al., 1981), and monoclonal antibodies (Nash and Aggarwal, 1986) have been shown to kill *Giardia* trophozoites. In experimentally infected mice, the secretion of *Giardia*-specific IgA antibodies is associated with parasite clearance (Snyder et al., 1985). Anti-parasite IgM antibodies, which we and others have identified in persons with symptomatic giardiasis (Goka et al., 1986; Nash et al., 1987; Janoff et al., 1988a), are capable of sensitizing *Giardia* in vitro for complement lysis by the classical pathway as well as by a unique pathway that requires C1 and factor B, but not C4 and C2 (Hill et al., 1984; Deguchi et al., 1987). Antibodies to *Giardia* also appear to augment cellular cytotoxic mechanisms. For example, cytotoxic activity for the parasite by mononuclear and polymorphonuclear phagocytes, which contain surface Fc receptors, is augmented by immune serum (Smith et al., 1983; Kaplan et al., 1985; Hill and Pearson, 1987), supporting the original opsonization studies of Radulescu and Meyer in which hyperimmune rabbit serum enhanced phagocytosis of *Giardia* by rabbit macrophages (Radulescu and Meyer, 1981).

5. Humoral immune responses in clinical studies

Most subjects infected with *Giardia* produce detectable levels of anti-parasite antibodies as noted above (see Epidemiologic Perspectives). However, the role of specific antibody to *Giardia* in determining the host's clinical response to infection has not been delineated. Is the presence of specific antibody more frequently associated with symptomatic *Giardia* infections or asymptomatic infections? Regarding the former, Ridley and Ridley (1976) found a strong correlation between the presence of malabsorption and of parasite-specific IgG antibodies, which were absent in asymptomatically infected subjects. However, using different antigens and antibody detection assays, other groups have failed to corroborate this observation (Visvesvara and Healley, 1979; Jokipii and Jokipii, 1982) (Table 1).

Regarding its role in asymptomatic infections, antibody may play a protective role in illness or serve as a marker of infection. Substantial epidemiologic data support a role for antibody in controlling or eradicating *Giardia* infections. First, populations in developing countries, where symptomatic *Giardia* infections are uncommon (Chavalittamrong et al., 1978; Gilman et al., 1988), show high levels of *Giardia*-specific antibody in serum (Gilman et al., 1985; Miotti et al., 1986; Janoff et al., 1990) and breast milk (Miotti et al., 1986; Nayak et al., 1987). Second, subjects with hypogammaglobulinemia have a high rate of chronic diarrhea, frequently due to *Giardia* (Ament and Rubin, 1972; Brown et al., 1972; Ajdukiewicz et al., 1972; Ament et al., 1973; Hermans et al., 1976; Hartong et al., 1979; Webster, 1980; LoGalbo et al., 1982; Hausser et al., 1983; Lederman et al., 1985) (Table 2). Among hypogammaglobulinemic subjects, *Giardia* is identified in up to 90% of those with chronic diarrhea, but only in approximately 10% of those without diarrhea (Table 2). Also, children with chronic diarrhea and giardiasis have an increased incidence of hypogammaglobulinemia (Perlmutter et al., 1985). Third, similar to the clinical response to infection of hypogammaglobulinemic patients, AIDS patients with giardiasis but without specific antibody often have acute symptomatic infections (Janoff et al., 1988a). In contrast, AIDS patients with giardiasis and with circulating *Giardia*-specific antibody appear to have symptoms unrelated to their infection with *Giardia*. These observations suggest a protective role for anti-trophozoite antibody in giardiasis.

Parasite-specific IgA may play a distinct role in defense against *Giardia*. IgA may be produced systemically or it may originate, in part, from local intestinal antibody production (Conley and Delacroix, 1987). In the murine model, intestinal IgA antibodies appear to be involved in parasite clearance (see Humoral Immune Responses in Experimental

TABLE 1
Prevalence of *Giardia*-specific antibodies

| Population | No. studied | Antigen/method | % Seropositive by antibody class ||| Ref. |
			Any	IgG	IgM	
Malabsorption with *Giardia*	36	Pre-cyst/IFA	91			Ridley et al., 1976
Malabsorption without *Giardia*	34		29			
Asymptomatic giardiasis	2		0			
Healthy subjects	17		0			
Malabsorption with *Giardia*	19	Cysts/IFA	95			Wright et al., 1977
Other enteric diseases	31		3			
Healthy controls 6	20		0			
Symptomatic giardiasis	20	Troph/IFA	95			Visvesvara et al., 1980
Healthy controls	19		0			
Acute giardiasis	12[a]	Troph/W. blot	92	92		Thorton et al., 1983
Healthy controls	10		20	20		
Acute giardiasis	18	Troph/IFA	100			Winiecka et al., 1984
Chronic giardiasis	52		50			
Asymptomatic giardiasis	10		70			
Healthy controls	40		13			
Asymptomatic giardiasis	92	Cysts/IFA	99	99		Haralabdis et al., 1984 (Greece)

Asymptomatic giardiasis	50	Troph/CF	36			Nacapunchai et al.,
		LIT	58			1986 (Thailand)
		IHA	30			
		ELISA	72			
Healthy controls	50	CF	12			
		LIT	40			
		IHA	8			
		ELISA	52			
Volunteers given:		Troph/ELISA				Nash et al., 1987
Giardia strain GS/M	10		100	60	100	70
Giardia strain Isr	5		0	0	0	0
Healthy adults	66	Troph/ELISA	9	6	2	2	Janoff et al., 1988
Acute giardiasis	27		89	67	41	78
Healthy homosexual men	20		55	50	5	25
AIDS patients with giardiasis	14		64	36	7	43

1. [a] Four immunocompromised persons are not included.
2. Adapted from (Janoff et al., 1988a). A positive test was defined as an optical density greater than the mean plus two deviations for the 66 immunocompetent control subjects.
3. Abbreviations: Troph – Trophozoite; W. Blot – Western Blot; ELISA – Enzyme-linked Immunosorbent Assay; IFA – immunofluorescent Antibody; CF – Complement Fixation; LIT – Lectin Immunotest; IHA – Indirect Hemagglutination.

Studies). In humans, an early study suggested that patients with symptomatic giardiasis had lower levels of intestinal IgA despite normal levels of serum IgA (Zinneman and Kaplan, 1972), but the methods of this study have been challenged and results have not been reproduced (Jones and Brown, 1974). A selective deficiency in IgA is not generally associated with higher rates or severity of enteric infections, perhaps due to compensatory increases in mucosal secretory IgM. In fact, rather than finding lower levels of total IgA among 27 subjects with symptomatic giardiasis in Denver, we found serum IgA levels were higher than in uninfected subjects, and no infected subject was IgA deficient (Janoff et al., 1988a). Nayak and colleagues have shown that protection of breast-fed Indian children against *Giardia* infection is dependent upon the presence of *Giardia*-specific IgA in breast milk (Nayak et al., 1987). In the intestine, IgA antibodies may modulate the local response to *Giardia* by inhibiting parasite adherence, tissue invasion, or, possibly, mucosal penetration of parasite antigens. Although in humans systemic IgA does not pass into the gut (Conley and Delacroix, 1987), parasite-specific IgA in serum may be the most sensitive indicator of infection. The most frequently identified isotype of anti-*Giardia* antibodies among acutely ill subjects with giardiasis is IgA (Table 2), also shown for persons exposed to an outbreak of waterborne giardiasis in Vermont (Birkhead et al., 1989) and villagers in Thailand (Janoff et al., 1990).

Antibodies to *Giardia* likely act in concert with cellular defense mechanisms. For example, cytotoxic activity for the parasite by mononuclear and polymorphonuclear phagocytes, which contain surface Fc receptors, is augmented by immune serum (Smith et al., 1983; Kaplan et al., 1985; Hill and Pearson, 1987), similar to the opsonization studies of Radulescu and Meyer noted above (Radulescu and Meyer, 1981). Thus, both cellular and humoral defense mechanisms likely contribute to the host response to *Giardia*, amplifying each other in a highly integrated manner to provide an extremely efficient mechanism for clearing this enteric pathogen.

TABLE 2

Prevalence of *Giardia* in persons with hypogammaglobulinemia

Persons with *G. lamblia* (%)		
Chronic diarrhea	No diarrhea	References
4/5 (80)		Brown et al., 1972
8/9 (89)	3/30 (10)	Ament et al., 1973
16/25 (64)	1/10 (10)	Hermans et al., 1976
7/16 (44) (adults)		Webster, 1980
1/5 (20) (children)		
10/30 (33)		Hausser et al., 1983
5/26 (19)		Perlmutter et al., 1985
2/10 (20)		Lederman and Winkelstein, 1985

* This table includes only population-based studies.

6. Giardia antigens

Several groups have investigated the antigenic determinants of *Giardia*. Smith and colleagues analyzed four geographically distinct human isolates cultivated in vitro (Smith et al., 1982a). Comparison of soluble antigens by sodium dodecyl sulfate-polyacrylamide gel electrophoresis (SDS-PAGE) preparations and immunoelectrophoresis (IEP) showed no significant differences between isolates. However, crossed IEP revealed an absence of one major antigen and several minor antigens in one or more isolates. Although enzyme-linked immunosorbent assay (ELISA) showed reproducibility of antigen detection between strains, variation among the four isolates was noted when 10 human sera from patients with acute *Giardia* infections were tested. These data suggested a humoral response directed to specific antigens and possibly antigenic variation between strains.

The location and composition of these antigens have been characterized by Nash and his colleagues (Nash et al., 1983). By radiolabeling axenized WB and Portland 1 (P-1) *Giardia* strains, these investigators showed that the antigens were cell-surface exposed proteins, the majority of which were released into the media as 'excretory-secretory products'. The proteins, a 'polydisperse' major accumulation in the 94-225 kDa range and a fairly consistent minor band at 16.5-21 kDa, could be precipitated by antisera from animals immunized with trophozoites of a homologous but not a heterologous strain. These studies suggest that individual *Giardia* isolates have similar molecular weight antigens that may be immunologically distinct.

Giardia antigens also were characterized by Einfeld and Stibbs (Einfeld and Stibbs, 1984) using the parallel techniques of crossed and rocket IEP and SDS-PAGE analysis as well as the same four *Giardia* isolates employed by Smith et al. (Smith et al., 1982a). This and other studies (Taylor and Wenman, 1987) identified a common 82 kDa protein that could be adsorbed with polyspecific and monospecific rabbit antisera. Whereas the 82 kDa antigen appears to be a group antigen of the four *Giardia* isolates tested, the antigens described by Nash and colleagues appeared similar to one another by molecular weight but were immunologically distinct. Nash and colleagues (Nash et al., 1985) also correlated the antigenic variation noted in the WB and P-1 strains with their DNA banding patterns produced by exposure of the DNA in 15 *Giardia* strains to restriction endonucleases and labeled DNA probes, supporting the concept that antigenic variation is a true genotypic expression and not a laboratory artifact.

Recently, Rosoff and Stibbs characterized a trophozoite-derived 65 kDa antigen in stools of patients with *Giardia* infections (Rosoff and Stibbs, 1986a,b). We have confirmed the presence of this 65 kDa antigen and have shown that it is recognized by sera from rabbits immunized with *Giardia* WB and P-1 strain trophozoites and with *Giardia* cysts, which were used for detection of *Giardia* antigens by crossed IEP and ELISA (Craft and Nelson, 1982; Janoff et al., 1989).

Significant progress also has been made in defining the antigens to which patients with *Giardia* infections respond. Edson and colleagues identified an 88 kDa surface protein which was recognized by sera from one patient following *Giardia* infection (Edson et al., 1986). No other surface antigens were described. In contrast, two groups of investigators have shown that several antigens are recognized by immune human sera. The immunodominant surface antigens identified in these studies migrated at 31 kDa and 30-34 kDa (Taylor and Wenman, 1987; Janoff et al., 1988a) and were the antigens most consistently recognized by persons with *Giardia*-specific antibody by ELISA (Janoff et al., 1988a). The reactivity of human sera with trophozoite antigens, particularly the common bands between 30 and 34 kDa, is shown in Fig. 1. These antigens, which most often appear as a doublet, may represent the disk cytoskeleton proteins referred to as 'giardin' by some investigators (Crossley and Holberton, 1983; Taylor and Wenman, 1987).

7. Role of immune response in determining the course of infection

In summary, we have described three features of the host-parasite relationship that may contribute to the variable clinical response to *Giardia* infections. These include the local intestinal environment, which may affect the growth of the organism; *Giardia* strains, which may reflect differences in pathogenicity; and mechanisms of the host immune response, which we have focused on in this chapter. How can these features and disparate elements of clinical and experimental data from human and animal models be reconciled into a unifying hypothesis?

When *Giardia* organisms enter the small intestine, local factors such as bile salts, intestinal mucus, or the presence of other organisms enhance or inhibit their initial growth. Intestinal enzymes, which may induce the expression of surface lectins that mediate mucosal adherence, facilitate colonization (Lev et al., 1986). Once infected, the individual may become ill, depending on the virulence of the strain or the presence of pre-existing immunity. In the absence of prior immunity, interaction of trophozoites with intestinal macrophages may initiate an immune response. This nonspecific interaction may eliminate the parasite via cytotoxic mechanisms, or macrophages may process trophozoite antigens leading to the induction of a specific antibody response. These antibodies may be directly cytotoxic for the parasite or promote antibody-dependent cytotoxicity with granulocytes, and possibly monocytes. This integrated immune response results in clearance of the organism and resolution of symptoms. However, how does this sequence of events explain the chronic, asymptomatic excretion of the parasite observed in recurrently exposed persons? Following the development of a specific immune response in the small intestine, antibodies, as have been described following cholera infection, may appear against yet to be described toxins from *Giardia*. Alternatively, cytotoxic antibodies directed to specific antigens, such as the cysteine-rich 170 kDa antigen, may induce subsets of the organism to mutate. These mutants may no longer bear the antigen and would therefore not be susceptible to antibody-dependent mechanisms of killing.

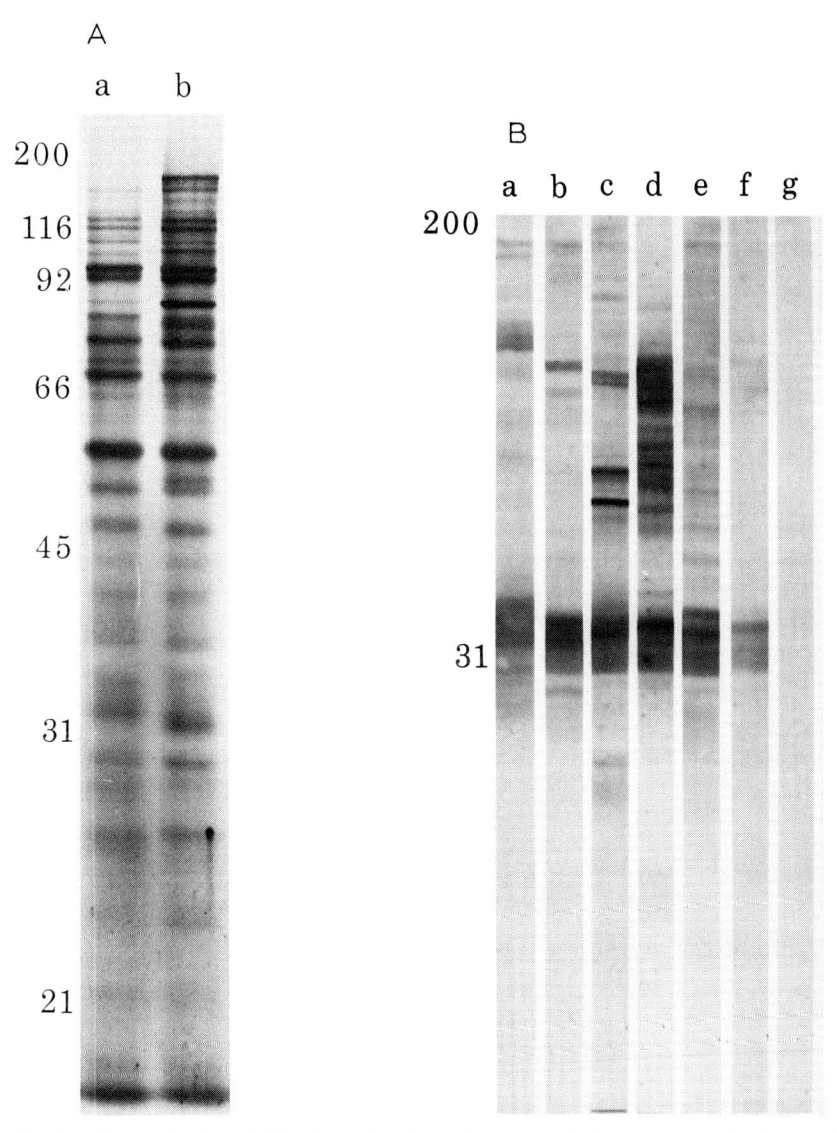

Fig. 1. Characterization of *Giardia* trophozoite antigens. A, gel electrophoresis showing whole WB strain trophozoites after (lane **a**) and before (lane **b**) being solubilized in a French pressure cell. The preparation in lane **a** was used in the immunoblotting and ELISA studies. Right, an immunoblot. After electrophoresis, the bands were electrophoretically transferred to nitrocellulose paper and reacted with sera from six patients with *Giardia* infection, three patients with AIDS (lanes **a-c**), three immunocompetent patients (lane **g**). Sera were diluted 1:50. The conjugate was horseradish peroxidase-conjugated *Staphylococcus aureus* protein A diluted 1:2000.

Recurrently exposed persons may therefore develop protective immunity to toxins or to pathogenic strains, thereby allowing chronic carriage of the organism without symptoms.

The above hypothesis is an attempt to integrate available information on the clinical and immunologic aspects of Giardia infections. However, many questions related to the host-parasite biology of Giardia remain. Is the intestinal environment in persons who develop clinical giardiasis different from that of persons who do not following similar exposure? What is the role of adherence and invasion in determining the establishment and clinical course of Giardia infections? Do trophozoites mutate in vivo? Is this mutation in response to antigen-specific antibody? What are the functionally important antigens? How are animal models relevant to understanding Giardia infections in man? Are intestinal phagocytic cells functionally active in the lumen of the intestine? How does Giardia cause illness?

An important consideration is whether efforts should be directed to vaccine development. Enteric disease is a major cause of morbidity and mortality among children in developing countries and, although most children in these areas appear to tolerate their Giardia infections well (Gilman et al., 1988), some chronic nutritional effects have been shown (Farthing et al., 1986b). However, children in developing countries are exposed to the parasite very early, when response to vaccine would be least effective. Immunocompromised patients, particularly those with hypogammaglobulinemia and AIDS, would likely respond poorly to vaccine (Janoff et al., 1988b), and these infections usually can be eradicated with available therapy. Vaccine development would be most beneficial for specific populations. These groups include persons likely to have infrequent, episodic exposure to Giardia, such as travelers and military personnel, who travel for limited stays to areas of high endemicity of Giardia. A rational basis for preventing these infections must be based on defining the mechanisms of the pathogenicity of and the immune response to Giardia.

References

Adam, R.D., Aggarwal, A., Lal, A.A., de la Cruz, V.F., McCutchan, T. and Nash, T.E. (1988) Antigenic variation of a cysteine-rich protein in Giardia lamblia. J. Exp. Med. 167, 109-118.
Aggarwal, A. and Nash, T.E. (1987) Comparison of two antigenically distinct Giardia lamblia isolates in gerbils. Am. J. Trop. Med. Hyg. 36, 325-332.
Aggarwal, A. and Nash, T.E. (1986) Lack of cellular cytotoxicity by human mononuclear cells to Giardia. J. Immunol. 136, 3486-3488.
Ajdukiewicz, A.B., Youngs, G.R. and Bouchier, I.A.D. (1972) Nodular lymphoid hyperplasia with hypogammaglobulinemia. Gut 13, 589-595.
Ament, M.E., Ochs, H.D. and Davis, D.D. (1973) Structure and function of the gastrointestinal tract in primary immunodeficiency syndromes: a study of 39 patients. Medicine 52, 227-248.
Ament, M.E. and Rubin, C.E. (1972) Relation of giardiasis to abnormal intestinal structure and function in gastrointestinal syndrome. Gastroenterology 62, 216-226.
Andrews, J.S., Jr. and Hewlett, E.L. (1981) Protection against infection with Giardia muris by milk containing antibody to Giardia. J. Infect. Dis. 143, 242-246.
Areekul, S. and Viravan, C. (1986) Prevalence of Giardia lamblia and its effect on hematological profile in asymptomatic school children. Southeast Asian J. Trop. Med. Publ. Hlth. 17, 96-100.

Barbour, A.G., Nichols, C.R. and Fukushima, T. (1976) An outbreak of giardiasis in a group of campers. Am. J. Trop. Med. Hyg. 25, 384-389.

Birkhead, G., Janoff, E.N., Vogt, R.L. and Smith, P.D.(1989) Elevated levels of immunoglobulin A to *Giardia lamblia* during a waterborne outbreak of gastroenteritis. G. Clin. Microbiol. 27, 1707-1710.

Black, R.E., Dykes, A.C., Sinclair, S.P. and Wells, J.G. (1977) Giardiasis in day-care centers: evidence of person-to-person transmission. Pediatrics 60, 486-491.

Boorman, G.A., Lina, P.H.C., Zurcher, C. and Nieuwerkerk, H.T.M. (1973) *Hexamita* and *Giardia* as a cause of mortality in congenitally thymus-less (nude) mice. Clin. Exp. Immunol. 15, 623-627.

Brandborg, L.L., Tankersley, C.B., Gottlieb, S. and Barancik, M. (1967) Histological demonstration of mucosal invasion by *Giardia lamblia* in man. Gastroenterology 52, 154-160.

Brodsky, R.E., Spencer, H.C., Jr. and Chultz, M.G. (1974) Giardiasis in American travelers to the Soviet Union. J. Infect. Dis. 130, 319-323.

Brown, W.R., Butterfield, D., Savage, D. and Tada, T. (1972) Clinical, microbiological, and immunological studies in patients with immunoglobulin deficiencies and gastrointestinal disorders. Gut. 13, 441-449.

Carlson, J.R., Heyworth, M.F. and Owen, R.L. (1986a) Response of Peyer's patch lymphocyte subsets to *Giardia muris* infection in BALB/c mice. I. T-cell subsets. Cell. Immunol. 97, 44-50.

Carlson, J.R., Heyworth, M.F. and Owen, R.L. (1986b) Response of Peyer's patch lymphocyte subsets to *Giardia muris* infection in BALB/c mice. II. B-cell subsets: enteric antigen exposure is associated with immunoglobulin isotype switching by Peyer's patch B cells. Cell. Immunol. 97, 51-58.

Chavalittamrong, B., Charoenvidhya, S., Tuchinda, P., Suntornpoch, V. and Chearskul, S. (1978) Prevalence of *Giardia lamblia* in children attending an out-patient department of Siriraj Hospital. Southeast Asian J. Trop. Med. Publ. Health 9, 51-54.

Clark, J.T. and Holberton, D.V. (1986) Plasma membrane isolated from *Giardia lamblia*: identification of membrane proteins. Eur. J. Cell Biol. 42, 200-206.

Conley, M.E. and Delacroix, D.L. (1987) Intravascular and mucosal immunoglobulin A: two separate but related systems of immune defense? Ann. Intern. Med. 106, 892-899.

Craft, J.C. and Nelson, J.D. (1982) Diagnosis of giardiasis by counterimmunoelectrophoresis of feces. J. Infect. Dis. 145, 499-504.

Crossley, R. and Holberton, D.V. (1983) Selective extraction with sarkosyl and repolymerization in vitro of cytoskeleton proteins from *Giardia*. J. Cell. Sci. 62, 419-438.

Deguchi, M., Gillin, F.D. and Gigli, I. (1987) Mechanism of killing of *Giardia lamblia* trophozoites by complement. J. Clin. Invest. 79, 1296-1302.

Duncombe, V.M., Bolin, T.D., Davis, A.E., Cummins, A.G. and Crouch, R.L. (1978) Histopathology in giardiasis: a correlation with diarrhea. Aust. NZJ Med. 8, 392-396.

Edson, C.M., Farthing, M.J.G., Thorley-Lawson, D.A. and Keusch, G.T. (1986) An 88 000 Mw *Giardia lamblia* surface protein which is immunogenic in humans. Infect. Immun. 54, 621-625.

Einfeld, D.A. and Stibbs, H.H. (1984) Identification and characterization of a major surface antigen of *Giardia lamblia*. Infect. Immun. 46, 377-383.

Farthing, M.J.G., Keusch, G.T., Carey, M.C. and Varon, S. (1985) Effects of bile and bile salts on growth and membrane lipid uptake by *Giardia lamblia*-possible implications for pathogenesis of intestinal disease. J. Clin. Invest. 76, 1727-1732.

Farthing, M.J.G., Pereira, M.E.A. and Keusch, G.T. (1986a) Description and characterization of a surface lectin from *Giardia lamblia*. Infect. Immun. 51, 661-667.

Farthing, M.J.G., Mata, L., Urrutia, J.J. and Kronmal, R.A. (1986b) Natural history of *Giardia* infection of infants and children in rural Guatemala and its impact on physical growth. Am. J. Clin. Nutr. 43, 395-405.

Gault, M.J., Gillin, F.D. and Zenian, A.J. (1987) *Giardia lamblia*: stimulation of growth by human intestinal mucus and epithelial cells in serum-free medium. Exp. Parasitol. 64, 29-37.

Gillon, J., Thamery, A.L. and Ferguson, A. (1982) Features of small intestinal pathology (epithelial cell kinetics, intraepithelial lymphocytes, disaccharidases) in primary *Giardia muris* infection. Gut 23, 498-506.

Gilman, R.H., Brown, K.H., Visvesvara, G.S., Mondal, G., Greenberg, B., Sack, R.B., Brandt, F. and Khan,

M.V. (1985) Epidemiology and serology of *Giardia lamblia* in a developing country: Bangladesh. Trans. R. Soc. Trop. Med. Hyg. 79, 469-473.

Gilman, R.H., Miranda, E., Marquis, G.S., Vestegui, M. and Martinez, H. (1988) Rapid reinfection by *Giardia lamblia* after treatment in a hyperendemic third world community. Lancet 1, 343-345.

Goka, A.K.J., Rolston, D.D.K., Mathan, V.I. and Farthing, M.J.G. (1986) Diagnosis of giardiasis by specific IgM antibody enzyme-linked immunosorbent assay. Lancet 2, 184-186.

Haralabdis, S.T. (1984a) Detection of antibodies against *Candida albicans* in *Giardia lamblia*-infected individuals. Acta Tropica 41, 303-304.

Haralabidis, S.T. (1984b) Immunodiagnosis of giardiasis by ELISA and studies on cross-reactivity between the anti-*Giardia lamblia* antibodies and some parasitic antigens and fractions. Ann. Trop. Med. Parasitol. 78, 295-300.

Hartong, W.A., Gourley, W.K. and Arvanitakis, C. (1979) Giardiasis: clinical spectrum and functional-structural abnormalities of the small intestinal mucosa. Gastroenterology 77, 61-69.

Hausser, C., Virelizier, J.L., Buriot, D., Griscelli, C. (1983) Common variable hypogammaglobulinemia in children. Clinical and immunologic observations in 30 patients. Am. J. Dis. Child. 137, 833-837.

Hermans, P.E., Diaz-buxo, J.C. and Stobo, J.D. (1976) Idiopathic late-onset immunoglobulin deficiency. Am. J. Med. 61, 221-237.

Heyworth, M.F. (1986) Antibody response to *Giardia muris* trophozoites in mouse intestine. Infect. Immun. 52, 568-571.

Heyworth, M.F., Kung, J.E. and Eriksson, E.C. (1986) Clearance of *Giardia muris* infection in mice deficient in natural killer cells. Infect. Immun. 54, 903-904.

Heyworth, M.F., Owen, R.L. and Jones, A.L. (1985) Comparison of leukocytes obtained from the intestinal lumen of *Giardia*-infected immunocompetent mice and nude mice. Gastroenterology 89, 1360-1365.

Heyworth, M.F., Carlson, J.R. and Ermak, T.H. (1987) Clearance of *Giardia muris* infection requires helper/inducer T lymphocytes. J. Exp. Med. 165, 1743-1798.

Hill, D.R., Burge, J.J. and Pearson, R.D. (1984) Susceptibility of *Giardia lamblia* trophozoites to the lethal effect of human serum. J. Immunol. 132, 2046-2052.

Hill, D.R. and Pearson, R.D. (1987) Ingestion of *Giardia lamblia* trophozoites by human mononuclear phagocytes. Infect. Immun. 55, 3155-3161.

Hoskins, L.C., Winawer, S.J., Broitman, S.A., Gottlieb, L.S. and Zamcheck, N. (1967) Clinical giardiasis and intestinal malabsorption. Gastroenterology 53, 265-279.

Hossain, M.M., Ljungstrom, I., Glass, R.I., Lundin, L., Stoll, B.J. and Huldt, G. (1983) Amoebiasis and giardiasis in Bangladesh: parasitological and serological studies. Trans. R. Soc. Trop. Med. Hyg. 77, 552-554.

Islam, A., Stoll, B.J., Ljungstrom, I., Biswas, J., Nazrul, H. and Huldt, G. (1983) *Giardia lamblia* infections in a cohort of Bangladeshi mothers and infants followed for one year. J. Pediatr. 102, 996-1000.

Istre, G.R., Dunlop, T.S., Gaspard, B. and Hopkins, R.S. (1984) Waterborne giardiasis at a mountain resort: evidence for acquired immunity. Am. J. Publ. Hlth. 74, 602-604.

Janoff, E.N., Smith, P.D. and Blaser, M.J. (1988a) Acute antibody responses to *Giardia lamblia* are depressed in patients with the acquired immunodeficiency syndrome. J. Infect. Dis. 157, 798-804.

Janoff, E.N., Douglas, J.M., Jr., Gabriel, M., Blaser, M.J., Davidson, A.J., Cohn, D.L. and Judson, F.N. (1988b) Class-specific antibody response to pneumococcal capsular polysaccharides in men with human immunodeficiency virus-1 infection. J. Infect. Dis. 158, 983–990.

Janoff, E.N., Taylor, D.N., Echeverria, P., Glode, M. and Blaser, M.J. (1990) *Giardia lamblia*-specific antibodies in healthy U.S. and Thai children. West. G. Med. 152, in press.

Janoff, E.N., Craft, J.C., Pickering, L.K., Novotny, T., Blaser, M.J., Knisley, C.V. and Reller, L.B. (1988c) Diagnosis of *Giardia lamblia* infections by detection of parasite-specific antigens. J. Clin. Microbiol. 27, 431–435.

Joe, L.K., Rukmono, B., Oemijati, S., Sahab, K., Newell, K.W., Hway, S.T. and Talogo, R.W. (1966) Diarrhoea among infants in a crowded area of Djakarta, Indonesia. Bull. WHO 34, 197-210.

Jokipii, A.M.M. and Jokipii, L. (1982) Serum IgG, IgA, IgM, and IgD in giardiasis: the most severely ill patients have little IgD. J. Infect. Dis. 5, 189-193.

Jones, E.G. and Brown, W.R. (1974) Serum and intestinal fluid immunoglobulins in patients with giardiasis. Am. J. Dig. Dis. 19, 791-796.

Kaplan, B.S., Uni, S., Aikawa, M. and Mahmoud, A.A.F. (1985) Effector mechanism of host resistance in murine giardiasis: specific IgG and IgA cell-mediated toxicity. J. Immunol. 134, 1975-1981.

Kawanishi, H., Saltzman, L.E. and Strober, W. (1983) Mechanisms regulating IgA class-specific immunoglobulin production in murine gut-associated lymphoid tissue. J. Exp. Med. 157, 433-450.

Keister, D.B. (1983) Axenic culture of *Giardia lamblia* in TY-S-33 medium supplemented with bile. Trans. R. Soc. Trop. Med. Hyg. 77, 487-488.

Knight, R. (1980) Epidemiology and transmission of giardiasis. Trans. R. Soc. Trop. Med. Hyg. 74, 433-436.

Lederman, H.M. and Winkelstein, J.A. (1985) X-linked agammaglobulinemia: an analysis of 96 patients. Medicine 64, 145-156.

Lev, B., Ward, H., Keusch, G.T. and Pereira, M.E.A. (1986) Lectin activation in *Giardia lamblia* by host protease. A novel host-parasite interaction. Science 232, 713.

Levinson, J.D. and Nastro, L.J. (1978) Giardiasis with total villous atrophy. Gastroenterology 74, 271-275.

LoGalbo, P.R., Sampson, H.A., Buckley, R.H. (1982) Symptomatic giardiasis in three patients with X-linked agammaglobulinemia. J. Pediatr. 101, 78-80.

Lopez, C.E., Dykes, A.C., Juranek, D.D., Sinclair, S.P., Conn, J.M., Christie, R.W., Lippy, E.C., Schulz, M.G. and Mires, M.H. (1980) Waterborne giardiasis: a community-wide outbreak of disease and high rate of asymptomatic infection. Am. J. Epidemiol. 112, 495-497.

Meyer, E.A. and Radulescu, S. (1984) In vitro cultivation of *Giardia* trophozoites. In: S.L. Erlandsen and E.A. Meyer (Eds.), *Giardia* and Giardiasis, pp. 99-108, Plenum Press, New York and London.

Miotti, P.G., Gilman, R.N., Santosham, M., Ryder, R.W. and Yolken, R.H. (1986) Age-related rate of seropositivity of antibody to *Giardia lamblia* in four diverse populations. J. Clin. Microbiol. 24, 972-975.

Mirelman, D. (1987) Ameba-bacterium relationship in amebiasis. Microbiol. Rev. 51, 272-284.

Moore, G.T., Cross, W.M., McGuire, D., et al. (1969) Epidemic giardiasis at a ski resort. N. Engl. J. Med. 281, 402-407.

Morecki, R. and Parker, J.G. (1967) Ultrastructural studies of the human *Giardia lamblia* and subjacent jejunal mucosa in a subject with steatorrhea. Gastroenterology 52, 151-164.

Nacapunchai, D., Tepmonkol, M., Tharavanij, S., Thammapalerd, N. and Subchareon, A. (1986) A comparative study of four methods for detecting antibody in asymptomatic giardiasis. Southeast Asian J. Trop. Med. Publ. Hlth. 17, 96-100.

Nash, T.E. and Aggarwal, A. (1986) Cytotoxicity of monoclonal antibodies to a subset of *Giardia* isolates. J. Immunol. 136, 2628-2632.

Nash, T.E., Gillin, F.D. and Smith, P.D. (1983) Excretory-secretory products of *Giardia lamblia*. J. Immunol. 131, 2004-2010.

Nash, T.E., Herrington, D.A., Losonsky, G.A. and Levine, M.M. (1987) Experimental human infections with *Giardia lamblia*. J. Infect. Dis. 156, 974-984.

Nash, T.E., McCutchan, T., Keister, D., Dame, J.B., Conrad, J.D. and Gillin, F.D. (1985) Restriction-endonuclease analysis of DNA from 15 *Giardia* isolates obtained from humans and animals. J. Infect. Dis. 152, 64-73.

Nayak, N., Ganguly, N.K., Walia, B.N.S., Wahi, V., Kanwar, S.S. and Mahajan, R.C. (1987) Specific secretory IgA in the milk of *Giardia lamblia*-infected and uninfected women. J. Infect. Dis. 155, 724-727.

Novotny, T., Hopkins, R., Shillam, P., Janoff, E.N. (1990) Prevalence of *Giardia lamblia* and risk factors for infection among children attending day-care facilities in Denver. Fuel. Health, REP. 1990, 105, in press.

Owen, R.L., Allen, C.L. and Stevens, D.P. (1981) Phagocytosis of *Giardia muris* by macrophages in Peyer's patch epithelium. Infect. Immun. 33, 591-601.

Owen, R.L., Nemanic, P.C. and Stevens, D.P. (1979) Ultrastructural observation in giardiasis in a murine model. I. Intestinal distribution, attachment, and relationship to the immune system of *Giardia muris*.

Gastroenterology 76, 757-769.

Perlmutter, D.H., Leichtner, A.M., Goldman, H. and Winter, H.S. (1985) Chronic diarrhea associated with hypogammaglobulinemia and enteropathy in infants and children. Dig. Dis. Sci. 30, 1149-1155.

Phillips, S.C., Mildvan, D., Williams, D.C., Gelb, A.M. and White, M.C. (1981) Sexual transmission of enteric protozoa and helminths in a venereal-disease clinic population. N. Engl. J. Med. 305, 603-606.

Pickering, L.K., Woodward, W.E. and DuPont, H.L. (1984) Occurrence of *Giardia lamblia* in children in day-care centers. J. Pediatr. 104, 522-526.

Polis, M.A., Tuazon, C.U., Alling, D.W. and Talmanis, E. (1986) Transmission of *Giardia lamblia* from a day care center to the community. Am. J. Publ. Hlth. 76, 1142-1144.

Radulescu, S. and Meyer, E.A. (1981) Opsonization in vitro of *Giardia lamblia* trophozoites. Infect. Immun. 32, 852-856.

Rendtorff, R.C. (1954) The experimental transmission of human intestinal protozoan parasites. II. *Giardia lamblia* cysts given in capsules. Am. J. Hyg. 59, 209-220.

Ridley, M.J. and Ridley, D.S. (1976) Serum antibodies and jejunal histology in giardiasis associated with malabsorption. J. Clin. Pathol. 29, 30-34.

Roberts-Thomson, I.C., Stevens, D.P., Mahmoud, A.A.F. and Warren, K.S. (1976a) Giardiasis in the mouse: an animal model. Gastroenterology 71, 57-71.

Roberts-Thomson, I.C., Stevens, D.P., Mahmoud, A.A.F. and Warren, K.S. (1976b) Acquired resistance to infection in an animal model of giardiasis. J. Immunol. 117, 2036-2037.

Roberts-Thomson, I.C. and Mitchell, G.G. (1978) Giardiasis in mice. I. Prolonged infections in certain mouse strains and hypothymic (nude) mice. Gastroenterology 75, 42-46.

Rosoff, J.D. and Stibbs, H.H. (1986a) Isolation and purification of a *Giardia lamblia*-specific stool antigen (GSA 65) useful in coprodiagnosis of giardiasis. J. Clin. Microbiol. 23, 905-910.

Rosoff, J.D. and Stibbs, H.H. (1986b) Physical and chemical characterization of a *Giardia lamblia*-specific antigen useful in the coprodiagnosis of giardiasis. J. Clin. Microbiol. 24, 1079-1083.

Saha, T.K. and Gosh, T.K. (1977) Invasion of small intestinal mucosa by *Giardia lamblia*. Gastroenterology 73, 402-405.

Smith, P.D. (1985) Pathophysiology and immunology of giardiasis. Ann. Rev. Med. 36, 295-307.

Smith, P.D., Elson, C.O., Keister, D.B. and Nash, T.E. (1982) Human host response to *Giardia lamblia*. I. Spontaneous killing by mononuclear leukocytes in vitro. J. Immunol. 128, 1371-1376.

Smith, P.D., Gillin, F.D., Brown, W.R. and Nash, T.E. (1981) IgG antibody to *Giardia lamblia* detected by enzyme-linked immunosorbent assay. Gastroenterology 80, 1476-1480.

Smith, P.D., Gillin, F.D., Kaushal, N.A. and Nash, T.E. (1982a) Antigenic analysis of *Giardia lamblia* from Afghanistan, Puerto Rico, Ecuador, and Oregon. Infect. Immun. 36, 714-719.

Smith, P.D., Gillin, F.D., Spira, W.M. and Nash, T.E. (1982b) Chronic giardiasis: studies on drug sensitivity, toxin production, and host immune response. Gastroenterology 83, 797-803.

Smith, P.D., Keister, D.B. and Elson, C.O. (1983) Human host response to *Giardia lamblia*: II. Antibody-dependent killing in vitro. Cell. Immunol. 82, 308-315.

Smith, P.D., Keister, D.B., Wahl, S.M. and Meltzer, M.S. (1984) Defective spontaneous but normal antibody-dependent cytotoxicity for an extracellular protozoan parasite, *Giardia lamblia*, by C3H/HeJ mouse macrophages. Cell. Immunol. 85, 244-251.

Snyder, D.P., Gordon, J., McDermott, M.R. and Underdown, B.J. (1985) Chronic *Giardia muris* infection in anti-IgM-treated mice. I. Analysis of immunoglobulin and parasite-specific antibody in normal and immunoglobulin-deficient animals. J. Immunol. 134, 4153-4162.

Snyder, D.P. and Underdown, B.J. (1986) Quantitative and temporal analyses of murine antibody response in serum and gut secretions to infection with *Giardia muris*. Infect. Immun. 52, 271-278.

Speelman, P. and Ljungstrom, I. (1986) Protozoal infections among expatriates in Bangladesh. Am. J. Trop. Med. Hyg. 35, 1140-1145.

Steffen, R., Rickenbach, M., Wilhelm, V., Helminger, A. and Shar, M. (1987) Health problems after travel to developing countries. J. Infect. Dis. 156, 84-91.

Stevens, D.A., Frank, D.P. and Mahmoud, A.A.F. (1978) Thymus dependency of host resistance to *Giardia muris* infection: studies in nude mice. J. Immunol. 120, 680-682.

Takano, J. and Yardley, J.H. (1964) Jejunal lesions in patients with giardiasis and malabsorption. An electron microscopic study. Bull. Johns Hopkins Hosp. 116, 413-469.

Tandon, B.N., Tandon, R.K., Satpathy, B.K. and Shriniwas (1977) Mechanism of malabsorption in giardiasis: a study of bacterial flora and bile salt deconjugation in upper jejunum. Gut 18, 176-181.

Taylor, G.D. and Wenman, W.M. (1987) Human immune response to *Giardia lamblia*. J. Infect. Dis. 155, 137-140.

Thornton, S.A., West, A.H., Du Pont, H.L., and Pickering, L.K. (1983) Comparison of methods for identification of *Giardia lamblia*. Am. G. Clin. Pathol. 80, 858–860.

Tomkins, A.M., Wright, S.G., Drasar, B.S. and James, W.P.T. (1978) Bacterial colonization of jejunal mucosa in giardiasis. Trans. R. Soc. Trop. Med. Hyg. 72, 33-36.

Underdown, B.J., Roberts-Thomson, I.C., Anders, R.F. and Mitchell, G.F. (1981) Giardiasis in mice: studies on the characteristics of chronic infection in C3H/He mice. J. Immunol. 126, 669-672.

Vinayak, V.K., Jain, P. and Naik, S.R. (1978) Demonstration of antibodies in giardiasis using the immunodiffusion technique with *Giardia* cysts as antigen. Ann. Trop. Med. Parasitol. 72, 581-582.

Visvesvara, G.S. and Healey, G.R. (1979) The possible use of an indirect immunofluorescent test using axenically grown *Giardia lamblia* antigens in diagnosing giardiasis. In: W. Jakubowski and J.C. Hoff (Eds.), Waterborne Transmission of Giardiasis. Environmental Protection Agency 600/9-79-001, pp. 53-63.

Visvesvara, G.S., Smith, P.D., Healy, G.R. and Brown, W.R. (1980) An immunofluorescence test to detect serum antibodies to *Giardia lamblia*. Ann. Intern. Med. 93, 802-805.

Webster, A.D.B. (1980) Giardiasis and immunodeficiency diseases. Trans. R. Soc. Trop. Med. Hyg. 74, 440-443.

William, D.C., Shookhoff, W.G., Feldman, M. and DeRamos, S.W. (1978) High rates of enteric protozoal infections in selected homosexual men attending a venereal disease clinic. Sex. Transm. Dis. 5, 155-157.

Winiecka, J., Kasprzak, W., Kociecka, W., Plotkowiak, J., Myjak, P. (1984) Serum antibodies to *Giardia intestinalis* detected by immunofluorescence using trophozoites as antigen. Tropenmed. Parasitol. 35, 20-22.

Wolfe, M.S. (1979) Giardiasis. Pediatr. Clin. N. Am. 26, 295-303.

Wright, S.G., Moody, A.H., Tomkins, A.M. and Ridley, D.S. (1977) Fluorescent antibody studies in giardiasis. Gut 18, A986.

Wright, S.G. and Tomkins, A.M. (1977) Quantification of the lymphocytic infiltration in jejunal epithelium in giardiasis. Clin. Exp. Immunol. 29, 408-412.

Wright, S.G. and Tomkins, A.M. (1978) Quantitative histology in giardiasis. J. Clin. Pathol. 31, 712-716.

Yardley, J.H., Takano, J. and Hendrix, T.R. (1964) Epithelial and other mucosal lesions of the jejunum in giardiasis. Jejunal biopsy studies. Bull. Johns Hopkins Hosp. 115, 389-406.

Zaki, A.M., DuPont, H.L., Elalmy, M.A., et al. (1986) The detection of enteropathogens in acute diarrhea in a family cohort population in rural Egypt. Am. J. Trop. Med. Hyg. 35, 1013-1022.

Zenian, A.J, and Gillin, F.D. (1987) Intestinal mucus protects *Giardia lamblia* from killing by human milk. J. Protozool. 34, 22-26.

Zinneman, H.H. and Kaplan, A.P. (1972) The association of giardiasis with reduced intestinal secretory immunoglobulins. Am. J. Digest. Dis. 17, 793-797.

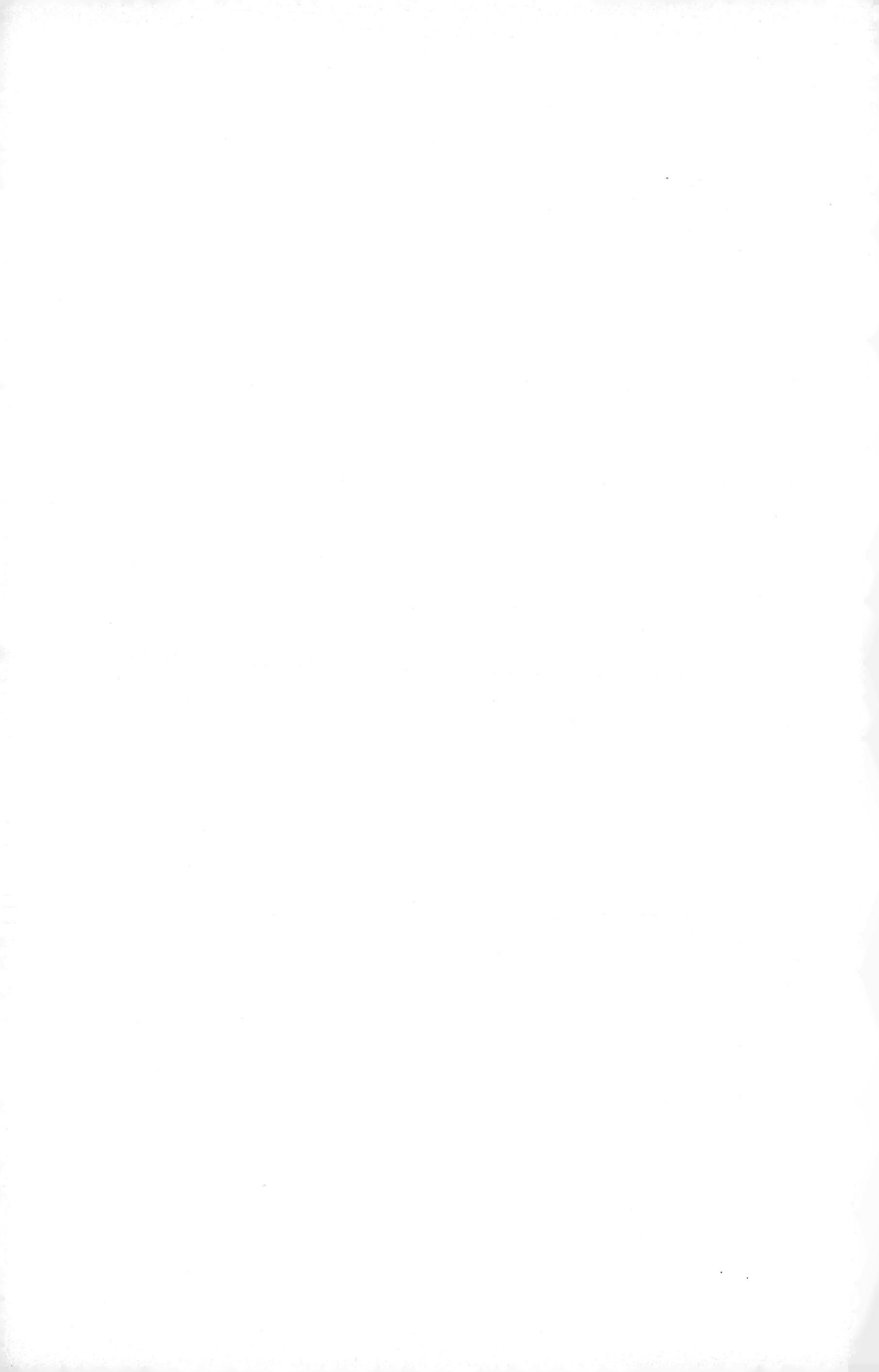

Giardiasis (E.A. Meyer, ed.)
© 1990 Elsevier Science Publishers B.V. (Biomedical Division)

14

Giardiasis in developing countries

ASMA ISLAM

International Centre for Diarrhoeal Disease Research, Dhaka, Bangladesh

1. Introduction	236
2. Prevalence	236
2.1. Geographical distribution	236
2.2. Age distribution	237
2.3. Urban and rural distribution	239
2.4. Seasonality	239
3. Susceptibility	240
3.1. Age and age groups	240
3.2. Sex	241
3.3. Socio-economic and environmental factors	241
3.4. Occupation and behaviour	242
3.5. Gastric acidity	242
3.6. Nutritional status	242
3.7. Diet	243
3.8. Immunity	244
3.9. Pregnancy	245
3.10. Travellers	245
4. *Giardia* infection and disease	246
4.1. *Giardia* as a cause of acute diarrhoea	246
4.2. *Giardia* as a cause of chronic diarrhoea	248
5. The interaction between *Giardia* infection and nutrition	249
5.1. Nutrient intake	249
5.2. Intestinal malabsorption	250
5.3. Digestive enzyme activity	252
6. Impact on child health	252
7. Transmission	254
7.1. Vehicles of transmission	254
7.1.1. Water	254
7.1.2. Food	255
7.1.3. Person-to-person transmission	255
8. Reservoirs	256
9. Control measures	257
10. Conclusion	259
References	260

1. Introduction

Giardiasis is a disease of the small intestine of man caused by the flagellate protozoan *Giardia duodenalis* (=*G. lamblia*, *G. intestinalis*). It is one of the most frequent isolated intestinal protozoa (Feachem et al., 1983) and is found world-wide in the traditional and transitional communities of the developing world (Moore et al., 1966; Melvin and Mata, 1971; Chuttani et al., 1973; Oyerinde et al., 1977; Islam et al., 1983; Miotti et al., 1986) as well as in industrialized and technologically sophisticated societies (Keystone et al., 1978; Craun, 1979). In the last 20 years there have been numerous reports which indicate that *Giardia* can be pathogenic to man. Recently, major advances have been made with regard to the identification and characterization of *Giardia* (Smith et al., 1981; Goka et al., 1986). In addition, immunological aspects have also been studied, a field which also includes the development of immunodiagnostic tests for giardiasis (Ungar et al., 1984; Green et al., 1985; Edson et al., 1986; Goka et al., 1986; Nash et al., 1987).

In developing countries giardiasis remains one of the important unresolved health problems. This is mostly due to: (1) the absence of simple but reliable diagnostic techniques; (2) the lack of a simple means to distinguish between asymptomatic and symptomatic infections; (3) unexplained immunological differences in various populations and (4) a lack of epidemiological information about the means by which infections are transmitted. In addition there is still much that is not known about the pathogenesis of intestinal disease, the natural history of infection, transmission and reinfection, and factors pertaining to host susceptibility in developing countries. This chapter will attempt to highlight some epidemiological issues related to the prevalence of giardiasis in developing countries, the disease spectrum, its transmission, control and the importance of the parasite.

For a detailed description of diagnostic techniques see chapter 10 and 11.

2. Prevalence

There is wide variation in the prevalence of *Giardia* infection between countries and within regions of the same country. Children are more commonly infected than adults. Social, environmental and climatic factors may influence the prevalence of infections.

2.1. Geographical distribution

The prevalence of *Giardia* infections worldwide was estimated in 1965 to be 7.2% (Belding, 1965). In a review of 24 published surveys, Quinn (1971) arrived at a prevalence in the United States of 7.4%. As shown in Table 1 the prevalence is much higher in developing countries, ranging from 5% in Indonesia to 43% in the Seychelles (Carney et al., 1977; Bilo and Bilo-Groen, 1983). In Bangladesh, various studies provide evidence of a wide variation in the prevalence of *Giardia* infection (Muttalib, 1970; Hossain, 1983; Gilman et al., 1985). Muttalib (1970) reported an infection rate of 21% on the basis of examining a single stool from an urban population. A prevalence rate of 13% in a periurban community comprising 358 people was reported on the basis of single stool examination employing the merthiolate iodine formalin technique (Gilman et al., 1985). Examination of a single stool from patients aged 5-9 years with diarrhea attending an urban hospital yielded an infection rate of 21% in Bangladesh (Hossain, 1983). Similar prevalence rates have also been found in India (20%), Thailand (21%), Guatemala (20%) and Zimbabwe (22%) (Dube et al., 1970; Areekul and Viravan, 1984; Farthing et al., 1986; Mason et al., 1986). Higher prevalence rates have also been reported from Egypt (35%) and Seychelles (43%) (Bilo and Bilo-Groen, 1983; Shukry et al., 1986). The variation in prevalence given in Table 1 could be due partly to the technique employed to diagnose *Giardia* as well as due to differences in the personal and environmental hygiene of the groups examined.

2.2. Age distribution

A high prevalence of giardiasis in children has been demonstrated in several studies (Oyerinde et al., 1977; Hossain et al., 1983; Zaki et al., 1983; Gilman et al., 1985). Table 2 shows the age-specific acquisition of *Giardia* in one study in Bangladesh (Gilman et al., 1985). In this study the prevalence of *Giardia* infection rapidly declined with increasing age: it was highest in 5-10-year-old children and rare after the age of 40. In the same study, a cohort of children were studied prospectively to estimate the number of newly acquired *Giardia* infections (Table 3). Over 40% of the children less than 7 years old acquired *Giardia* within 18 months; acquisition rates did not change with age. Data on the age-specific prevalence have also been reported from urban Nigeria where the

TABLE 1

Prevalence of *Giardia* in developing countries

Location	Prevalence (%)	Population studied	Reference
Bangladesh	21	–	Muttalib et al., 1970
Bangladesh	13	358	Gilman et al., 1985
Bangladesh	21	2246[c]	Hossain et al., 1983
Guatemala	20	45	Mata et al., 1978
Nigeria	8	2099[b]	Oyerinde et al., 1977
Thailand	21	179[a]	Areekul and Viravan, 1984
Seychelles	43	1000[b]	Bilo and Bilo Groen, 1983
India	20	–	Dube et al., 1970
Egypt	35	145[d]	Shukry et al., 1986
Saudi Arabia	9.9	5200	Kasim and Elhelu, 1983
Indonesia	5	1945	Carney et al., 1977
Zimbabwe	22	480[a]	Mason et al., 1986

[a] 7-19-year-old school children; [b] all age groups; [c] 5-9-years-old; [d] infants; – not known.

TABLE 2
Infection and age-specific prevalence of antibodies to *Giardia lamblia* (G.l.) in two Bangladesh villages: Nandipara (NP) and Meheran

	Nandipara					Meheran [a,b]		
Age (years)	Total No. of subjects	Stool positive for G.l.		No. of subjects seropositive for G.l.[c]		Total No. of subjects	No. of subjects seropositive for G.l.[c]	
		N	% of total	N	% of total		N	% of total
0<1*	5	0	0	2	40	20	4	20
1<2	17	2	11	4	24	35	10	29
2<5	50	5	10	7	14	46	15	33
5<10	89	19	21	31	35			
10<20	77	10	13	35	45			
20<40	80	8	10	27	34			
40+	40	2	5	18	45			
Total	358	46	13	124	35	101	29	29

[a] Stool examinations not performed in Meheran. A single stool specimen was examined in NP.
[b] Only subjects aged 0–3 years sampled.
[c] Due to different starting dilutions, a positive titre was 1/32 for Meheran village and 1/40 for N.P.
[d] There was a significant difference in the prevalence rates among the age groups tested (0–4.9, 5–9.9, 10–19.9, and 20+) by chi-square analysis ($P<0.05$).
* Nine children were under 6 months of age, one from NP and 8 from Meheran. In NP, one subject from each of the 2–<5 and 20–<40 <40+ age groups and two subjects from the 5–<10 age groups did not have their stool examined. From Gilman et al. (1985), with permission.

TABLE 3
The number of Bangladeshi (Nandipari village) children with consecutive examination periods (3–monthly) positive for *Giardia lamblia* (G.l.) in stool[a]

Age (years)	Children examined (N)	No. (%) of children with positive consecutive stool examinations				All examinations negative
		1 G.l.	2 G.l.	3 G.l.	4 G.l.	G.l.
0–<1	20	4 (20%)	2 (15%)	0	0	13 (65%)
1–<2	21	8 (38%)	7 (33%)	0	1 (5%)	5 (24%)
2–<5	50	17 (34%)	6 (12%)	2 (4%)	3 (6%)	22 (44%)
5–6	26	7 (27%)	5 (19%)	5 (19%)	0	9 (35%)
Total	117	36 (31%)	20 (17%)	7 (3%)	4 (3%)	49 (42%)

[a] Only children with specimens available for at least four consecutive periods included in analysis. All children observed prospectively for one year. From Gilman et al. (1985), with permission.

peak prevalence approached 14% in 1-5 year-old children. After that age the prevalence declined to approximately 5% and continued at that level among most adult age groups (Oyerinde et al., 1977). In a recent survey in an Egyptian village the prevalence of *Giardia* in stools from subjects with diarrhea was 31%; however, curiously, 57% of 2-4-year-old children with diarrhea excreted *Giardia* (Zaki et al., 1983). In Northern Nigeria, the prevalence of giardiasis rose from 1% in 0-3-month-old infants to 11% in 2-3-year-old children and declined to 8% in adults (Tomkins, 1981). A study in the Gambia has shown that the age-specific prevalence of giardiasis rose from 1% in infants (under 1 year) to 24% in children (3-4 years) and the age-specific prevalence declined to 16% in those over 40 years old (Bray and Harris, 1977). Thus it is evident that infections with *Giardia* are often acquired in early life, and that this is reflected by highest antibody prevalence throughout infancy and childhood as observed in Bangladeshi and Peruvian children (Gilman et al., 1985; Miotti et al., 1986). The high prevalence rate in young children may be related to lack of immunity and a greater risk of infection.

2.3. Urban and rural distribution

The prevalence of giardiasis may differ between rural and urban settings. By screening a single stool specimen from patients attending both urban and rural diarrheal treatment centres, higher prevalence of *Giardia* was seen in urban children compared with rural children (Hossain et al., 1983). This finding is further substantiated by a study in Zimbabwe which reported a significant difference ($P < 0.001$) between the prevalence of *Giardia* in urban children compared with rural children: 22.0% versus 11.6% (Mason et al., 1986).

These findings suggest that a high population density and overcrowding may contribute to a high prevalence of giardiasis.

2.4. Seasonality

A striking seasonal pattern has been described for some infectious diseases, notably cholera and rotavirus (Stoll et al., 1982; Khan et al., 1983), but little evidence is available on any seasonality in *Giardia* infections. A unique longitudinal study of 45 Guatemalan children studied from birth for the first 3 years of life, revealed that the prevalence rates tended to be highest in the cooler and wetter months, when climatic conditions are known to favour cyst survival (Jarroll et al., 1980; Farthing et al., 1986). A survey of *Giardia* infections was conducted in five regions of Saudi Arabia for the months of January–December 1980 (Kasim and Elhelu, 1983); the highest prevalence of giardiasis (16%) was noted in the cool month of September. In Bangladesh, hospital-based surveillance of 1873 patients attending Dhaka Hospital of the International Centre for Diarrhoeal Disease Research, Bangladesh between January to December 1986, screened for enteric pathogens, found *Giardia* to be more common in the month of August and September – (8.1-6.6.%) coinciding with the rainy season (Fig. 1) (Alam et al., personal

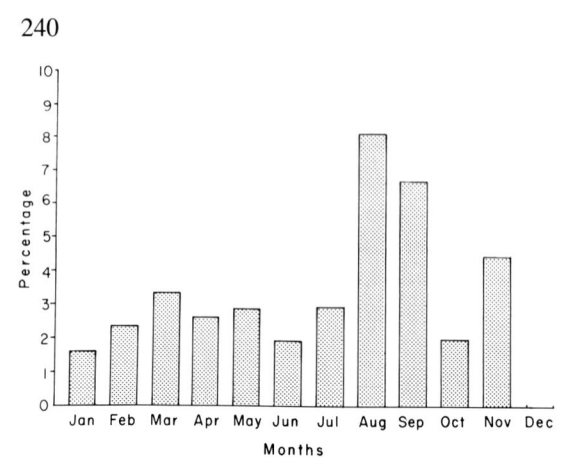

Fig. 1. Seasonal distribution of isolation of *Giardia* in diarrheal patients attending ICDDR, B.

communication). However, another longitudinal study in a rural area of Bangladesh did not demonstrate any striking seasonality of infections with *Giardia* (Black et al., 1983).

3. Susceptibility

Susceptibility to *Giardia* infection is likely to be influenced by age, sex, socio-environmental conditions, occupation, gastric acidity, nutritional status, pregnancy and host immunity.

3.1. Age and age groups

In Bangladesh, where giardiasis is endemic, infections with *Giardia* are acquired early in life. A prospective study of 33 infant mother pairs observed that 42% of the infants and 82% of the mothers were infected with *Giardia* at some time during the study. Infants became infected as early as three months of age and always developed diarrhea (Islam et al., 1983).

In Guatemala, two out of 45 infants studied from birth were found to have *Giardia* in their stools during the first week of life (Farthing et al., 1986). Unknown factors related to age influence host susceptibility to clinical disease after infection is acquired. Infants and children under 10 years are more susceptible to *Giardia* infection, and acute illness is more common in children than in adults. Infected adults are more often asymptomatic.

In general it appears that in countries where *Giardia* is endemic, infections are acquired at an early age. This first infection usually causes disease but results in a degree of immunity which may protect people from further disease, although they may become reinfected. This may explain why symptomatic infections in adults are uncommon.

3.2. Sex

Differences which have been observed in the prevalence of infections with *Giardia* between sexes remain unexplained. In Saudi Arabia the prevalence of infection has been shown to be higher in males (64%) than in females (36%) (Kasim and Elhelu, 1983), possibly a result of a different rate of exposure to the parasites. In contrast, *Giardia* infection rates of 8% in male and 7.4% in female have been reported from a survey of intestinal parasites in Lagosian population of 2099 comprising 43% males and 57% females (Oyerinde et al., 1977). Yet another survey conducted in 10 villages of Central and South Sulawesi, Indonesia reported an equal prevalence of giardiasis (4% in male and 5% in female) in South Sulawesi and 8% and 6% in central Sulawesi (Carney et al., 1977).

3.3. Socio-economic and environmental factors

The prevalence of infections with *Giardia* in many developing countries varies inversely with socio-economic status, and is highest where sanitation and sanitary practices are substandard and where faecal contamination of the environment is common (Knight, 1980; Miotti et al., 1986). Prevalences are especially high among poor communities and disadvantaged ethnic groups. The prevalences of *Giardia* among poor children aged 6 months to 16 years in Glasgow (Scotland) were 13% in native Scots, 10% in Asians, 1% in Africans and 1% in Chinese (Goel et al., 1977). Reports from developed countries have documented outbreaks in institutions such as asylums, orphanages, and homes for the retarded where good hygiene is difficult to maintain [Mathews et al., 1919 (cited by Burke et al., 1977); Yoeli et al., 1972; Thacker et al., 1979]. A study in Saudi Arabia revealed a lower infection rate (2%) among people living in urban areas where sanitary conditions were good, in contrast to relatively higher rates of infection (7-14%) in people of the rural areas with inadequate sanitary and hygienic conditions (Kasim and Elhelu, 1983; Miotti et al., 1986). Inadequate hygienic conditions are evidenced by animals and pets having free access to the main living area and may influence the higher incidence rate (Zaki et al., 1986). Although the same socio-environmental conditions may be true in the majority of developing countries, but in contrast the fact lies that giardiasis in American campers or in overseas travellers is predominantly a disease of affluent individuals (Babb et al., 1971; Barbour et al., 1976). However, a more recent study from Zimbabwe found that providing piped water as not associated with a reduced prevalence of *Giardia* infections (Mason et al., 1986). Further studies are necessary to understand socio-environmental factors contributing to giardiasis in developing countries where population density is high and increasing, when the majority of people living in rural areas do not have access to sanitary latrines and when people still defaecate indiscriminately.

3.4. Occupation and behaviour

Certain occupations predispose people to *Giardia* infections and higher rates have been reported in sewage and irrigation workers, thereby raising the prevalence in adult males (Knight, 1980). Young children defaecate indiscriminately throughout their homestead. In these environments, excreta disposal habits and facilities are unhygienic and lacking. Thus the possibility of faecal oral transmission of infection is increased.

3.5. Gastric acidity

The importance of gastric acid in nonspecific resistance to bacterial enteric infection is well known but remains unproven with respect to parasitic infections such as *Giardia* (Giannella et al., 1973). Nevertheless, a report by Hass and Bucken (1967) from a developed country showed that out of 50 patients with giardiasis, 42% were hypochlorhydric and 12% were achlorhydric, suggesting that disturbances in gastric acid production may predispose people to *Giardia* infection. In addition, patients who have had a gastrectomy are known to be prone to infection with *Giardia* perhaps because of a reduced gastric acid production (Yardley et al., 1974). It is likely that normal gastric acidity ordinarily provides a significant barrier to the establishment of an infection with *Giardia*. Although *Giardia* is primarily a duodenal parasite, some achlorhydric patients may harbour the parasite in their gastric content (Yardley et al., 1967). This could only happen if the stomach's pH is between 6.4 and 7.1, the optimum pH required for survival of *Giardia* trophozoites (Hass and Bucken, 1967). In contrast, when an appropriate host ingests mature cysts the excystation process is induced, presumably by acidic conditions during gastric passage (Bingham and Meyer, 1977).

Achlorhydria is associated with blood group A. One study indicated a greater susceptibility to *Giardia* infection in people with this blood group as reported by Paulsen (1977) but subsequent studies have not confirmed this association.

A reduced secretion of gastric acid also occurs as a consequence of malnutrition and the impairment of this nonspecific defense may increase susceptibility to infections with *Giardia*. In addition, malnutrition may also suppress immunity. However, little evidence is available to support or refute this hypothesis.

3.6. Nutritional status

In India a study has shown that there is no significant difference in the prevalence of disease between well-nourished and malnourished children (Walia et al., 1986). This observation is in contrast to the generally believed predisposition of malnourished people to *Giardia* infections (Gracey, 1973), and the findings of Mata et al. (1972) that 9 out of 13 severely malnourished children had *Giardia* infection. In Bangladesh, 51% of severely malnourished hospitalized children at a nutrition unit had acquired *Giardia* infections (Gilman et al., 1985). Moreover, highest prevalence rates of IgG antibody to

Giardia were noted in Peruvian children who were being treated for malnutrition (Miotti et al., 1986).

It is uncertain whether giardiasis is an important contributor to malnutrition or whether malnutrition predisposes to prolonged giardiasis because of a suppressed immune response. It has been stated that patients with hypogammaglobulinaemia and agammaglobulinaemia have overt gastrointestinal symptoms and a higher frequency of steatorrhea compared to patients with normal serum immunoglobulin levels (Ament et al., 1972, 1973; Webster et al., 1980). Both hypochlorhydria and pancreatic enzyme deficiency predispose to giardiasis and these two factors are present in protein-energy malnutrition (Jain et al., 1986). Therefore, it may be suggested that there is an association between high prevalence of *Giardia* infection and malnutrition. Nutritional status may impair both nonspecific and specific defenses against infection so it seems reasonable that there is an association between giardiasis and malnutrition.

3.7. Diet

The rate of *Giardia* infection in mice fed protein as the only nutrient is lower than that in animals fed a carbohydrate rich diet (Schneider, 1961). Furthermore, glucose is known to stimulate glycogen utilization and oxygen consumption in *Giardia* (Smith, 1978). Based on these observations Kasim (1983) commented that the high prevalence of giardiasis in Saudi Arabia may be attributed to the population's staple diet, consisting of carbohydrate rich foods. However, hygienic practices may be more important. The consumption of raw vegetables may contribute to acquiring *Giardia* infections (Panicker and Krishnamoorthi, 1978) as vegetables may become contaminated with the cysts of *Giardia*, in polluted water used for washing and refreshing the vegetables, and in human excreta in fertilizing vegetable gardens.

The role of breast milk in modulating giardiasis has recently been investigated both in animals and humans. Andrews and Hewlett (1981) showed that suckling mice are protected against *Giardia muris* if they are fed milk from immune mothers containing specific IgA antibody to *Giardia*. In a study of humans, infection with *Giardia* was acquired by three infants who were totally breast-fed (two of them drank milk containing antibodies to *Giardia* at the time they acquired infections (Islam et al., 1983). But infection with *Giardia* was less common in infants younger than 6 months, an age when many are totally breast-fed; this might be related to protection associated with breast-feeding or to decreased exposure to *Giardia* in the breast-fed children (Islam et al., 1983). *Giardia* is rapidly killed by exposure to normal human milk in vitro (Gillin et al., 1983). However, the lethal effect of human milk does not appear to be dependent on secretory immunoglobulin, rather by an enzyme, bile salt-stimulated lipase. A more recent study has confirmed that normal human milk kills *Giardia* trophozoites in vitro and that this killing is due to the release of free fatty acids from milk triglycerides by the action of the bile salt-stimulated lipase on human milk (Reiner et al., 1986).

3.8. Immunity

The influence of host immunity on infection and on modulating the clinical course of giardiasis remains undefined. In some hosts, the infection may be short-lived and spontaneously self-limited (Danciger and Lopez, 1975). In others, giardiasis may range from a short, clinically innocuous infection to a prolonged, debilitating illness (Hoskins et al., 1967). There remains no explanation for the striking variability of clinical illness during these infections. Nevertheless, protective immunity is suggested by the self-limiting nature of most infections and also by the lower prevalence of giardiasis in adults in areas where the disease is endemic compared with symptomatic infections in travellers to the same areas who are newly exposed (Babb et al., 1971).

The role of a humoral response to *Giardia* as detected by *Giardia* antibodies after infection in humans is not well understood. The evidence for and against the role of secretory antibodies in protecting against infection has been elucidated by few epidemiological and serological studies (Islam et al., 1983; Gilman et al., 1985; Miotti et al., 1985, 1986). Islam et al. (1983) demonstrated serum antibodies IgG against *Giardia* in 45% of mothers who excreted *Giardia* (± 2 months) in a prospective community-based study of 33 mothers. This finding was similar to that of Gilman et al. (1985) who also observed that 39% of subjects with *Giardia* in their stools had IgG antibodies to *Giardia*. Both these findings suggest a poor correlation between infection and the presence of these antibodies. In a prospective study from both of infant-mother pairs, the majority of infected mothers (86%) had no symptoms (Islam et al., 1983). This may be explained by the development of a partial immunity which protects against disease but not against infection. In contrast, significant concentrations of antibodies were not detected in any of the sera from infants, and the acquisition by infants of their first infection was associated with gastrointestinal symptoms. On the other hand, in Peru the prevalence of serum IgG antibodies to *Giardia* was found to be highest throughout infancy and childhood (Miotti et al., 1986). However, the study did not examine the correlation between symptoms and serum antibodies. Although IgG antibody responses to *Giardia* infections have been demonstrated in malnourished hospitalized children in both Bangladesh and Peru, their roles in protecting against disease have not been evaluated (Gilman et al., 1985; Miotti et al., 1986).

Secretory IgA to *Giardia* (sIgA) has been demonstrated in breast milk from women in Bangladesh (73%) and Mexico (77%), indicating a high incidence of infection in these populations (Islam et al., 1983; Miotti et al., 1985). Infants in these areas may thus acquire antibodies from their mothers by way of breast milk. This may explain why infection with *Giardia* is uncommon in infants younger than 6 months. This theory is confirmed by the observation of Mata (1978) in a study of 45 Guatemalan children, who found that, during exclusive breast feeding, infection with *Giardia* was uncommon and asymptomatic.

3.9. Pregnancy

In cholera, pregnant women are thought to be more susceptible to clinical illness (Hirchhorn et al., 1969), but there is a paucity of epidemiological studies with regard to pregnancy and giardiasis. It has been shown that *Giardia*-infected female mice which have ceased to pass parasites in their stools again shed *Giardia* cysts during pregnancy and lactation (Stevens et al., 1978). Some evidence for a similar situation in humans comes from a study in Bangladesh. Of the 33 Bangladeshi women studied, 18 were followed during their pregnancies starting 3 months before delivery, and 44% of these pregnant women excreted *Giardia* cysts, trophozoites or both at least once during their pregnancies. The excretion of *Giardia* by pregnant women was compared with the excretion of parasites by 11 non-pregnant, non-lactating women and with 29 non-pregnant, lactating women. There was a significant difference in the overall excretion of *Giardia* between non-pregnant, lactating women and non-pregnant, non-lactating women (Ljungstrom et al., 1987). Further studies of *Giardia* infection during pregnancy and lactation are needed to understand the differences between animals and humans as well as comparison between pregnant and lactating women in developed and developing countries where hosts are subjected to greater changes of infection and where nutritional and socio-environmental conditions are different.

3.10 Travellers

Giardia infection is one of the several causes of travellers' diarrhea. Speelman and Ljungstrom (1986) studied 251 expatriates living in Bangladesh over a 1-year period. The prevalence and incidence of *Giardia* was found to be 5.2 and 11.8%, respectively. Children of 10 or younger and newcomers were most frequently infected. Of the infected expatriates, 37% experienced diarrhea.

Lopez et al. (1978) reported a high incidence of diarrhea in a group of approximately 1400 Americans who travelled in October 1976 to the Portuguese island of Madeira. Of the 859 travellers who responded to the survey, 39% experienced diarrhea, and in 42% of these cases the diarrhea lasted longer than 1 week. Of all travellers surveyed, 33% developed a combination of symptoms suggesting giardiasis, with a median incubation period of 4 days. Of 58 ill patients whose stools were examined for parasites, *Giardia* was recovered from 27 (47%). It is possible that newcomers or travellers visiting areas where *Giardia* is endemic are more likely to have symptomatic infections compared with indigenous people because of their lack of immunity due to previous exposure to the parasite.

4. Giardia: infection and disease

Giardia infection is more commonly found in children than adults but it has not always been regarded as a cause of illness. Clinical and epidemiological studies have indicated that the infection is associated with a wide range of symptoms ranging from mild, watery diarrhea to chronic diarrhea and florid malabsorption. In some, the disease may be fatal (Shukry et al., 1986). However, a larger proportion of infected individuals may remain asymptomatic, ranging from 20-84%. Case-control studies have indicated similar infection rates ranging from 16-86% in individuals who had diarrhea compared with those who did not (Table 4). Infected infants develop symptoms at a relatively higher rate compared with children and adults, probably because of their first exposure to the parasite (Islam et al., 1983). It is not well understood why an infection with Giardia is self-limited and asymptomatic in some people but causes severe disease with malabsorption and growth faltering in others. This variable host-pathogen interaction could be due to differences between strains of Giardia or due to difference in the immune response of the host (Smith et al., 1981). The difference between infection and disease is important for epidemiological studies.

4.1. Giardia as a cause of acute diarrhea

Prevalence rates in various studies in developing countries indicate that Giardia accounts for 2-44% of cases of acute diarrhea (Table 5). The prevalence of Giardia as a cause of diarrhea may be underestimated in developing countries because in most of these studies a diagnosis is usually made by examining microscopically only a single stool sample and this may reduce the actual prevalence by as much as 50% compared with other diagnostic techniques (Kamath and Murugasu, 1974). Table 5 summarizes the prevalence of Giardia in patients with acute diarrhea in several developing countries. The variations in findings within countries such as Bangladesh, India and Costa Rica may be due to the difference

TABLE 4
Giardia infection with and without diarrhea

Location	Age	Population studied	Symptomatic (%)	Population studied	Asymptomatic (%)	Reference
India	< 6 yr	159	16.3	159	83.6	Walia et al., 1986
Guatemala	1–5 yr	101	29[a]	110	26[a]	Pierce et al., 1962
Thailand	1–19 yr	–	–	179	21[a]	Areekul and Viravan, 1984
Zimbabwe	2 –< 6 yr	236	39[a]	192	20[a]	Nathoo et al., 1985
Egypt	All ages	3080	44[a]	703	56[a]	Zaki et al., 1986
Bangladesh	Infant	33	86	–	–	Islam et al., 1983

[a] Control studies; –, not studied

TABLE 5
Percentage, prevalence of *Giardia* in acute diarrheal patients

Country	Prevalence (%)	No. studied	References
Bangladesh[b]	6 (all ages)	2246	Stoll et al., 1982
Bangladesh[a]	2 (all ages)	8139	Black et al., 1980
Bangladesh[b]	18 (adult)	182	Rabbani et al., 1982
India[b]	11 (children)	1551	Gupta and Mehta, 1973
India[b]	16.5 (children)	455	Walia et al., 1986
Egypt[b]	35 (infant)	148	Shukry et al., 1986
Egypt[a]	44 (all ages)	3080	Zaki et al., 1986
Costa Rica[b]	4.5 (children)	888	Mata et al., 1983
Costa Rica[a]	11.5 (children)	347	Moore et al., 1966
Brazil[a]	6.7 (all ages)	150	Guerrant et al., 1983
Guatemala[a]	13 (children)	45	Farthing et al., 1986
Zimbabwe[a]	15 (children)	46	Mason et al., 1985

[a] Rural; [b] Urban.

in the composition of the sampled population with regard to age and urban/rural settings. Another factor affecting these prevalence rates may be the fact that only the presence of the vegetative form of *Giardia* was regarded as indicating an acute infection (Black et al., 1980). Despite the limitations of such reports, it appears that *Giardia* accounts for up to 20% of acute episodes of diarrhea in young children in Bangladesh where it ranks seventh of all identified organisms responsible for acute diarrhea (Stoll et al., 1982). The high rate of occurrence of *Giardia* (35-44%) in Egypt may be due to the high asymptomatic carriage rate of the parasite in this population (Shukry et al., 1986; Zaki et al., 1986).

The pattern of diarrhea associated with *Giardia* infections in young children in Guatemala appears to change during the first 3 years of life (Farthing et al., 1986). In this study a cohort of 45 children were studied prospectively for the first 3 years of life with particular attention to diarrheal disease and physical growth. The study showed that the prevalence of giardiasis rose progressively during the 3 years with a peak in the final year of over 20%. With the exception of episodes during the first 6 months, 50% or more of *Giardia* infections were accompanied by diarrhea. In addition it was also observed that approximately half of these diarrheal episodes lasted less than 2 weeks. However, 28% of *Giardia* episodes in the first year of life lasted six weeks or more. It was further observed that 30-50% of the *Giardia* infections occurred in the absence of intestinal symptoms (Fig. 2).

In contrast, asymptomatic infections with *Giardia* were found much more commonly (75-92%) in preschool children in India (Walia et al., 1986). The difference between the studies in Guatemala and India could be due to the fact that children were relatively older in India and only cysts of *Giardia* were regarded as indicating infection; vegetative forms were not found. In Central America Moore et al. (1966) reported a prevalence rate of 11.5-36.8% in preschool children of similar age group with diarrhea; a similar prevalence

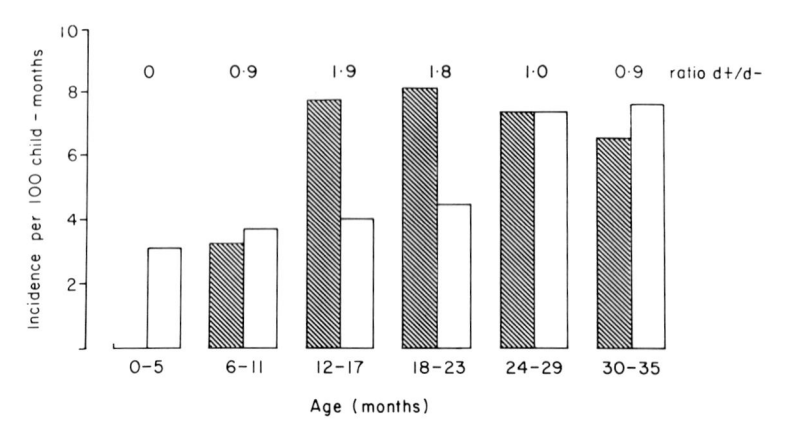

Fig. 2. Association of diarrheal illness with *Giardia* infections during the first 3 years of life; *Giardia* episodes with (d+) and without (d−) diarrhea.

was found in children without diarrhea. However, all these studies were liable to exclude the role of other enteric pathogens in addition to *Giardia* as causes of the diarrhea.

4.2. Giardia *as a cause of chronic diarrhea*

It is now quite evident that *Giardia* stands out as a significant cause of chronic diarrhea in both adults and children (Guardiola-Rotger et al., 1964; Chuttani et al., 1973). In India in the early seventies, the prevalence of *Giardia* was substantially higher in patients with chronic diarrhea than with acute diarrhea, ranging from 11-26% (Gupta and Mehta, 1970; Walia, 1971; Chuttani et al., 1973). Recently *Giardia* was found to be present in 13% of 150 children with chronic diarrhea attending a clinic in Vellore in southern India (Mathan et al., 1986). A study reported from Puerto Rico reported data from two similar groups of 72 children – one group with chronic diarrhea, the other a healthy control. Children with chronic diarrhea had a substantially higher prevalence of *Giardia* compared with the control group (Guardiola-Rotger et al., 1964).

So far there are very few reports on *Giardia* as a cause of chronic diarrhea with PEM. The most striking report is from Guatemala, where *Giardia* was found to be the most common pathogen in 9 out of 13 severely malnourished children with chronic diarrhea (Mata et al., 1972). This finding was further substantiated by another recent study in Costa Rica in which *Giardia* was detected in the small intestine of 38% of malnourished children with chronic diarrhea using a string test (Lopez et al., 1978). Table 6 summarises the prevalence of *Giardia* as a cause of chronic diarrhea.

TABLE 6

Giardiasis as a cause of chronic diarrhea[a]

Location	Subjects studied	Prevalence %	References
Puerto Rico	72	32	Guardiola-Rotger et al., 1964
India	62	19	Gupta and Mehta, 1970
India	200	26	Walia et al., 1971
India	62	26	Chuttani et al., 1973
Guatemala	22	38	Mata et al., 1976[b]
Bangladesh	563	20	Ali, 1981
Zimbabwe	16	44	Mason and Nathoo, 1985
India	150	15	Mathan, 1986

[a] Diarrhea persisted for > 2 weeks; [b] *Giardia* found in small intestine with severe protein energy malnutrition.

5. The interaction between Giardia infection and nutrition

The interaction between *Giardia* infection and nutrition can be studied in individuals by clinical investigation or in communities by field surveys. Most clinical studies to date have involved certain aspects: food intake, absorption of nutrients, functional disturbances of gastric and jejunal enzyme secretion and morphological changes in the gut. There are still too few longitudinal studies of individuals that could improve our understanding regarding the nutritional impact of giardiasis (Rowland et al., 1977; Farthing et al., 1986).

5.1. Nutrient intake

It is evident that anorexia plays an important role in the interaction between infection and nutrition. Acute diarrhea due to cholera, rotavirus, *Shigella* and enterotoxigenic *Escherichia coli* appear to reduce the intake of energy by one third below requirements (Sarker et al., 1982; Molla et al., 1983). A decreased food intake during parasitic disease including *Giardia* has been well documented in developed countries (Moore et al., 1969; Jokipii and Jokipii, 1974; Crompton, 1984; Rosenberg, 1984). It is likely that nausea, vomiting and abdominal distention, which have been reported in most patients with giardiasis in developed countries, may lead to a decreased food intake (Brodskey et al., 1974; Moore et al., 1969). However, there are few studies of food intake during giardiasis reported from developing countries. Gupta (1973) demonstrated a poor appetite in 29% of Indian children with giardiasis. The low percentage of anorectic children could possibly be due to the fact that only cysts in the stool were considered to confirm a diagnosis of giardiasis. Hence further studies are needed to determine the food intake pattern in *Giardia*-infected patients. A recent community based study in the Gambia, West Africa, indicated that even when food was provided in abundance, children with protracted diarrhea associated with giardiasis obtain only two thirds of their energy requirement (Tomkins, 1983). Successful therapy was followed by an increase in food intake.

Recently in Bangladesh, a hospital-based study was performed to see the intake and absorption of nutrients in children with giardiasis during acute diarrhea and after recovery. Reduction in intake of food could not be established in those children which may be explained by the varied clinical spectrum of the disease. Moreover, fever, which was thought to be an important factor in the metabolic and nutritional disturbances, was not present in any of the children in this study (Molla et al., 1986) as it was in another study (Brodsky et al., 1974).

5.2. Intestinal malabsorption

Malabsorption in giardiasis has been reported from many countries (Amini et al., 1963; Antia et al., 1966; Alp and Hislop, 1969; Moore et al., 1969; Tewari and Tandon, 1974; Meyer and Jarroll, 1980). In reviewing malabsorption due to *Giardia*, a number of problems arise. Since multiple parasitic infections are common, ascribing malabsorption in single parasites such as *Giardia* may be difficult. The lack of appropriate socio-economic data and an age-matched population makes it difficult to determine the incidence of malabsorption in giardiasis. In addition, coexistence of malnutrition in infected people, diverse selection criteria and the variable severity of infection are also important factors. Despite these limitations, various aspects of nutrient malabsorption in patients with giardiasis have been studied (Table 7). Most people studied were symptomatic. Barbieri et al. (1970) did, however, study 11 Brazilian children who were symptom-free and found that 82% of the children had fat malabsorption and 27%

TABLE 7
Malabsorption of nutrients in giardiasis

Location	No. of subjects	D-xylose	Lactose	Fat	Vit B_{12}	Vit A	Reference
Argentina	20	–	–	25	–	–	Cantor et al., 1976
Brazil	11	27	–	82	–	–	Barbieri et al., 1970
India	30	23	–	50	6	–	Tewari and Tandon, 1974
Cuba	50	62	27	34	–	–	Rabassa et al., 1975
India	63	4	–	27	–	–	Tandon et al., 1977
India	4	79	–	50	–	100	Mahalanabis et al., 1979
Thailand	57	–	–	–	–	35	Chavalittamrong et al., 1980
Israel	8	50	–	41	–	–	Judd et al., 1983
Brazil	33	–	56	–	–	–	Jove et al., 1983

% subjects with abnormal results

–, not investigated.

had malabsorption of D-xylose. However, the study did not attempt to discover other possible causes of malabsorption. A recent study from Bangladesh (Molla et al., 1986) has attempted to determine the effect of *Giardia* on absorption of fat, nitrogen, carbohydrate, and energy derived from familiar food in children aged 1-10 years. The study failed to demonstrate any malabsorption during acute or recovery (post-treatment) stages of the disease. However, there were several possible explanations why the study was unable to demonstrate malabsorption; (i) study children were from older age groups and were not susceptible to absorption defects associated with giardiasis, (ii) immunity against *Giardia* might be present, (iii) possible low parasite load and trophozoites/cysts not sufficient to demonstrate malabsorption.

It could be postulated that the repeated exposure of people to *Giardia* leads to a moderation of the difference of any disease in a way similar to that found in experimental animals (Roberts-Thomson et al., 1976; Stevens et al., 1978; Kanwar et al., 1985). Malabsorption of D-xylose and fat is well documented during giardiasis in between 25 to 80% of subjects in developing countries. D-xylose absorption studies have been found normal in one Indian study (Gupta and Mehta, 1973) which indicates that malabsorption is probably not enterogenic. However, the validity of the D-xylose test as an indicator of absorption potential is now in question as D-xylose can be metabolised by some intestinal bacteria (Cook, 1980). There is a paucity of knowledge of vitamin B_{12} absorption in giardiasis. However, Tewari and Tandon (1974) documented malabsorption of vitamin B_{12} in 6% of children with giardiasis. The prevalence of vitamin B_{12} malabsorption was found to be very high (50%) in Caucasians who had acquired the infection during overland travels in Asia, Africa, and India (Butler et al., 1973; Wright et al., 1977). Malabsorption of D-xylose and fat was also present in 57 and 38%, respectively, in 40 symptomatic patients with giardiasis in that study. There was significant improvement of absorption after anti-*Giardia* therapy.

In India Mahalanabis et al. (1979) demonstrated malabsorption of vitamin A, along with D-xylose and fat in 4 children. In another study, 35% of Thai children with giardiasis and 22.6% of normal children showed vitamin A concentrations lower than 20 μg/dl. However, an impaired absorption of vitamin A did not improve or return to normal for at least 3 weeks after treatment with anti-*Giardia* drugs (Chavalittamrong et al., 1980). An impaired absorption of vitamin A is likely to be related to morphological changes in the mucosa of the proximal small intestine. Accelerated small intestinal cell turnover has been demonstrated in the mouse model (Ferguson et al., 1980); this may relate to mucosal exfoliation.

Although iron malabsorption in giardiasis has been reported from a study in a developed country (DeVizia et al., 1985), reports from developing countries are still lacking. However, the results of haemoglobin, haematocrit and serum iron values in 37 asymptomatic cases of giardiasis in comparison with 142 uninfected cases did not show any significant difference (Areekul and Viravan, 1984).

Nutrient loss in a stool during giardiasis has not been investigated in developing countries. An apparent-protein losing enteropathy has been reported in one case (Sherman and

Lieban, 1980) but whether a protein-losing enteropathy actually exists during giardiasis remains to be explored.

5.3. Digestive enzyme activity

There is little information in the literature on the digestive enzyme status in giardiasis, particularly in children in developing countries. One study attempted to examine the activity of digestive enzymes, particularly in relation to pancreatic function, in 25 Indian children with symptomatic giardiasis (Gupta and Mehta, 1973). Pancreatic lipase and trypsin were found to be lower in activity in the infected group in comparison with controls. The concentration of fat and N_2 in the stools were found to be greater in the group with giardiasis in comparison with the controls. The loss of fat in the stool correlated with the alteration in lipase activity, thus suggesting a possible explanation for the steatorrhea which commonly occurs during giardiasis (Gupta and Mehta, 1973). Disaccharidase deficiency in giardiasis has also been documented in developed countries (Ament et al., 1972) but not yet in developing countries. In another study an attempt was made to correlate histological changes with mucosal enzyme activity in 10 Israeli children with giardiasis (Judd et al., 1983). It was observed that except for a lactase deficiency, disaccharidase activities correlated poorly with the severity of mucosal damage shown by a biopsy. Steatorrhea was not found in children with abnormal biopsies. Thus it was concluded that absorptive defects did not necessarily correlate with morphological changes associated with giardiasis (Judd et al., 1983; Jove et al., 1983).

6. Impact on child health

It is now well established that recurrent gastrointestinal infections may lead to retarded growth of infants and children. The majority of reports indicate that giardiasis in children, particularly those less than 5 years old, may significantly interfere with growth and normal development (Cole and Perkin, 1977; Mata et al., 1978; Gupta and Urrutia, 1982; Farthing et al., 1986). Most hospital-based studies have been performed in developed countries, and involved relatively few patients (Veghelyi, 1938; Boe and Rinvik, 1943; Cortner, 1959; Court and Anderson, 1959; Burke, 1975; Pugh and Newton, 1980). The reports generally relate to children whose symptoms were sufficiently severe to warrant a visit to a physician and therefore had giardiasis.

Although *Giardia* is highly prevalent in developing countries, the impact of infection on child growth and development has not been investigated at a community level. There are very few community based studies to report on the effect of *Giardia* infections on physical growth during infancy and childhood. The only prospective longitudinal study in a rural community that has attempted to study the question, is the work of Mata on the children of Santa Maria Cauque, a village in highland Guatemala (Farthing et al., 1986).

This study showed that the mean number of *Giardia* infections per child increased from 0.7 in the first year to 3.6 in the third year. The report also showed that 50% of infections were associated with diarrhea. The majority of these episodes (50%) were short – less than 2 weeks in duration. However, in the first year of life a sufficient proportion of episodes (28%) lasted from more than 2-6 weeks, then progressively decreased during 2nd and 3rd years. Growth measurements during the second year of life showed that children who suffered giardiasis lasting 2 weeks or more tended to have lower median weight and height velocities. Children with diarrhea associated with *Giardia* infections had a significantly lower median height velocity (50-60% NCHS) than those children who had *Giardia* episodes without diarrhea (75% NCHS standard; P <0.05). Weight velocities were similar in children with or without diarrhea. These observations suggest that both the duration of *Giardia* infections and their association with diarrheal illness were factors associated with growth retardation. Although simultaneous infection with other enteropathogens occurred in many children, the findings suggest that *Giardia* infection may have independent deleterious effects on child growth (Farthing et al., 1986). The analysis of the Guatemalan study has its limitation as it was not specifically designed to examine the effect of a single pathogen on growth. A recent study from India reported that the persistence of *Giardia* infection in preschool children did not significantly impair annual weight increment (Walia et al., 1986). The difference may be that this study involved relatively older and asymptomatic children.

Another study in Guatemala has attempted to demonstrate the nutritional impact of giardiasis and ascariasis on child growth by a prospective placebo controlled study of periodic parasitic eradication (Gupta et al., 1982). The study randomly allocated 159 children 2 to 5 years of age to twice monthly treatment of one of four treatment regimens: (i) placebo, (ii) piperazine, (iii) metronidazole or (iv) metronidazole + piperazine. During the year of the study, growth and parasite loads were determined at regular intervals. In the groups receiving metronidazole, a significant increase in height (average 1 cm) was observed, and a fall in the prevalence of *Giardia* from 21.5 to 2.5% at the end of the study. Similar findings were reported from Africa in hospital settings where malnourished children with giardiasis were treated with anti-*Giardia* therapy; children receiving metronidazole showed a significant gain in weight after therapy (Okiahealam, 1983). It is difficult to assess the nutritional impact of *Giardia* in these children with any certainty because metronidazole is not a specific treatment and will eradicate many intestinal anaerobic infections. Thus the entire growth-promoting effect of anti-*Giardia* therapy cannot be ascertained. However, the result of these studies suggest that *Giardia* infections contribute to the development of malnutrition in the children and that treatment for *Giardia* may result in improved growth and development (Gupta and Urrutia, 1982).

Rowland et al. (1977) studied the growth of 152 Gambian children followed prospectively from 3 months to 3 years of age. The impact of a variety of infections, including gastroenteritis and giardiasis on child growth was assessed. Although reductions occurred in weight velocity during giardiasis the magnitude of the effect failed to achieve statistical significance.

Another longitudinal study of children from Gambia and from Uganda, investigating the relationships between growth and different types of infection, was reported by Cole and Parkin in 1977. Significant reduction was noted in weight velocity ($P < 0.05$) due to giardiasis as well as to gastroenteritis and malaria.

While much attention has been focused on symptomatic giardiasis, the impact of the parasite on growth has not been adequately studied in asymptomatic individuals living in unsanitary conditions in developing countries where giardiasis is endemic. Attempts should be made to evaluate and compare the impact of asymptomatic and symptomatic *Giardia* infection on growth and development. Some community-based studies indicate that giardiasis in children, particularly those under 5 years of age, may significantly interfere with growth and normal development. Studies on the impact of giardiasis have concentrated on people with severe symptomatic disease. However, little work has been done on less severe infections or even on the difference between the effect on the human host of symptomatic and asymptomatic infections.

7. Transmission

Infection follows the ingestion of as few as 10 viable cysts of *Giardia* (Rendtorff and Holt, 1954). Infection can be spread by water, food and directly from person to person by the fecal-oral route, particularly between children (Black et al., 1977). In developed countries, venereal spread has been reported in homosexual males (Schemerin et al., 1978). Epidemiological information about transmission in developing countries is sadly deficient.

7.1. Vehicles of transmission

7.1.1. Water

Based on epidemiological evidence, contaminated water appears to be the principal vehicle of transmission of *Giardia*. In developed countries, waterborne outbreaks of giardiasis have occurred primarily in areas where water supplies were contaminated either by a failure of filtration systems or by direct contamination of water supplies with sewage. Prospective epidemiological studies of travellers to the Soviet Union indicate an association between giardiasis and the consumption of tap water in Leningrad which appears to have been inadequately treated (Brodsky et al., 1974). Davis and Ritchie (1948) provided some early epidemiological evidence of the waterborne transmission of *Giardia* when they studied 150 American occupants of a Tokyo apartment building between December 1946 to January 1947. The outbreak was attributed to sewage contamination of the building's water supply. *Giardia* was isolated from 86% of the occupants who experienced diarrhea with abdominal discomfort. Water contaminated with sewage was incriminated in an epidemic at a ski resort in Aspen, Colorado (Moore et al., 1969).

Very few epidemiological investigations and reports exist about water as a mode of transmission of giardiasis in developing countries. In many developing countries rapid urban growth is often associated with a deterioration in the quality of water supplies, which coupled with an ineffective sewage system, may maintain infections. In Egypt transmission of *Giardia* cysts via piped water has also been reported (Khairey et al., 1982). In India most cities use untreated sewage and waste water containing large number of eggs or cysts of intestinal parasites for irrigation of crops. This lack of adequate sewage treatment not only poses risk of contaminating drinking water supplies but may result in the contamination of farm produce (Panicker and Krishnamoorthi, 1978).

7.1.2. Food
Although community wide waterborne outbreaks of giardiasis are now common in developed countries, foodborne giardiasis was also reported by Osterholm (1981) in a farming community in south-western Minnesota. Contamination of food by food handlers who practice substandard hygienic practices may play a role in the transmission of disease in developing countries. In Santiago, Chile, Reyes et al. (1972) examined three fecal samples each from 107 food handlers who worked in locations where foods were prepared and found *Giardia* in 15.9% of the studied population. In 1975, Reyes and Munoz reported that 206 food handlers working in one private and 4 governmental hospitals also in Santiago had serial stool examinations. Of all these apparently healthy subjects, 128 (62.1%) were found to have protozoa and/or helminth infections; *Giardia* accounted for 8.7%. In a similar study by Dall'Orso et al. (1975) in Concepcion, Chile, stool examinations of 169 food handlers revealed that 7.7% were positive for *Giardia*. The food handlers may act as reservoirs of infection for the transmission of disease. It may be mentioned that infected children in sharing their food with their friends or their younger brother and sisters may also transmit the cysts. The possibility of transmission of *Giardia* from feces to food by flies also has been reported from India (Gupta et al., 1972).

7.1.3. Person-to-person transmission
Person-to-person transmission has been strongly implicated in nurseries, schools, and other childrens institutions in developed countries (Black et al., 1977; Keystone et al., 1978). Black et al. (1977) reported a prevalence of *Giardia* in day care children to be significantly higher than the 2% in age-matched children not in day care centers. Furthermore, epidemiological data suggested the fecal-oral transmission of the parasite from child to child in the day-care centers and from infected children to other family members at home. In developing countries, transmission is much more likely to be by the fecal-oral route, especially in conditions of poverty, overcrowding and where water supply and sanitation are inadequate.

A recent study in Zimbabwe suggests that the direct spread of *Giardia* from person-to-person through the use of communal toilets occurs in urban children (Mason et al., 1986). However, in Bangladesh a cohort study of 33 mothers and their infants did not establish evidence for transmission of *Giardia* from mothers to their infants; the rate of infection of infants and mothers appeared to be independent (Table 8).

8. Reservoirs

Although the chief host of the *Giardia* which infect man *is* man, there is some evidence

TABLE 8
Giardia in 33 infant-mother pairs observed for 10 to 15 months, Nandipara, 1981–1982

| Stool findings || Maternal antibody findings ||
Infant	Mother	Serum titre ≥ 20	Milk titre ≥ 5
++	−	+	++
+	−	++	−
++	−	+	−
+	+	+	−
++	+	+	−
++	+	−	+
++	+	+	++
+	+	++	++
++	++	−	++
++	++	+	++
++	++	−	+
++	+	−	++
+	++	−	++
+	++	−	−
−	−	−	−
−	−	−	+
−	−	−	++
−	+	−	++
−	+	++	++
−	++	+	+
−	+	+	++
−	++	+	++
−	++	−	−
−	++	−	−
−	+	++	++
−	+	−	+
−	++	+	−
−	+	−	+
−	+	−	++
−	++	−	++
−	+	−	+
−	++	−	++
−	++	+	+

−, Negative; +, positive; ++, positive more than once.

that humans may acquire, these infections from animals. It thus may be a zoonosis (Woo, 1984). *Giardia* cysts, obtained from several species of animals, have been shown to be capable of initiating human infections. *Giardia* from humans has been transmitted to the rat, gerbil, guinea pig, beaver, dog, cat, raccoon, bighorn, mouflon and pronghorn (Davies and Hibler, 1979; Meyer and Radulescu, 1980). The possibility that *Giardia* from animals may infect humans was strengthened with the discovery that the watershed of one affected city's water supply harbored beavers (Davies and Hibler, 1979). Beavers have been incriminated as a reservoir of infection for hikers who drink water from streams contaminated with beaver feces. Recently, *Giardia* trophozoites were found at necropsy in a great blue heron suggesting another potential source of infection (Georgi et al., 1986). These studies have established that *Giardia* cysts from beavers are infective to humans but the extent to which animals are responsible for endemic and epidemic human disease remains unclear (Roberts-Thomson et al., 1976).

In the past, relatively little attention has been paid to the possibility that reservoir hosts for *Giardia* might exist, but recent studies (Davies and Hibler, 1979; Woo, 1984) suggest that at least some strains of *Giardia* are not highly host specific and that infected lower animals cannot be excluded as possible reservoirs in developing countries where animals such as dogs, cats, cattle, and pigs live in close proximity to human dwellings (Zaki et al., 1986; Bilo and Bilo-Groen, 1983).

The role of asymptomatic carriers as a potential reservoir of *Giardia* infections needs to be evaluated. A substantial proportion of asymptomatic carriers may continuously contaminate the environment with *Giardia* cysts because they are less likely to seek treatment than those with symptomatic disease. A case report of a 2-year-old girl who over a 10-month period had 3 episodes of *Giardia* which did not respond to treatment with metronidazole, prompted the investigators to examine patient's family (father, mother, and a cousin) who were all found to be symptomless carriers. The entire family was treated and cured and so also the patient's symptoms disappeared. This evidence strongly supports the need to detect and treat symptomless *Giardia* carriers (Pancorbo et al., 1985).

9. Control measures

Recognizing that infections with *Giardia* often result from ingesting viable cysts in contaminated water and food, may help to devise control measures. Such measures should be directed towards (1) preventing the contamination of water and food with cysts, (2) destroying or removing cysts which manage to reach water or food, (3) reducing the number of clinically asymptomatic chronic cyst passers, and (4) improving personal hygiene to reduce the risks of person-to-person transmission.

Preventing the contamination of water or food with cysts depends on the availability and use of safe fecal waste disposal systems, the treatment of human feces used as fertilizers to kill cysts, and protecting sources of drinking water from contamination with infected material, whether derived from humans or potential animal reservoirs. In developing countries, many opportunities remain for human sewage to contaminate the water supply. This may occur in the local community stream or when the supply is contaminated by household practices after the water is obtained for family use (Anonymous, 1981). Nevertheless, the major contribution to contamination is the indiscriminate defecation habits of many people in developing countries because they do not have latrines. Although there are many improved methods available for water and waste management systems, in practice it is a process which needs a certain level of social, economic and educational development in order to be successful (Anonymous, 1981). To avoid contamination of food, eating only cooked or peeled foods should be advised.

Killing or removing of cysts from water supplies can be accomplished by disinfection and filtration systems (Logsdon et al., 1979; Jarroll et al., 1980). However, in the context of many developing countries it may be an impractical approach because piped drinking water is not provided to the population at large. Since drinking water is a significant source of *Giardia* infection, heating the water to boiling has been shown to kill the cysts instantaneously (Bingham and Meyer, 1979). However, in developing countries the cost of fuel is a major limiting factor in the use of this otherwise simple method of water purification.

All people with identified symptomatic giardiasis and asymptomatic cyst passers should be treated to eliminate reservoirs of infection. An aggressive reduction of the human enteric reservoir throughout a community not only reduces sources for community spread e.g., in contaminating water supplies, but also reduces opportunities for immediate person to person spread.

Improved personal hygiene will reduce person to person spread of giardiasis. Health benefits can be achieved by improved personal hygiene, by better preparation and storage of food and water, hand washing, and by controlling of insects which may become contaminated with infected human stools and secondarily contaminate food or water within the household (Keusch, 1985).

Of all the control measures outlined, the treatment of symptomatic and asymptomatic cyst passers seems to be effective on a temporary basis (Stevens, 1985). However, treatment regimens for asymptomatic cysts passers still need to be defined.

A vaccine if it could be developed would have a role in protecting groups of the population most vulnerable to giardiasis. Two such high risk groups are travellers and children residing in areas where *Giardia* is endemic. Vaccination protocols have resulted in resistance to *Giardia muris* in mice (Roberts-Thomson and Mitchell, 1979) and recently an 88 kDa *Giardia* surface protein has been reported to be a potentially important immunogen in humans (Edson et al., 1986).

10. Conclusion

Giardia is one of the most commonly identified intestinal pathogens in the world and is an important cause of disease in children of the developing countries. Where *Giardia* is endemic, the age-specific prevalence has its peak in children aged less than 10 and declines thereafter; this might be explained by acquired immunity differences in host response, and by sanitation and behavioral factors that change exposure to infection. Research on *Giardia* over the last 40 years has yielded rapid diagnostic techniques to detect *Giardia* antigen in stool and antibodies in blood but they cannot differentiate between asymptomatic infection and disease. Serological tests still remain to be validated as a diagnostic technique for use with individual patients. Nonetheless, research has not progressed to develop an effective, safe, single-dose treatment for asymptomatic cyst passers, probably the major contributors to the transmission of this disease. The treatment of giardiasis with anti-*Giardia* therapy has clearly shown the positive impact on growth and development of children (Gupta and Urrutia, 1982). But we still do not understand why a substantial proportion of infected people pass cysts, yet are asymptomatic. The precise mechanism of immunity to *Giardia* is also unclear. There are many other unknowns, notably the epidemiological and immunological determinants which affect the pathogenesis and transmission of the disease.

Understanding the biology of the parasite and the mechanism of the host's protective response will lead to strategies to control *Giardia*. Although improvements in sanitary conditions and water supplies are believed to interrupt transmission of the disease, it is an expensive endeavour and a slow process, and it is doubtful whether this will take place in the near future. Efforts to control individual infections can be expected to be successful only on a temporary basis while waiting for the development of vaccine against *Giardia*. A vaccine will require further work on the kinetics of the antibody response to primary infections, as well as studies to ascertain whether distinct strains of the parasite exist with different pathogenic potentials (Smith et al., 1981). The poor prospect for a vaccine in the foreseeable future leaves control of this disease in the short run to the immediate treatment of all diagnosed cases to reduce long-term morbidity in developing countries.

Acknowledgements

The author expresses her sincere appreciation to Dr Andrew Hall and Dr S.A. Sarker for their help in revising the manuscript. Thanks are due to Dr R.N. Mazumder and Mr A.R. Patwary for their technical assistance in the preparation of this manuscript. The author also acknowledges the support of Library and Publication Branch of ICDDR, B.

References

Ali, S. (1981) Incidence of amoebiasis and giardiasis in recurrent diarrhoea and therapeutic study with shorter course nitroimidazole. Bangladesh Med. J. 10, 23-28.
Alp, M.H. and Hislop, I.G. (1969) The effect of *Giardia lamblia* infestation on the gastro-intestinal tract. Aust. Ann. Med. 18, 232-237.
Ament, M.E. and Rubin, C.E. (1972) Relation to giardiasis to abnormal intestinal structure and function in gastrointestinal immunodeficiency syndromes. Gastroenterology 62, 216-226.
Ament, M.E., Ochs, H.D. and Davis, S.D. (1973) Structure and function of the gastrointestinal tract in primary immunodeficiency syndromes, a study of 39 patients. Medicine 52, 227-248.
Amini, F. (1963) Giardiasis and steatorrhoea. J. Trop. Med. Hyg. 66, 190-192.
Anonymous (1981) The International Drinking Water Supply and Sanitation Decade Directory. Published by World Water magazine in collaboration with the WHO., U.K.
Andrews, J.S. Jr. and Hewlett, E.L. (1981) Protection against infection with *Giardia muris* by milk containing antibody to *Giardia*. J. Infect. Dis. 143, 242-246.
Antia, F.P., Desai, H.G., Jeejeebhoy, K.N., Kane, M.P. and Borkar, A.V. (1966) Giardiasis in adults. Incidence, symptomatology and absorption studies. Indian J. Med. Sci. 20, 471-477.
Areekul, S. and Viravan, C. (1984) Prevalence of *Giardia lamblia* and its effect of hematological profile in asymptomatic school children. Southeast Asian J. Trop. Med. Publ. Health 15, 429-430.
Babb, R.R., Peck, O.C. and Vescia, F.G. (1971) Giardiasis: a cause of traveller's diarrhoea. J. Am. Med. Assoc. 217, 1359-1361.
Barbieri, D., DeBrito, T., Hoshino, O., Nascimento, O.B., Martins-Campos, J.V., Quarentei, G. and Marcondes, E. (1970) Giardiasis in childhood: absorption tests and biochemistry, histochemistry, light and electron microscopy of jejunal mucosa. Arch. Dis. Child. 45, 466-472.
Barbour, A.G., Nichols, C.R., Fukushima, T. (1976) An outbreak of giardiasis in a group of campers. Am. J. Trop. Med. Hyg. 25, 384-389.
Bray, R.S. and Harris, W.G. (1977) The epidemiology of infection with *Entamoeba histolytica* in the Gambia, West Africa. Trans. R. Soc. Trop. Med. Hyg. 71, 401-407.
Beal, C.B., Viens, P., Grant, R.G.L. and Hughes, J.M. (1970) A new technique for sampling duodenal contents. Am. J. Trop. Med. Hyg. 19, 349-352.
Belding, D.L. (1965) Textbook of Parasitology, 3rd edit. Appleton, New York, pp. 126.
Bilo, H.S. and Bilo-Groen, C.E. (1983) Worm, *Giardia* and amoebic infestations on Praslin, Seychelles. Trop. Geogr. Med. 35, 179-180.
Bingham, A.K. and Meyer, E.A. (1977) *Giardia* excystation can be induced in vitro in acidic solutions. Nature (London) 277, 301-302.
Black, R.E., Merson, M.H. and Brown, K.H. (1983) Epidemiological aspects of diarrhoea associated with known enteropathogens in rural Bangladesh. In: L.C. Chen and N.S. Scrimshaw (Eds.), Diarrhea and Malnutrition: Interactions, Mechanisms and Interventions. Plenum Press, New York, pp. 73-86.
Black, R.E., Dykes, A.C., Senclair, S.P. and Wells, J.G. (1977) Giardiasis in day-care centres: evidence of person-to-person transmission. Pediatrics 60, 486-491.
Black, R.E., Merson, M.H., Rahman, A.S.M.M., Yunus, M., Alim, A.R.M.A., Huq, I., Yolken, R.H. and Curlin, G.T. (1980) A two-year study of bacterial, viral, and parasitic agents associated with diarrhoea in rural Bangladesh. J. Infect. Dis. 142, 660-664.
Boe, J. and Rinvik, R. (1943) Infection with lamblia intestinalis in children: its clinical significance and treatment. Acta Pediatr. 31, 125-146.
Brodsky, R.E., Spencer, H.C. and Schultz, M.G. (1974) Giardiasis in American travellers to the Soviet Union. J. Infect. Dis. 130, 319-323.
Bulletin of the World Health Organization (1980) Parasite-related diarrhoeas. Report of WHO Scientific Working Group, pp. 819-830.

Burke, J.A. (1975) Giardiasis in childhood. Am. J. Dis. Child. 129, 1304-1310.
Burke, J.A. (1977) The clinical and laboratory diagnosis of giardiasis. CRC Crit. Rev. Clin. Lab. Sci. 373-391.
Butler, T., Middleton, F.G., Earnest, D.L. and Strickland, G.T. (1973) Chronic and recurrent diarrhea in American servicemen in Vietnam: an evaluation of etiology and small bowel structure and function. Arch. Intern. Med. 132, 373-377.
Cantor, D., Biempica, L., Toccalino, H. and O'Donnell, J.C. (1967) Small intestine studies in giardiasis. Am. J. Gastroenterol. 47, 134-141.
Carney, W.P., Van Peenen, P.F.D., See, R., Hagelstein, E. and Lima, B. (1977) Parasites of man in remote areas of central and south Sulawesi, Indonesia. Southeast Asian J. Trop. Med. Hyg. 8, 380-389.
Chavalittamrong, B., Sunlornpoch, V., Siddhikal, C. (1980) Vitamina A concentration in children with giardiasis. South Am. J. Trop. Med. Public Health 11, 245-249.
Chhuttani, P.N., Sehgal, A.K., Mysorker, N.R., Sarin, R.K. and Guleria, S.S. (1973) A search for hill diarrhoea at Simla (India). Indian J. Med. Res. 61, 1039-1047.
Cole, T.J. and Parkin, J.M. (1977) Infection and its effect on the growth of young children: a comparison of the Gambia and Uganda. Trans. R. Soc. Trop. Med. Hyg. 71, 196-198.
Cook, C.G. (1980) Breath hydrogen after oral xylose in tropical malabsorption. Am. J. Clin. Nutr. 33, 555-560.
Cortner, J.A. (1959) Giardiasis: a cause of coeliac syndrome. Am. J. Dis. Child. 98, 311-316.
Court, J.M. and Anderson, C.M. (1959) The pathogenesis of *Giardia lamblia* in children. Med. J. Aust. 46, 436-438.
Craft, J.C. and Nelson, J.D. (1982) Diagnosis of giardiasis by counterimmunoelectrophoresis of feces. J. Infect. Dis. 145, 499-504.
Craun, G.F. (1979) Waterborne giardiasis in the United States: a review. Am. J. Public Health 69, 817-819.
Crompton, D.W.I. (1984) Influence of parasitic infection in food intake. Fed. Proc. 43, 239-245.
Dall'Orso, L.M., Pinilla, N., Parra, G. and Bull, F. (1975) Intestinal parasites and commensal protozoa in foodhandlers from the central area of the city of Concepcion, Chile. Bol. Chil. Parasitol. 30, 30-31.
Danciger, M. and Lopez, M. (1975) Number of *Giardia* in the feces of infected children. Am. J. Trop. Med. Hyg. 24, 237-242.
Davies, R.B. and Hibler, C.P. (1979) Animal reservoirs and cross-species transmission of *Giardia*. In: W. Jakubowski and J.C. Hoff (Eds.), Waterborne Transmission of Giardiasis. US Environmental Protection Agency, Ohio, pp. 104-126.
Davis, C. and Ritchie, L.S. (1948) Clinical manifestations and treatment of epidemic amebiasis occurring in occupants of the Mantetsu apartment building, Tokyo, Japan. Am. J. Trop. Med. 28, 817-823.
DeVizia, B., Poggi, V., Vajro, P., Cucchiara, S., Acampora, A. (1985) Iron malabsorption in giardiasis. J. Pediatr. 107, 75-78.
Dube, S.K., Mehta, S., Walia, B.N.S. and Grewal, M.S. (1970) Giardiasis in children: effect on the small bowel functions. P.G.I. 1, 33.
Edson, C.M., Farthing, M.J.G., Thorley-Lawson, D.A. and Keusch, G.T. (1986) An 88 000-Mr *Giardia lamblia* surface protein which is immunogenic in humans. Infect. Immun. 54, 621-625.
Farthing, M.J.G., Mata, L.J., Urrutia, J.J. and Kronmal, R.A. (1984) Giardiasis: impact on child growth. In: J.A. Walker-Smith and A.S. McNeish (Eds.), Diarrhoea and Malnutrition in Childhood. Butterworths, London, pp. 68-78.
Farthing, M.J.G. (1984) Giardiasis: pathogenesis of chronic diarrhoea and impact on child growth and development. In: E. Lebenthal (Ed.), Chronic Diarrhea in Children, Raven Press, New York, pp. 253-267.
Farthing, M.J., Mata, L., Urrutia, J.J. and Kronmal, R.A. (1986) Natural history of *Giardia* infection of infants and children in rural Guatemala and its impact on physical growth. Am. J. Clin. Nutr. 43, 395-405.
Feachem, R.G., Bradley, D.J., Garelick, H. and Mara, D.D. (1983) Sanitation and Disease, Health Aspects of Excreta and Wastewater Management. John Wiley & Sons, Chichester.
Ferguson, A., Gillon, J. and Al-Thawery, D. (1980) Intestinal abnormalities in murine giardiasis. Trans. R. Soc. Trop. Med. Hyg. 74, 445-448.
Georgi, M.E., Carlisle, M.S. and Smiley, L.E. (1986) Giardiasis in a great blue heron (Ardea Herodias) in New

York state: another potential source of waterborne giardiasis. Am. J. Epidemiol. 123, 916-917.

Giannella, R.A., Brottman, S.A., Zamcheck, N. (1972) The gastric barrier to micro-organisms in man: in vivo and in vitro studies. Gut 13, 251-256.

Giannella, R.A., Brottman, S.A. and Zamcheck, N. (1973) Influence of gastric acidity on bacterial and parasitic enteric infections. Ann. Int. Med. 78, 1271-1276.

Gillin, F.D., Reiner, D.S. and Wang, C.S. (1983) Human milk kills parasitic intestinal protozoa. Science 221, 1290-1292.

Gilman, R.H., Brown, K.H., Visvesvara, G.S., Mondal, G., Greenberg, B., Sack, R.B., Brandt, F. and Khan, M.U. (1985) Epidemiology and serology of *Giardia lamblia* in a developing country: Bangladesh. Trans. R. Soc. Trop. Med. Hyg. 79, 469-473.

Goel, K.M., Shanks, A., McAllister, T.A. and Follett, E.A.C. (1977) Prevalence of intestinal parasitic infestation, salmonellosis, brucellosis, tuberculosis, and hepatitis B among immigrant children in Glasgow. Br. Med. J. 1, 676-679.

Goka, A.K.J., Rolston, D.D.K., Mathan, V.I. and Farthing, M.J.G. (1986) Diagnosis of giardiasis by specific IgM antibody enzyme-linked immunoabsorbent assay. Lancet 2, 184-186.

Gracey, M. (1973) Enteric disease in young Australian aborigines. Aust. NZ J. Med. 3, 576-579.

Green, E.L., Miles, M.A. and Warhurst, D.C. (1985) Immunodiagnostic detection of *Giardia* antigen in faeces by a rapid visual enzyme-linked immunosorbent assay. Lancet 2, 691-693.

Guardiola-Rotger, A., Kander, E., Munoz, A., Lopez, V.A., Gadea, D.E. and Funkenbusch, M.J. (1964) Studies on diarrhoeal disease. J. Pediatr. 65, 87-91.

Guerrant, R.L., Kirchhoff, L.V., Shields, D.S., Nations, M.K., Leslie, J., de Sousa, M.A., Araujo, J.G., Correia, L.L., Sauer, K.T., McClelland, K.E., Trowbridge, F.L. and Hughes, J.M. (1983) Prospective study of diarrheal illnesses in northeastern Brazil: patterns of disease, nutritional impact, etiologies and risk factors. J. Infect. Dis. 148, 986-997.

Gupta, M.C. and Urrutia, J.J. (1982) Effect of periodic antiascaris and antigiardia treatment on nutritional status of preschool children. Am. J. Clin. Nutr. 36, 79-86.

Gupta, R.K. and Mehta, S. (1973) Giardiasis in children: a study of pancreatic functions. Indian J. Med. Res. 61, 743-748.

Gupta, S.P. and Mehta, S. (1970) Chronic diarrhoea: an etiological study. Indian Pediatr. 7, 625-627.

Gupta, S.R., Rao, C.K., Biswas, H., Krishnaswami, A.K., Wattal, B.L. and Raghavan, N.G.S. (1972) Role of the house-fly in the transmission of intestinal parasitic cysts/ova. Indian J. Med. Res. 60, 1120-1125.

Hass, J. and Bucken, E.W. (1967) Zum Krankheitswert der Lamblien Infektion. Dtsch. Med. Wochenschr. 92, 1869-1871.

Hirschhorn, N.A., Chowdhury, A.K.M. and Lindenbaum, J. (1969) Cholera in pregnant women. Lancet 1, 1230-1232.

Hossain, M.M., Ljungstrom, I., Glass, R.I., Lundin, L., Stoll, B.J. and Huldt, G. (1983) Amoebiasis and giardiasis in Bangladesh: parasitological and serological studies. Trans. R. Soc. Trop. Med. Hyg. 77, 552-554.

Hoskins, L.C., Winawer, S.J., Broitman, S.A., Gottlieb, L.S. and Zamcheck, N. (1967) Clinical giardiasis and intestinal malabsorption. Gastroenterology 53, 265-279.

Islam, A., Stoll, B.J., Ljungstrom, I., Biswas, J., Nazrul, H. and Huldt, G. (1983) *Giardia lamblia* infections in a cohort of Bangladeshi mothers and infants followed for one year. J. Pediatr. 103, 996-1000.

Jain, M.K., Bhui, P.S., Mehta, N.J., Taskar, S.P., Sane, S.Y. and Mehta, A.P. (1986) The role of pancreas: pancreatic function in malnourished children. In: J.A. Walker-Smith and A.S. McNeish (Eds.), Diarrhoea and Malnutrition in Childhood. Butterworths, London, pp. 142-146.

Jarroll, E.L., Bingham, A.K. and Meyer, E.A. (1980) *Giardia* cyst destruction: effectiveness of six small-quantity water disinfection methods. Am. J. Trop. Med. Hyg. 29, 8-11.

Jokipii, L. and Jokipii, A.M.M. (1974) Giardiasis in travellers: a prospective study. J. Infect. Dis. 130, 295-299.

Jove, S., Fangundes-Neto, U., Wehba, J., Machado, N.L. and Silvia Patricio, F.R. (1983) Giardiasis in childhood and its effect on the small intestine. J. Pediatr. Gastroenterol. Nutr. 2, 472-477.

Judd, R., Deckelbaum, R.J., Weizman, Z., Granot, E., Ron, N. and Okon, E. (1983) Giardiasis in childhood: poor clinical and histological correlations. Israel J. Med. Sci. 19, 818-823.

Kamath, K.R. and Murugasu, R. (1974) A comparative study of four methods for detecting *Giardia lamblia* in children with diarrhoeal diseases and malabsorption. Gastroenterology 66, 16-21.

Kanwar, S.S., Ganguli, N.K., Wali, B.N.S. and Mahajan, R.C. (1985) Acquired resistance to *Giardia lamblia* infection in mice. Trop. Geogr. Med. 37, 32-36.

Kasim, A.A. and Elhelu, M.A. (1983) Giardiasis in Saudi Arabia. Acta Trop. 40, 155-158.

Keusch, G.T. (1985) Control of intestinal protozoal infections: realities and opportunities. In: C. Chagas and G.T. Keusch (Eds.), The Interaction of Parasitic Diseases and Nutrition. Pontificiae Academiae Scientiarvm Scripta Varia, 61, pp. 285-299.

Keystone, J.S., Krajden, S. and Warren, M.R. (1978) Person-to-person transmission of *Giardia lamblia* in day-care nurseries. Can. Med. Assoc. 119, 241-258.

Khairey, A.E.M., El Sebai, O., Gawad, A.A. and El Attar, L. (1982) The sanitary condition of rural drinking water in a Nile Delta village. I. Parasitological assessment of 'Zir' stored and direct tap water. J. Hyg. 88, 57-61.

Khan, M.U., Shahidullah, M., Ahmed, W.U., Purification, D. and Khan, M.A. (1983) The eltor cholera epidemic in Dhaka in 1974 and 1975. Bull WHO 61, 653-659.

Knight, R. (1980) Epidemiology and transmission of giardiasis. Trans. R. Soc. Trop. Med. Hyg. 74, 433-436.

Ljungstrom, I., Stoll, B. and Islam, A. (1987) *Giardia* infection during pregnancy and lactation (correspondence). Trans. R. Soc. Trop. Med. Hyg. 81, 161.

Logsdon, G.S., Symons, J.M. and Hoye, R.L. (1979) Water filtration techniques for removal of cysts and cyst methods. In: W. Jakubowski and J.C. Hoff (Eds.), Waterborne Transmission of Giardiasis. US Environmental Protection Agency, Ohio, pp. 240-256.

Lopez, M.E., Mata, L., Lizano, C. and Gambox, F. (1978) Infection duodeno-jejunal en el nini con desnutricion energetico-proteinica. Rev. Med. Hosp. Nal. Ninos. (Costa Rica) 13, 53-62.

Lopez, C.E., Juranek, D.D., Sinclair, S.P. and Schultz, M.G. (1978) Giardiasis in American travellers to Madeira Island, Portugal. Am. J. Trop. Med. Hyg. 27, 1128-1132.

Mahalanabis, D., Simpson, T.W., Chakraborty, M.L., Ganguli, C., Bhattacharjuee, A.K. and Mukherjee, K.L. (1979) Malabsorption of water miscible vitamin A in children with giardiasis and ascariasis. Am. J. Clin. Nutr. 32, 313-318.

Mason, P.R. and Nathoo, K.J. (1985) Giardiasis, diarrhoea, and malnutrition. Afr. J. Med. 31, 125-126.

Mason, P.R., Patterson, B.A. and Loewenson, R. (1986) Piped water supply and intestinal parasitism in Zimbabwean school children. Trans. R. Soc. Trop. Med. Hyg. 80, 88-93.

Mata, L.J. (1978) The Children of Santa Maria Cauque. MIT Press, Cambridge, USA.

Mata, L., Simhon, A., Padilla, R., del Mar Gamboa, M., Vargas, G., Hernandez, F., Mohs, E. and Lizano, C. (1983) Diarrhea associated with rotaviruses, enterotoxigenic *Escherichia coli*, *Campylobacter* and other agents in Costa Rican children, 1976-1981. Am. J. Trop. Med. Hyg. 32, 146-153.

Mata, L.J., Mejicanos, M.L. and Jimenez, F. (1972) Studies on the indigenous gastrointestinal flora of Guatemalan children. Am. J. Clin. Nutr. 25, 1380-1390.

Mathan, V.I. (1986) Chronic diarrhoea: malabsorption and the role of viruses. In: J.A. Walker-Smith and A.S. McNeish (Eds.), Diarrhoea and Malnutrition in Childhood. Butterworths, London, pp. 97-102.

Mathews, J.R. and Smith, A.M. (1919) The spread and incidence of intestinal protozoal infections in the population of Great Britain IV. Asylum patients. V. University and school cadets. Ann. Trop. Med. Parasitol. 13, 19.

Melvin, D.M. and Mata, L.J. (1971) Intestinal parasites in a Mayan-Indian village of Guatemala. Rev. Lat. Microbiol. 13, 15-19.

Meyer, E.A., Radulescu, S. (1980) *Giardia* and giardiasis. Adv. Parasitol. 17, 1-14.

Meyer, E.A. and Jarroll, E.L. (1980) Giardiasis. Am. J. Epidemiol. 111, 1-12.

Miotti, P.G., Gilman, R.H., Santosham, M., Ryder, R.W. and Yolken, R.H. (1986) Age-related rate of seropositivity of antibody to *Giardia lamblia* in four diverse populations. J. Clin. Microbiol. 24, 972-975.

Miotti, P.G., Gilman, R.H., Pickering, L.K., Ruiz-Palacios, G., Park, H.S. and Yolken, R.H. (1985) Prevalence of serum and milk antibodies to *Giardia lamblia* in different populations of lactating women. J. Infect. Dis. 152, 1025-1031.

Molla, A.M., Molla, A., Sarker, S.A. and Rahaman, M.M. (1983) Food intake during and after recovery from diarrhea in children. In: L.C. Chen and N.S. Scrimshaw (Eds.), Diarrhea and Malnutrition: Interactions, Mechanisms, and Interventions. Plenum Press, New York, pp. 113-123.

Molla, A., Molla, A.M. and Sarker, S.A. (1986) Malabsorption in enteric infection, a nutritional cost in children with diarrhoea. In: C. Chagas and G.T. Keusch (Eds.), Study Week On The Interaction of Parasitic Diseases and Nutrition, October 22-26, 1985. Pontificiae Academiae Scientiarvm, Citta del Vaticano 61, 71-80.

Moore, G.T., Cross, W.M., McGuire, D., Mollohan, C.S., Gleason, N.N., Healy, G.R. and Newton, L.H. (1969) Epidemic giardiasis at a ski resort. N. Engl. J. Med. 281, 402-407.

Moore, H.A., De La Cruz, E., Vargas-Mendez, O. and Perez, F.I. (1966) Diarrheal disease studies in Costa Rica. II. The prevalence of certain enteric organisms and their relationship to diarrhea. Am. J. Public Health. 56, 442-451.

Muttalib, M.A. (1970) Helminthiasis: problem of E. Pakistan. Pak. Med. Rev. 5, 191-202.

Nash, T.E., Herrington, D.A. and Levine, M.M. (1987) Usefulness and enzyme-linked immunosorbent assay for detection of *Giardia lamblia* antigen in feces. J. Clin. Microbiol. 25, 1169-1171.

Nathoo, K.I., Mason, P.R., Trijssenaar, F.J., Lyons, N.F. and Tewana, S.A. (1986) Microbial pathogens associated with diarrhoea in children admitted to Harare Hospital for rehydration. Central Afr. J. Med. 32, 118-123.

Okeahialam, T.C. (1983) Growth of Nigerian children with marasmus after hospital treatment. J. Natl. Med. Assoc. 75, 75-80.

Osterholm, M.T., Forfang, J.C., Ristinen, T.L., Dean, A.G., Washburn, J.W., Godes, J.R., Rude, R.A. and McCullough, J.G. (1981) An outbreak of foodborne giardiasis. N. Engl. J. Med. 304, 24-28.

Oyerinde, J.P.O., Ogunbi, O. and Alonge, A.A. (1977) Age and sex distribution of infections with *Entamoeba histolytica* and *Giardia intestinalis* in the Lagos population. Int. J. Epidemiol. 6, 231-234.

Pancorbo, J.M.C., Munoz, M.T.G. and Badia, J.L.S. (1985) Giardiasis: treatment of carriers. Lancet 2, 951.

Panicker, P.V.R.C. and Krishnamoorthi, K.P. (1978) Elimination of enteric parasites during sewage treatment processes. IAWPC Tech. Annual-V, 130-138.

Paulsen, O. (1977) Blood group A and giardiasis. Lancet 2, 984.

Pierce, V., Ascoli, W., de Leon, R. and Gordon, J.E. (1962) Studies of diarrheal disease in Central America. III. Specific etiology of endemic diarrhea and dysentery in Guatemalan children. Am. J. Trop. Med. Hyg. 11, 395-400.

Quinn, R.W. (1971) The epidemiology of intestinal parasites of importance in the United States. South Med. Bull. 59, 29-30.

Pugh, R.J. and Newton, R.W. (1980) Giardiasis in infancy and childhood. Practitioner 224, 393-397.

Rabassa, E.B., Arbelo, T.F., Guillot, C.C. and Gonzales, E.S. (1975) Malabsorcion por *Giardia lamblia*. Rev. Cub. Pediatr. 47, 247-263.

Rabbani, G.H., Gilman, R.H., Islam, A. and Froelich, J. (1982) Comparison of string-test and stool examination in the diagnosis of strongyloidiasis and giardiasis in gastroenteritis patients. Asian Med. J. 25, 695-700.

Radulescu, S., Iancu, L., Simionescu, O. and Meyer, E.A. (1976) Serum antibodies in giardiasis. J. Clin. Pathol. 29, 863.

Rendtorff, R.C. and Holt, C.J. (1954) The experimental transmission of human intestinal protozoan parasites. II. *Giardia lamblia* cysts given in capsules. Am. J. Hyg. 59, 209-220.

Reyes, H., Olea, M. and Hernandez, R. (1972) Enteroparasitoses in foodhandlers in the public health sector east of Santiago. Bol. Chil. Parasitol. 27, 115-116.

Reyes, H. and Munoz, V. (1975) Intestinal parasitosis in hospital handlers. Rev. Med. Child. 103, 477-479.

Reiner, D.S., Wang Chi-Sung and Gillin, F.D. (1986) Human milk kills *Giardia lamblia* by generating toxic lipolytic products. Infect. Dis. 154, 825-832.

Roberts-Thomson, I.C., Stevens, D.P., Mahmood, A.A.E. and Warren, K.S. (1976) Acquired resistance to

infection in an animal model of giardiasis. Immunology 117, 2036-2037.
Roberts-Thomson, I.C. and Mitchell, G.F. (1979) Protection of mice against *Giardia muris* infection. Infect. Immun. 24, 971-973.
Rosenberg, I.H. and Bowman, B.B. (1984) Impact of intestinal parasites on digestive function in humans. Nutr. Parasitol. Infect. Fed. Proc. 43, 246-250.
Rosenthal, P. and Liebman, W.M. (1980) Comparative study of stool examinations, duodenal aspiration, and pediatric entero-test for giardiasis in children. Pediatrics 96, 278-279.
Rowland, M.G.M., Cole, T.J. and Whitehead, R.E. (1977) A quantitative study into the role of infection in determining nutritional status in Gambian village children. Br. J. Nutr. 37, 441-450.
Sarker, S.A., Molla, A.M., Karim, A.K.M.M. and Rahman, M.M. (1982) Calorie intake in childhood diarrhoea. Nutr. Rep. Int. 26, 581-590.
Schmerin, M.J., Jones, T.C. and Klein, H. (1978) Giardiasis: association with homosexuality. Ann. Intern. Med. 88, 801-803.
Schneider, C.C. (1961) *Giardia muris* II. The influence of nutrition and other factors on the course of infection. Z. Tropenmed. Parasitol. 12, 365-385.
Sherman, P. and Lieban, W.M. (1980) Apparent protein-losing enteropathy associated with giardiasis. Am. J. Dis. Child. 134, 893-894.
Shukry, S., Zaki, A.M., Dupont, H.L., Shoukry, I., el Tagi, M. and Hamed, S. (1986) Detection of enteropathogens in fatal and potentially fatal diarrhea in Cairo, Egypt. Clin. Microbiol. 24, 959-962.
Smith, J.A. (1978) Glucose utilization and related metabolism of *Giardia felis* trophozoites. University of Oregon Medical School. Thesis (submitted).
Smith, P.D., Gillin, F.D., Brown, W.R. and Nash, T.E. (1981) IgG antibody to *Giardia lamblia* detected by enzyme-linked immunosorbent assay. Gastroenterology 80, 1476-1480.
Smith, P.D., Gillin, F.D., Kaushal, N.A. and Nash, T.E. (1981) Antigenic analysis of *Giardia lamblia* from Afghanistan, Puerto Rico, Ecuador and Oregon. Infect. Immun. 36, 713-719.
Speelman, P. and Ljungstrom, I. (1986) Protozoal enteric infections among expatriates in Bangladesh. Am. J. Trop. Med. Hyg. 35, 1140-1145.
Stevens, D.P. (1982) Giardiasis: host-pathogen biology. Rev. Infect. Dis. 4, 851-858.
Stevens, D.P. (1985) Selective primary health care: strategies for control of disease in the developing world. XIX. Giardiasis. Rev. Infect. Dis. 7, 530-535.
Stevens, D.P., Frank, D.M. and Mahmoud, A.A.F. (1978) Thymus dependency of host resistance to *Giardia muris* infection: studies in nude mice. J. Immunol. 120, 680-682.
Stoll, B.J., Glass, R.I., Huq, M.I., Khan, M.U., Holt, J.E. and Banu, H. (1982) Surveillance of patients attending a diarrhoeal disease hospital in Bangladesh. Br. Med. J. 285, 1185-1188.
Tandon, B.N., Tandon, R.K., Satpathy, B.K., Shriniwas. (1977) Mechanism of malabsorption in giardiasis: a study of bacterial flora and bile salt deconjugation in upper jejunum. Gut 18, 176-181.
Tewari, S.G. and Tandon, B.N. (1974) Functional and histological changes of small bowel in patients with *Giardia lamblia* infestation. Indian J. Med. Res. 62, 689-695.
Thacker, S.B., Simpson, S., Gordon, T.J., Wolfe, M. and Kimball, A.M. (1979) Parasitic disease control in a residential facility for the mentally retarded. Am. J. Public Health 69, 1279-1281.
Tomkin, A.M., Drasar, B.S., Bradley, A.K. and Williamson, W.A. (1978) Bacterial colonization of jejunal mucosa in giardiasis. Trans. R. Soc. Trop. Med. Hyg. 72, 33-36.
Tomkin, A.M. (1983) Nutritional cost of protracted diarrhoea in young Gambian children. Gut 24, A495.
Tomkins, A. (1981) The significance of intestinal parasites in malnourished populations. Parasitology 82, 38-40.
Ungar, B.L.P., Yolken, R.H., Nash, T.E. and Quinn, T.C. (1984) Enzyme-linked immunosorbent assay for the detection of *Giardia lamblia* in fecal specimens. J. Infect. Dis. 149, 90-97.
Veghelyi, P.V. (1938) Giardiasis in children. Am. J. Dis. Child. 56, 1231-1241.
Visvesvara, G.S., Smith, P.D., Healy, G.R. and Brown, W.R. (1980) An immunofluorescence test to detect serum antibodies to *Giardia lamblia*. Ann. Intern. Med. 93, 802-805.
Vizia, B.D., Poggi, V.P., Cucchiara, S. and Acampora, A. (1985) Iron malabsorption in giardiasis. J. Pediatr.

75-78.

Walia, B.N.S., Gupta, S.P., Meheta, S. and Agarwal, K.C. (1971) Chronic diarrhoea in North Indian children. Indian J. Med. Res. 59, 1448-1453.

Walia, B.N.S., Ganguly, N.K., Mahajan, R.C., Kumar, D., Madan, I.J., Gambhir, S.K. and Kanwar, S.S. (1986) Morbidity in preschool *Giardia* cyst excretors. Trop. Geogr. Med. 38, 367-370.

Webster, A.D.B. (1980) Giardiasis and immunodeficiency syndromes. Trans. R. Soc. Trop. Med. Hyg. 74, 440-441.

Woo, P.K. (1984) Evidence for animal reservoirs and transmission of *Giardia* infection between animal species. In: S.L. Erlandsen and E.A. Meyer (Eds.), *Giardia* and Giardiasis. Plenum Press, New York, pp. 341-364.

Wright, S.G., Tomkins, A.M. and Ridley, D.S. (1977) Giardiasis: clinical and therapeutic aspects. Gut 18, 343-350.

Yardley, J.H., Takano, J. and Hendrix, T.R. (1964) Epithelial lesions of the jejunum in giardiasis: jejunal biopsy studies. Johns Hopkins Med. J. 115, 389-406.

Yardley, J.H. and Bangless, T.M. (1967) Giardiasis. Gastroenterology 52, 301-304.

Yoeli, M., Most, H., Hammond, J. and Scheinesson, G.P. (1972) Parasitic infections in a closed community: results of a 10-year survey in Willowbrook state school. Trans. R. Soc. Trop. Med. Hyg. 66, 764-776.

Zaki, A.M., El-Alamy, M. and DuPont, H.L. (1983) Acute diarrhea in rural Egyptian population (abstract). In: Proceedings of the Annual Meeting of the American Society of Tropical Medicine and Hygiene. San Antonio, December.

Zaki, A.M., Dupont, H.L., El-Alamy, M.A., Arefat, R.R., Amin, K., Awad, M.M., Bassiouni, L., Imam, I.Z., El-Malik, G., El-Marsafie, A., Mohieldin, M.S., Naguib, T., Rakha, M.A., Sidaros, M., Wasef, N., Wright, C.E. and Wyett, R.G. (1986) The detection of entero-pathogens in acute diarrhea in a family cohort population in rural Egypt. Am. J. Trop. Med. Hyg. 35, 1013-1022.

Giardiasis (E.A. Meyer, ed.)
© 1990 Elsevier Science Publishers B.V. (Biomedical Division)

15

Waterborne giardiasis

GUNTHER F. CRAUN[1]

U.S. Environmental Protection Agency, 26 West Saint Clair, Cincinnati, OH 45268, U.S.A.

1. Introduction	267
2. Waterborne giardiasis in travelers	270
3. Endemic waterborne giardiasis	271
4. Waterborne outbreaks of giardiasis	272
4.1. United States 1965-85	272
4.2. Other countries	283
5. *Giardia* cysts in drinking water	284
6. Conclusions	288
References	290

1. Introduction

Although much is still to be learned about *Giardia* and its transmission, our knowledge has improved dramatically over the past several decades. Few now question that *Giardia* is an intestinal pathogen in both children and adults (Editorial, 1980). *Giardia* infects humans throughout the world, in arctic locations (e.g., Canadian Yukon and Greenland) and temperate and tropical climates (Jakubowski, 1988), and it is the most frequently identified parasite in the United States (Anonymous, 1978) and Britain (Editorial, 1980). In the United States *Giardia* has been found to infect 2 to 20% of the population, depending on community and age group studied (Benenson, 1980). In a 1976 survey of 55 state and territorial laboratories by CDC, *Giardia* was found in 3.8% of 414 820 stool specimens examined (Anonymous, 1978).

---

[1]This chapter was written by Gunther F. Craun in his private capacity. No official support or endorsement by the Environmental Protection Agency, or any other agency of the Federal Government is intended or should be inferred.

Giardiasis is transmitted fecal-orally by contact with infected individuals, contaminated drinking water (Craun, 1984; Craun and Jakubowski, 1987) or food (Osterholm et al., 1981). Frequently reported are outbreaks in day-care centers (Black et al., 1977; Keystone et al., 1978; Sealy and Schuman, 1983) and infections in campers and backpackers, travelers outside the United States, and homosexuals (Schmerin et al., 1978; Stevens, 1982). *Giardia* can infect a wide variety of wild and domestic animals, and both humans and animals can be important sources (primary or intermediary) of *Giardia* contamination of water supplies. Although it is not clear that *Giardia* cysts from all of these animal sources can infect humans, human infectivity is suggested from experimental studies showing that animals can be infected by cysts from human sources (Jakubowski, 1988).

It is difficult to quantify the relative significance of each mode of transmission, but an important source of *Giardia* infection is contaminated water. In the United States *Giardia* is the most commonly identified pathogen in waterborne outbreaks (Table 1). During the period 1971-85, *Giardia* was identified in 92 (18%) waterborne outbreaks resulting in 24 124 (22%) cases of illness. An etiologic agent was determined in 251 waterborne outbreaks reported during this period, and *Giardia* was responsible for 49% of the cases of illness and 37% of the outbreaks with an established etiology.

Although incomplete epidemiologic investigation and reporting make it difficult to determine the significance of the waterborne transmission of giardiasis in the United States accurately, the waterborne route of transmission seems to be more important for this protozoan than for other more commonly recognized waterborne pathogens. Some 58 504 cases of giardiasis were optionally reported from all causes during 1976-80 (Craun, 1986b). The cases of giardiasis associated with waterborne outbreaks during this

TABLE 1

Etiology of waterborne outbreaks reported in the United States, 1971–85

Illness	Number of outbreaks
Gastroenteritis, undefined	251
Giardiasis	92
Chemical poisoning	50
Shigellosis	33
Hepatitis A	23
Gastroenteritis, viral	20
Campylobacteriosis	11
Salmonellosis	10
Typhoid	5
Yersiniosis	2
Gastroenteritis, toxigenic *E. coli*	1
Cryptosporidiosis	1
Cholera	1
Dermatitis	1
Amebiasis	1
Total	502

period represent 25% of these optionally reported cases. In comparison, since 1951 in the United States, generally less than 2% of all reported cases of typhoid fever, salmonellosis, shigellosis, or infectious hepatitis have occurred in waterborne outbreaks in the United States (Craun, 1986a).

The waterborne transmission of *Giardia* was suggested as early as 1946 in an epidemiologic investigation of an outbreak of amebiasis attributed to sewage contamination of a water supply in a Tokyo apartment building (Davis and Ritchie, 1948). *Entamoeba histolytica* and *Giardia* were recovered from 64% and 77% of the occupants, respectively; *Giardia* was isolated from 86% of the occupants who experienced diarrhea with abdominal discomfort and had stools that were negative for *E. histolytica*. In 1954 infection was established in volunteers who ingested drinking water containing a small number of cysts (Rendtorff, 1954). A survey during an outbreak of 50 000 cases of gastroenteritis in Portland, Oregon, from October 1954 to March 1955 (Veazie, 1969; Meyer, 1973) revealed that *Giardia* was detectable in the majority of individuals with a chronic syndrome of 14.8 days average duration characterized by abdominal discomfort, diarrhea, loss of appetite, nausea, and in severe cases weight loss (Veazie et al., 1979). Of the known possible etiologic agents of such a syndrome, only *Giardia* was identified in clinical specimens. This finding, however, did not prevent controversy among investigators concerning this organism's pathogenicity and its role in the outbreak. The source of infection and mode of transmission were never satisfactorily determined although drinking water was suspected; Portland uses an unfiltered surface water source with disinfection as the only treatment (Craun, 1979).

The first well documented waterborne outbreak of giardiasis in the United States occurred in Aspen, Colorado, in 1965-66 (Moore et al., 1969). The outbreak was investigated when a physician developed characteristic symptoms of giardiasis after returning from a ski holiday at Aspen, and a stool examination yielded *Giardia* cysts but no bacterial pathogens. A survey of 1094 skiers who had vacationed in Aspen during December 1965 to January 1966 found at least 123 had developed similar symptoms. *Giardia* was considered the etiologic agent because of its association with the illness, the absence of other pathogens, and the response of individuals to treatment. Approximately half of the city's water came from a small mountain stream and half from three wells. Each water source was chlorinated, but the stream water was not filtered. Intermittent coliform contamination was detected in water samples during the outbreak. The stream received no obvious sewage discharges. Fluorescent and detergent tracers placed in the sewage system were detected in two of the wells suggesting sewage contamination from leaking sewer mains. *Giardia* cysts were also isolated from the leaking sewage. A parasitologic survey of Aspen residents showed a difference in prevalence of *Giardia* infection between the area of the city served by the wells (6.9%) and the area served by the stream (3.7%), but this difference was found not to be statistically significant. In retrospect it is possible that even though no obvious human sewage pollution was found, the stream could have been contaminated with *Giardia* cysts from animal sources, hikers, or campers. Although not considered at the time, this contamination could have resulted in a higher than normal prevalence of infection for the area served by the stream, thus contributing to an inability to observe a statistical significance.

It was not until the past two decades that the role of *Giardia* in waterborne diseases has become apparent. This was recognized most dramatically in the United States after (1) the occurrence of several large waterborne outbreaks in community water systems, and (2) increased reports of infection in American tourists to the Soviet Union, and backpackers and campers using untreated stream water.

2. Waterborne giardiasis in travelers

Reports of giardiasis in American travelers to the Soviet Union in the 1970s generally increased the recognition, investigation, and reporting of this disease in the United States. The first reports appeared in persons accompanying the U.S. Olympic Boxing Team on a tour of the Soviet Union in February and March 1970, and in a group of scientists visiting the Soviet Union in May of the same year; Leningrad was implicated as the site of acquisition of the infection, and tap water was the probable mode of transmission (CDC, 1970; Walzer et al., 1971; Brodsky et al., 1974). Additional retrospective and prospective epidemiologic studies of American and other tourists served to confirm an association between giardiasis in the travelers and the consumption of tap water in Leningrad (Johnson, 1972; Anderson et al., 1972; Jokipii, 1972; Forssell et al., 1972; Aust Kettis and Magnius, 1973; Fiumara, 1973; CDC, 1974; 1975; Gendel, 1974; Jokipii and Jokipii, 1974; Martin and Martin, 1975). In two studies where tap water consumption was quantified, the risk of infection was found to increase with the amount of water consumed (Brodsky et al., 1974; CDC, 1975). The strongest evidence for an association between giardiasis and consumption of tap water in Leningrad was provided by two prospective studies which included the examination of stool specimens prior to and after travel to Leningrad by staff members of the National Aeronautics and Space Administration (Brodsky et al., 1974) and Finnish students (Jokipii and Jokipii, 1974). Although it was not possible to obtain data directly on water supplies in Leningrad, limited information was available to question the effectiveness of water treatment to remove and inactivate *Giardia* cysts (Craun, 1984).

A waterborne outbreak of giardiasis was also reported in American travelers to the Portuguese island of Madeira in October 1976, but this appeared to be an isolated event rather than an ongoing problem such as in Leningrad (CDC, 1977). A retrospective survey of a group of 1400 tourists who had become ill on their return from the island showed drinking water was statistically associated with illness; 27% of 859 respondents developed an illness resembling giardiasis, and *Giardia* was identified from 27 of 58 patients who had a stool examination. The drinking water was reportedly chlorinated, but information on water sources, chlorine levels, operation, or other treatment was not available. A follow-up survey of Americans traveling to Madeira in the spring of 1977 showed that less than 4% developed an illness compatible with giardiasis.

3. Endemic waterborne giardiasis

Studies in Colorado (Wright et al., 1977), Minnesota (Weiss et al., 1977), Washington (Harter et al., 1982; Frost et al., 1983), New Hampshire (Chute et al., 1985, 1987), and Utah (Laxter, 1985) have suggested that consumption of untreated drinking water is an important cause of endemic infection in the United States. A 1973 survey of 256 Colorado residents having *Giardia*-positive stools, when compared to 256 controls matched by age, gender, race, and place of residence, showed a higher proportion of cases in those who visited Colorado mountains (69% vs. 47%), camped overnight (38% vs. 18%), and drank untreated mountain water (50% vs. 17%). Bacteriologic examination of 16 mountain streams in areas with no permanent human habitation showed fecal coliform contamination in each stream; the highest concentration occurred between June and August, a seasonal pattern which correlated with the monthly distribution of human *Giardia* infections. A 1975 survey of 78 Minnesota residents having *Giardia*-positive stools and no history of recent foreign travel showed that 63% had consumed untreated water during the period of study and 46% had not been out of the state in the 2 months before onset of symptoms. Unfortunately, an appropriate control group was not included for comparison. Results of a case-control study of 349 Washington State residents having *Giardia*-positive stools during July 1978 to March 1980 and 349 controls matched by age and gender showed nursery school exposure for children, foreign travel to Third World countries for adults, and consumption of untreated water in Washington State for all age groups to be associated with a higher risk of acquiring infection (Frost et al., 1983). Consumption of untreated water occurred more frequently among adult males but was observed in both genders and in all age groups; it occurred throughout the year but was more common during the summer. A survey of intestinal parasites conducted in two Washington counties found a 7.1% *Giardia* prevalence among 518 children, one to three years of age (Harter et al., 1983). No statistically significant difference in prevalence of infection was found by source (surface or well) of domestic drinking water; however, only one of 37 (2.7%) children residing in a home using filtered surface water was found to be infected with *Giardia* compared with 10 of 175 (6.9%) children residing in homes using unfiltered surface water. A statistically significant increased prevalence of infection was also found in children who had a history of drinking untreated surface water from streams or lakes during recreational activities. Results of a case-control study of 171 giardiasis patients identified through the Hitchcock Clinic laboratory in New Hampshire during January, 1977 to June, 1984 and 684 controls matched by age and gender showed increased risks of acquiring giardiasis associated with travel outside the United States, family member with diagnosed giardiasis, family member in a day-care program, camping, and use of a shallow well or surface water for individual, household water supply. Individuals with giardiasis were more likely to use shallow well or surface water sources for their household water supply [oddsratio (OR), 2.1; 95% confidence interval (CI), 1.3,3.2) rather than any other water sources, drilled well or municipal. The risk of giardiasis associated with the household use of shallow well or surface water sources was slightly higher (OR 2.6; 95% CI 1.6,4.3) when compared only with the household use of municipal water sources. Shallow well sources, a previously unrecognized risk factor for endemic giardiasis, are reportedly common in northern New England and are frequently open to surface water contamination. The 18% etiologic fraction found to be attributable to the use of shallow well or surface water sources suggests they may have a significant impact on endemic giardiasis. A questionnaire survey of 383 Utah National Guard members showed that 15% had symptoms suggestive of giardiasis and that the guardsmen were at risk of contracting giardiasis by drinking contaminated water during field exercises in the state (Laxter, 1985). It was found that 62% of the 58 guardsmen who showed symptoms had supplemented the water supply provided during the exercises with untreated water from lakes, streams, and a cattle watering trough.

4. Waterborne outbreaks of giardiasis

4.1. United States 1965-1985

Since 1965, 95 waterborne outbreaks and 24 541 cases of giardiasis have been reported (Craun, 1984, 1986c) in the United States (Table 2). Most (56%) of these outbreaks were reported during the past five years. The outbreaks reported are those in which drinking water was epidemiologically implicated as the vehicle of transmission of the illness. In addition to outbreaks caused by consumption of water intended for drinking or domestic purposes, the statistics include outbreaks caused by consumption of water from nonpotable sources, by swimmers or divers, and from creeks by backpackers and campers.

Waterborne giardiasis outbreaks were reported in 22 states but occurred primarily in the

TABLE 2

Waterborne outbreaks of giardiasis in the United States, 1965–85

Time period	Community water systems		All water systems	
	Outbreaks	Cases	Outbreaks	Cases
1965-70	2	157	3	176
1971-75	5	4942	13	5136
1976-80	17	12148	26	14416
1981-85	38	4144	53	4813
	62	21391	95	24541

TABLE 3
Location of waterborne outbreaks of giardiasis in the United States, 1965–85

State	Outbreaks	Cases of illness
Colorado	34	6258
Washington	7	1363
Utah	6	1432
Pennsylvania	5	4314
New Hampshire	5	898
Oregon	5	255
New York	4	4948
Montana	4	1135
Vermont	4	96
Alaska	3	315
Idaho	3	124
Virginia	3	40
California	2	154
Florida	2	10
Arizona	1	2000
Massachusetts	1	703
Nevada	1	342
New Mexico	1	100
Wisconsin	1	25
Illinois	1	15
New Jersey	1	9
Tennessee	1	5
Totals	95	24541

mountainous regions of the Northeast, West, and Northwest (Table 3). Over 90% of the outbreaks and cases occurred in 17 northeastern, western, and northwestern states. Water supplies in these areas are usually obtained from streams or reservoirs not contaminated by wastewater discharges. The quality of these surface water sources is generally good and the watersheds are often sparsely populated or protected by various restrictions on recreation, development, and human activities. As a result water treatment has been minimal. Because turbidity is generally low, treatment for surface water sources consists primarily of disinfection without filtration. Maintaining continuous, adequate disinfection has not received as much attention as in areas where treatment of surface water generally consists of coagulation, sedimentation, and filtration in addition to disinfection.

Although large outbreaks of giardiasis have been reported, outbreaks have generally occurred in small community water systems and noncommunity water systems (Table 4). Community water systems are defined as water supplies serving communities, subdivisions, or trailer parks having at least 15 connections or 25 year-round residents. The noncommunity water systems must serve an average of 25 individuals for 60 or more days and include camps, parks, resorts, and institutions which maintain their own water supply. Individual water systems are used by residents in areas without community systems or

TABLE 4

Waterborne outbreaks of giardiasis in various types of water systems in the United States, 1965–85

Type of system	Outbreaks	Cases of illness
Community	62	21391
Noncommunity	21	2964
Individual or recreational	12	186
Totals	95	24541

persons traveling outside of populated areas (e.g. backpackers, campers). Grouped with the individual systems for analysis and considered as miscellaneous outbreaks are those caused by use of nonpotable sources or ingestion of water while swimming or diving. Not included in these statistics are a number of single cases of giardiasis in backpackers which were reported in an anecdotal manner and not investigated epidemiologically.

Colorado has reported 34 waterborne outbreaks of giardiasis, more than any other state, but this may reflect primarily increased surveillance and investigation (Hopkins et al., 1985; Harter et al., 1985). The reporting of waterborne outbreaks is voluntary, and more waterborne outbreaks have occurred than are reported to the Environmental Protection Agency (EPA) and Centers for Disease Control (CDC). While the reporting of waterborne outbreaks has generally improved since 1971, many factors influence the degree to which outbreaks are recognized, investigated, and reported in any single year. These include the number of affected individuals, whether the disease is reportable, the type of water system, and interest in the problem and capabilities for recognition and investigation at the state and local level. For example, officials in Pennsylvania, Colorado, and Washington generally increased their waterborne disease surveillance activities during the 1970s, and together these states were responsible for reporting 31% of all waterborne outbreaks during the period 1971-80. During the previous 20-year period, only 8% of all waterborne outbreaks were reported by these states (Craun, 1986a).

It is difficult to estimate the number of waterborne outbreaks which are not recognized, investigated, and reported. One estimate (Craun and McCabe, 1973) based on data from 1946-70 suggested that about one third of the waterborne outbreaks in noncommunity water systems and about one half of those in community water systems are reported. A study (Barker, 1974) of improved surveillance and investigation of foodborne outbreaks in the state of Washington indicated that only one of ten foodborne outbreaks had been recognized, investigated, and reported. The results of this study may be applicable to the reporting of waterborne outbreaks because of similarities in the recognition and investigation of foodborne and waterborne outbreaks, and this figure could represent a maximum estimate of underreporting for small community and noncommunity water systems.

Outbreaks in community water systems, which number about 59000 and serve about 180 million people, are probably the most likely to be reported. Outbreaks in noncommunity systems, which number about 240000 and serve about 20 million people, primarily travelers, are the next most likely to be reported. It is difficult to recognize and investigate an outbreak in travelers because they may become ill after leaving the area where the illness was contracted, and the illness may be reported to several different health authorities. Unless the outbreak is large or attracts widespread attention, knowledge may be lacking of similar cases outside the immediate area and a common source may not be suspected. Even if a common source is suspected, it may be difficult to investigate. The publicity associated with recent giardiasis outbreaks in travelers, however, has resulted in a greater recognition of the possibility of common source outbreaks in travelers, and health departments and physicians are more suspicious when an illness such as giardiasis is diagnosed after vacation or travel. Outbreaks in individual water systems, which serve about 30 million people, are least likely to be reported. Many health departments lack the authority or have insufficient resources to conduct water quality surveillance programs for individual water systems, and sporadic reports of disease in rural areas may be inadequately investigated. Reportable diseases such as typhoid fever are likely, however, to be investigated even when a single case is reported. Increased epidemiologic investigations are anticipated for suspected outbreaks of giardiasis, as more states now require its reporting. Prior to 1980, giardiasis was optionally reported in most states, and reporting was required in only eight states. At present some 38 states list giardiasis as a reportable disease (Jakubowski, 1988). Active surveillance of reportable diseases may help detect outbreaks. For example, only ten cases of shigellosis initiated an investigation which uncovered an outbreak of some 1200 illnesses in a community of 6500 persons in Florida in 1974 (Weisman et al., 1976). If local health authorities had not been conducting shigellosis surveillance, the initial ten cases might never have been recognized as an unusual occurrence, and a waterborne outbreak as large as this might have gone undetected.

During a three-year period of intensive surveillance for waterborne disease in Colorado in 1980-83, eighteen waterborne outbreaks were documented; *Giardia* was the etiologic agent in nine of these outbreaks (Hopkins et al., 1985). Only six waterborne outbreaks had been reported during the previous three years when the health department had a passive surveillance system with responsibility for follow-up of water-related disease and complaints divided among three separate sections. In general, increased disease surveillance and follow-up in Colorado were found to be more effective in detecting waterborne outbreaks than increased surveillance and follow up of water quality problems (Hopkins et al., 1985; Harter et al., 1985). Activities important for effective surveillance included educational outreach programs to local health agencies, physicians, and the public and the designation of one individual to whom all water-related complaints and health department inquiries were directed. Colorado participated with Washington and Vermont in an evaluation of the effectiveness of nine active and one enhanced passive surveillance activities in detecting waterborne outbreaks. The active methods included routine review and follow-up of coliform monitoring results, illness surveys and pathogen testing of water samples in systems with water quality problems, investigation of laboratory cases of giardiasis and other waterborne pathogens, and surveillance of illness in schools, parks, camps, and industries. The passive surveillance system normally employed by states is based on voluntary reporting with little or no effort devoted to soliciting specific illness reports which may be related to contaminated drinking water. The passive surveillance system was enhanced during the study by ensuring the services of a full-time epidemiologist and part-time engineer or microbiologist for the investigation of suspected waterborne outbreaks and expanded support for laboratory analysis. During this two-year evaluation the number of waterborne outbreaks in public water systems increased in Colorado but not in Washington or Vermont when compared with the previous two-year period. In all states, intensive surveillance of water systems with coliform violations did not reveal enteric illness among water users. In Colorado, the daily monitoring and follow-up of positive coliform tests failed to uncover any gastroenteritis outbreaks in the affected communities. Coliform bacteria were elevated in only ten of the waterborne outbreaks reported in all states. The presence of coliforms failed to predict illness in the community, and the absence of coliforms did not assure safe drinking water. While in some instances coliforms may be indicative of water contamination or water treatment failure, these data suggest they are a less reliable indicator of health risk and may be ineffective in preventing waterborne outbreaks. The failure of coliforms to predict outbreaks has also been noted in previous studies (Craun, 1978; Batik et al., 1983).

The collection of epidemiologic data on laboratory diagnosed cases of giardiasis in Colorado resulted in the investigation and identification of only one waterborne outbreak of giardiasis during the two-year evaluation of surveillance methods (Harter et al., 1985). Frost et al. (1983), however, found significant underreporting of waterborne giardiasis in Washington. A follow-up of 883 individual cases of giardiasis reported from July 1978 to March 1980 showed that 275 cases were possibly due to common-source outbreaks: six clusters of at least 8 cases involved 70 individuals and 79 smaller clusters involved a total of 205 cases. None of the 85 clusters of cases had previously been investigated or reported as outbreaks. Some 23 clusters were felt to be of waterborne origin, primarily related to the consumption of untreated stream water by hikers, campers, game workers, and loggers while on an outing as a group or during their work.

Waterborne outbreaks of giardiasis have affected both visitors and permanent residents, and a seasonal trend is suggested for outbreaks among visitors (Table 5). Outbreaks in noncommunity water systems, which primarily serve visitors, were reported most frequently during the summer months. This implies either increased contamination of noncommunity water supplies or use of these supplies by larger numbers of susceptible individuals during the summer. Miscellaneous outbreaks and outbreaks in individual water systems, which have affected campers, backpackers, swimmers, and divers, also occurred most frequently during the summer, when these recreational activities are most prevalent. Outbreaks in community water systems did not show a clear seasonal trend, but a slightly higher occurrence was noted during the fall. This higher occurrence may be related to increased contamination of watersheds due to the influx of hikers and campers or less effective water treatment during this period; however, more data are needed to make this determination.

Although most outbreaks (71%) and most cases (84%) were attributed to contaminated

TABLE 5

Seasonal distribution of waterborne outbreaks of giardiasis in the United States, 1965–85

Month	Number of outbreaks in		
	Community systems	Noncommunity systems	Individual systems; miscellaneous
January	6	1	0
February	3	2	0
March	4	1	0
April	4	1	2
May	4	1	1
June	6	4	1
July	5	3	2
August	4	3	1
September	5	3	4
October	8	1	1
November	8	0	0
December	5	1	0
Total	62	21	12

surface water, a few outbreaks (12%) occurred when groundwater became contaminated (Table 6). In most instances groundwater was found to be contaminated by human sewage, but in two outbreaks surface water downstream from a beaver dam contaminated a well water source and spring, respectively. Few communities use surface water without treatment, and the twelve outbreaks (13%) attributed to the use of contaminated, untreated surface water were reported primarily in other than community water systems, resulting in a small number of cases of giardiasis (Table 6). The majority of outbreaks (42%) and cases (52%) occurred in surface water systems where disinfection was the only treatment (Table 6). Two of the largest outbreaks attributed to inadequate disinfection as the only treatment of surface water occurred in Rome, New York, with 350 laboratory confirmed cases and an estimated 4800-5300 cases during November 1974 to June 1975 and Bradford, Pennsylvania, with 3500 cases during September to December 1979. In Rome, chloramine was used for disinfection (Craun, 1984). The watershed was sparsely populated, but the presence of human settlements suggested the water supply could have been contaminated by human sewage. Prior to the beginning of the outbreak, higher than normal coliform counts (up to 4600/100 ml) were observed in the untreated water; however, results of routine bacteriological sampling of disinfected water in the distribution system showed no evidence of a widespread problem. From November 1974 to June 1975 an average of 66 samples were collected each month; all had been negative for coliforms except four samples on February 25. No coliforms were detected in water samples collected from the distribution system during the outbreak investigation at 13 locations, and only at two locations were 1 and 3 coliforms/100 ml found (Shaw et al., 1977). *Giardia* was isolated from the raw water source. In Bradford, three impoundments served as water sources

TABLE 6
Waterborne giardiasis outbreaks in the United States classified by type of water system and cause of outbreak, 1965–85

Water source and treatment/deficiency	Community systems		Noncommunity and individual systems; miscellaneous	
	Outbreaks	Cases	Outbreaks	Cases
1. Surface water source				
Clorination only	31	12082	9	709
Filtration	15	7440	–	–
Untreated	1	79	11	243
2. Contamination of distribution system	5	1533	2	2006
3. Groundwater source				
Untreated	3	56	3	15
Chlorination only	4	155	1	32
4. Consumption of water from nonpotable tap, contaminated cistern, or while swimming, diving	–	–	6	126
5. Insufficient information	3	46	1	19
Totals	62	21391	33	3150

(CDC, 1980; Lippy, 1981). The city owned the impoundments and watersheds and prohibited recreational activities. Although chlorination was provided, it was interrupted, and it was considered ineffective because of the method used to adjust feed rates. Turbidities in excess of 10 NTU were recorded on many occasions. Heavy rains prior to the outbreak contributed to high turbidity and numerous complaints of muddy water. Turbidity standards were exceeded but were not required to be reported because of a waiver granted by EPA. The coliform standard was not exceeded until a month prior to the outbreak, when three of twenty water samples from the distribution system were found positive for coliforms; at the time the validity of these results was questioned. In September and October 1979 more routine water samples collected from the distribution system were positive for coliforms, but they stimulated the collection of check samples rather than corrective action. The outbreak investigation began at the end of October, not because of the water quality problems but when *Giardia* was found in stool specimens from ten of fifteen residents with diarrheal illness. *Giardia* cysts were also isolated from the water source and beavers on the watershed.

More recently a large outbreak of 703 confirmed and 3800 estimated cases occurred during November 1985 to January 1986 in Pittsfield, Massachusetts (Kent et al., 1988). Again a surface water supply was involved and chlorination was the only treatment. In Pittsfield the incidence of illness peaked about two weeks after an auxiliary surface water reservoir was placed into service. This reservoir had not been used for three years. As the flow from this reservoir was increased in mid-November complaints of turbid water were received from many areas of the city. Turbidity was attributed to reversals in flow of water which caused the suspension of sediments in water mains. An epidemiologic study showed that persons with giardiasis drank more water than persons without illness and that the attack rate of giardiasis for residents of areas supplied by the auxiliary reservoir was 14.3/1000 compared with 7.0/1000 in areas that received no water from this reservoir. *Giardia* cysts were detected in water samples from the auxiliary reservoir; cysts were also detected but at lower concentrations in the two other surface water reservoirs. Beavers and muskrats in the area were found to be infected with *Giardia* and may have contributed to the contamination of the reservoirs. The beavers and muskrats may have originally been infected from a human source, since trophozoites found in laboratory animals inoculated with the extract from the auxiliary reservoir resembled trophozoites of human rather than beaver origin. It could not be determined whether the reservoir had also been directly contaminated by human sewage. There was no evidence of sewage contamination of any of the reservoirs, but signs of human activity were found near the shore of the auxiliary reservoir in officially restricted areas. *Giardia* cysts isolated from clinical specimens during the outbreak were found to cause infection when inoculated in both beavers and muskrats, and the cysts shed by these animals also resembled *Giardia* typically of human origin.

Although the water from each reservoir was disinfected, the chlorinator at the auxiliary reservoir had malfunctioned during the entire month of November. Records of free chlorine residuals showed levels of between 0 to 0.5 mg/l after 15 min contact time at the auxiliary reservoir in November compared with an average chlorine residual of 2 mg/l during December. Water from the other two reservoirs during both months showed an average chlorine residual of 2 to 3 mg/l with a 15 min contact time. Water temperature was 5°C and pH was 7.4, and it is not clear that the malfunctioning chlorinator contributed to the outbreak, since the chlorine concentrations and contact times which were normally provided are insufficient to inactivate 99.9% of *Giardia* cysts in water at this temperature and pH (EPA, 1987). During October results from 80 routine water samples from the distribution system showed that the coliform standard had not been exceeded. However, in November, five days after the episode of turbid water, five of seventeen water samples were found to contain coliforms greater than 5/100 ml. Check samples were taken daily for the next seven days, but apparently no attempt was made at this time to determine the cause of contamination and take corrective action (e.g., repair or adjust the chlorinator). Coliforms continued to be found in the check samples; after two days, all samples were negative except at one location which continued to yield 8 to 41 coliforms/100 ml until the defective chlorinator was repaired on December 1.

In outbreaks in unfiltered surface water systems, disinfection was inadequate for various reasons, primarily because of insufficient chlorine concentration and contact time. In only a few outbreaks was disinfection interrupted, but in many outbreaks no residual chlorine was detected in the system, even though disinfection was continued. In some instances, increased turbidity was noted prior to the outbreak, and this may have been associated with *Giardia* contamination or may have interfered with disinfection. In a few outbreaks, coliform organisms were detected prior to the outbreak. However, in many outbreaks neither the turbidity limit nor the coliform limit was exceeded, and in several outbreaks water samples were negative for coliforms prior to the outbreak. Most often the chlorine concentration and contact time were sufficient to inactivate coliforms but insufficient to inactivate *Giardia* cysts.

Disinfection with chlorine can inactivate *Giardia* cysts but only if the water consistently has low concentrations of substances which can cause turbidity, create a chlorine demand, or interfere with the disinfection process. Also provided must be a sufficient concentration of chlorine and contact time, as determined from laboratory and field studies[1], for various operating parameters such as water temperature and pH. It is important that heavy or overwhelming contamination, whether brief or intermittent, not deplete the chlorine residual.

Since *Giardia* cysts are resistant to the low chlorine concentrations and contact times normally applied in water treatment practices, it is important to decrease the sole reliance on disinfection for cyst inactivation. Both water filtration theory and laboratory experiments indicate that *Giardia* cysts can be removed by rapid granular media filters if effective chemical pretreatment is accomplished prior to filtration (Logsdon et al., 1981, 1985; Wickramanayake, 1986). Effective pretreatment includes coagulation, flocculation, and settling prior to filtration or if the settling process is not used, the addition of appropriate chemicals for conditioning the water or filter media. Slow sand or diatomaceous earth filtration can be used successfully for cyst removal; proper maintenance and operation are necessary to achieve 99.9% removal. Since the filtration process is the only barrier for the removal of cysts in rapid rate direct sand, slow sand, and diatomaceous earth filtration plants where sedimentation is not part of the treatment, it is important to verify that the raw water quality is appropriate for filtration without sedimentation. Properly operated water filtration plants can clarify water, making disinfection more effective and can remove *Giardia* cysts, leaving fewer in the water for disinfection to inactivate.

In the United States surface water sources are used by an estimated 155 million people in 6000 community water systems, 23% of which provide unfiltered drinking water to some 21 million people. Currently under consideration by the Environmental Protection Agency to reduce the risk of waterborne infectious disease, especially giardiasis, are criteria by which state regulatory agencies will determine when filtration will be required for public water systems using surface water sources (EPA, 1987). Colorado has required all surface waters to be disinfected and filtered since 1977; this includes coagulation, flocculation, and sedimentation (Hopkins et al., 1985).

Ineffective filtration of surface water has been responsible for 16% of the outbreaks and 30% of disease caused by this organism. The first waterborne outbreak of giardiasis

---

[1] For example, at 5°C and pH 6.0, 2 mg/l HOCl residual for 61 min or 1 mg/l HOCl residual for 108 minutes contact time is required for 99.9% inactivation of *Giardia* cysts (EPA, 1987).

involving a filtered water supply occurred in Camas, Washington, in the spring of 1976 resulting in 600 cases of giardiasis in a population of 6000 (Kirner et al., 1978; Dykes et al., 1980; Craun, 1984). Prior to the outbreak, failure of the chlorination equipment occurred, and a number of deficiencies were found in the condition and operation of the pressure filters, including ineffective chemical pretreatment. It was reported that the treated water produced by the treatment plant had met both turbidity and coliform standards prior to and during the outbreak. A second outbreak in a filtered water supply occurred in Berlin, New Hampshire in the spring of 1977 resulting in 750 cases (Lippy, 1978; Lopez et al., 1980; Craun, 1984). An engineering evaluation revealed faulty construction of a common wall separating filtered and unfiltered water; it allowed unfiltered water to bypass the modern, conventional treatment plant. Again routine bacterial samples collected in the distribution system prior to the outbreak showed that the coliform standard had not been exceeded. A free chlorine residual was not maintained in the distribution system even though finished water at the treatment plants contained chlorine residuals of 0.3 to 0.7 mg/l. The largest outbreak in a filtered water supply resulted in an estimated 5000 cases of giardiasis in visitors and residents of Vail, Colorado, during March and April 1978 (CDC, 1978; CDC, 1980; Craun, 1984). The source of the outbreak was traced to a sewer line obstruction and leakage of sewage into Gore Creek; the water was filtered and chlorinated, but no chemical pretreatment was provided. Once again, routine bacteriologic sampling of the water distribution system in the previous year did not show that the coliform limit was exceeded. It was reported by the Colorado State Department of Health that turbidity of the filtered water frequently exceeded standards and that filter breakthrough occurred prior to the outbreak, resulting in turbidity values of 3 NTU. Research has shown that turbidity or passage of floc through the filter could be accompanied by *Giardia* cysts (Logsdon, personal communication).

A waterborne giardiasis outbreak at Aspen Highlands, Colorado, in November 1981 affected a small number of people but is important because it offered evidence for acquired immunity to *Giardia* and is one of the few waterborne giardiasis outbreaks in which a clear dose-response relationship was found for water consumption and clinical illness (Istre et al., 1984). An attack rate of 42% was found among persons who drank six or more glasses of water per day, and residents who had lived in the area for more than two years had a lower attack rate for illness than short-term residents. *Giardia* cysts were isolated from raw and treated water samples, and beavers were suspected as the source of contamination. Engineers dismantled the water treatment facility to determine flaws in its design and operation. Examination revealed several deficiencies, including a fixed-rate chlorinator that could not keep pace with increasing demand, lack of pretreatment by chemical coagulation, erosion of the dual media filter, and the presence of sand from the filter in the clear well.

Another relatively small outbreak of 342 confirmed cases of giardiasis in Pennsylvania during December 1983 and January 1984 is important because it occurred in a surface water system that received full conventional treatment and routinely met water quality standards (Akin and Jakubowski, 1986). The water plant was some 80 years old and operational deficiencies were noted in filtration. An unusually high demand for water had left an insufficient volume of water for filter backwashing, and turbidity breakthrough occurred because of long filter runs. Turbidity increased to 2.80 NTU from a weekly average of 0.24 to 0.90 NTU, but the turbidity standard apparently was not exceeded. A free chlorine residual of 1.0 to 1.3 mg/l was maintained, and the system continued to meet coliform standards.

Outbreaks which have occurred in filtered water supplies emphasize the necessity for proper chemical pretreatment and the importance of good design, careful installation, and conscientious operation of treatment facilities. Several outbreaks have also illustrated operating problems which may occur in pressure filter systems, and it should be noted that while pressure filters are routinely used to remove iron and manganese, they are not generally recommended for microbiological treatment (Great Lakes – Upper Mississippi River Board of Sanitary Engineers, 1976).

A small but significant (14%) number of cases of giardiasis resulted from outbreaks caused by contamination of water mains through cross-connections, damage of mains, and repair of mains (Table 6). The largest outbreak of this type, 2000 cases at a private campground in Arizona, occurred when sewage-contaminated water entered the drinking water system through a direct cross-connection between the potable water system and a pipe carrying sewage effluent for irrigation (Lippy, 1981; Starko et al., 1986; Craun, 1986c). Many of the affected individuals were from different health jurisdictions, and the outbreak was recognized only because visitors to the campground reported their illness to local authorities who then contacted the state agencies; this resulted in a multi-state investigation (Akin and Jakubowski, 1986). Routine water sampling of the system prior to the outbreak failed to indicate the potential problem because samples were collected from sites which were not representative of the entire water system. The cross-connection was located through fluorescein dye studies. In Tooele, Utah, 1272 cases occurred when contamination entered a water transmission line which had been damaged by mud slides and flooding due to heavy rains; routine water samples were positive for coliforms prior to this outbreak, as the contamination entered the water system just downstream from one of the water sources (CDC, 1983). Contaminated water during the repair of a water main was identified as the cause of 41 cases of giardiasis in another outbreak which occurred in Utah (Craun, 1986c). Cases were confined to the families located downstream from the repair site. The water main had been neither flushed nor chlorinated after repair and discolored, malodorous water was reported by residents when the water service was restored. The remaining giardiasis outbreaks of this type occurred after (1) contamination entered a community water system through backsiphonage due to low water pressure, (2) the backsiphonage of sewage into a camp water system through an improperly operating water valve, and (3) the loss of pressure within a community water system resulted in the pumping of sewage from a barge into the potable water system through several cross-connections. It is not unusual for water systems experiencing such outbreaks to report negative coliform results from routine water samples collected prior to the outbreak. Contamination from cross-connections generally affects a small area of the water system for a relatively short period of time, and water samples may not be collected in that part of the system or may not be collected frequently enough to detect the contamination. Unless the contamination is large or continuous, water samples collected during the epidemiologic investigation may also be negative for coliforms when the contaminant is rapidly flushed through the system. The presence of a chlorine residual in the water distribution system may also affect the detection of coliform contamination, as it may be sufficient to inactivate coliforms but not *Giardia*.

4.2. Other countries

The first recognized waterborne outbreak of giardiasis in Western Europe occurred in Mjovik, a small community in southwest Sweden (Neringer et al., 1987). The village obtained water from a drilled well which was aerated and filtered but not disinfected. Blockage of the village sewer caused a backflow of sewage which flooded the water treatment plant through a direct connection with the sewer system. The well was also contaminated by sewage leakage through an electric cable tubing. An epidemiologic study showed a high incidence of illness in the village compared with other areas which received chlorinated water from another treatment plant. The epidemic curve suggested a single common-source outbreak without secondary cases; however, the outbreak was of multiple etiology: one unidentified agent with a short incubation period and *Giardia* with a longer incubation period. During the first few days after the water contamination, 454 persons (76% of the population) became ill with gastroenteritis. At least 56 cases of giardiasis occurred several weeks later.

The first recognized waterborne outbreak of giardiasis in the United Kingdom occurred in 1985 when 108 laboratory-confirmed cases were reported between June 3 and August 11 in Bristol (Jephcott et al., 1986). Epidemiologic evidence indicated that the infection was spread by the municipal water system which was reportedly chemically pretreated, filtered, and disinfected. Half the city is supplied with water directly from the treatment plant and no cases were detected over the greater part of this area. Most cases were reported in the south of the city in a localized area supplied by water from a distribution storage reservoir. Routine bacteriological monitoring showed no contamination of either water leaving the treatment plant or the reservoir. Neither coliforms nor *Giardia* were detected in water samples collected from the distribution system of the localized area during the epidemiologic investigation. However, on two occasions the water mains had been opened for repair. A strong association was found between illness and consumption of water during the first week of July when the mains were opened. It was suspected that contamination of the water supply occurred downstream of the reservoir when the main were opened either by direct contamination during the repairs or backsiphonage from pressure changes associated with the repair.

In Canada, suspected waterborne outbreaks have occurred at Banff and Edmonton, Alberta (Wallis et al., 1986). Over 800 people were infected during the Edmonton outbreak with the disease centered around one of the city's water treatment plants. In the outbreak which occurred in Banff in the winter of 1982, infected beavers were found in the creek which supplied the town with water (Wilson et al., 1982). *Giardia* cysts isolated from beaver feces during the outbreak were inoculated orally in Mongolian gerbils and produced a pattern of infection similar to that found when the gerbils were inoculated with human isolates; it was suggested that the organism which infected the beavers was biologically similar to human *Giardia* (Faubert et al., 1983). Most municipal water systems in British Columbia are not filtered and in some instances are not disinfected (Isaac-Renton et al., 1987). Three documented waterborne outbreaks of giardiasis have occurred within the past five years in British Columbia (Isaac-Renton et al, 1987); one of these was reported at 100 Mile House (Wallis et al., 1986). All water systems used surface water without filtration, and *Giardia*-positive beavers were found in the water sources. In two outbreaks, *Giardia*-positive muskrats were found in the same water source. In the most recent outbreak of 200 laboratory-confirmed cases, two of three muskrats and three of twelve beavers trapped on the watershed tested positive. The outbreaks occurred at various times of the year: during spring, early autumn, and early winter. Because of the widespread infection in beavers and other mammals, poorly protected or unrestricted use of watersheds, and lack of adequate water treatment in this Canadian province, Isaac-Renton et al. (1987) warn of the high risk of waterborne transmission of giardiasis.

It should be remembered that contaminated water is not the only means of transmission of *Giardia*, and an epidemiologic study must be conducted to establish a mode of transmission. Since giardiasis is spread by the fecal-oral route of exposure, the waterborne route of transmission cannot be assumed whenever there is an unusual occurrence of giardiasis. Although contaminated drinking water was initially thought to be responsible for a presumed epidemic of giardiasis in 1986 in Coffs Harbour on the north coast of New South Wales, Australia, a survey provided no evidence that giardiasis was the etiologic agent (Walker et al., 1986). The finding of bacterial and viral pathogens in 18% of the children indicated other organisms could have been responsible for symptoms that were ascribed to *Giardia*, and it was pointed out that a diagnosis of giardiasis cannot be made on the basis of symptoms alone. Further investigation of a giardiasis outbreak in Mount Isa in northwest Queensland suggested person-to-person transmission rather than transmission by water (Boreham and Phillips, 1986).

5. Giardia cysts in drinking water

Giardia exists in a trophozoite and a cyst stage. *Giardia* are not free-living protozoa, and they must reproduce in a host. In addition to humans, a number of wild and domestic animals have been found infected. It is generally accepted from morphological differences that three species exist: *G. agilis* infecting amphibians (frogs and tadpoles); *G. muris* infecting rodents and birds; *G. duodenalis* (the organism in man also referred to as *G. lamblia*) infecting a wide variety of mammals including man and dog (Thompson, 1983).

Excystation takes place in the infected host after viable cysts are ingested. The resultant trophozoites reside in the upper small intestine where they multiply to large numbers; some move down the intestinal tract. Encystation takes place during this downward movement, and the environmentally resistant *Giardia* cysts can enter water supplies through animal or human fecal contamination. Water is not a suitable medium for growth of *Giardia* but it has a great potential for transmitting giardiasis, since only a small number of cysts is required to produce infection (Rendtorff, 1954). The numbers of cysts which enter water supplies decrease due to die-off and dilution, but cysts are known to remain viable for long periods of time in cold waters. They have been found to survive for three months in water at a temperature of 4°C, but only four days at 37°C (Meyer and Jarroll, 1980).

Estimates of the numbers of cysts in sewage suggest that raw sewage could contain 960 000 to 24 000 000 cysts/100 l when 1 to 25% of the population are infected (Akin and Jakubowski, 1986). Samples of raw sewage from several sewage treatment plants in Pennsylvania showed 124 200 cysts/100 l, but the numbers of cysts actually contained in the raw sewage could have been higher because the efficiency of the methods to detect and enumerate cysts ranged from 6 to 28%. Effluents from three of seven sewage treatment plants in Sangamon County, Illinois, were found to contain 1 to 1200 cysts/100 l (McHarry, 1984). Estimates of the numbers of cysts from several streams in Washington where animals would likely be the primary source of contamination were calculated using beaver population on the watershed, *Giardia* prevalence, stool size, cysts per stool, and stream flows (Akin and Jakubowski, 1986). During maximum flow the estimated numbers in six streams ranged from 0.4×10^{-4} to 2.5×10^{-4} cysts/100 l, but during minimum stream flows the numbers ranged from 0.3 to 64.8 cysts/100 l. Although there is considerable uncertainty in these estimates, they do indicate that a few infected animals could contaminate a small stream. In Pittsfield, Massachusetts, 7.4 to 21.1 cysts/100 l were found in water samples from the auxiliary surface water source associated with the recent waterborne giardiasis outbreak; 1.9 and 2.4 cysts/100 l were obtained from each of the other reservoirs (Kent et al., 1988). In an examination of data from a limited number of water sources (Akin and Jakubowski, 1986) the numbers of cysts in water supplies were found to range from 0.013 to 180 cysts/100 l. In the Sierra Nevada, California, *Giardia* cysts were detected in 22 (45%) stream water samples collected at sites downstream from areas of high recreational use and in 5 (17%) samples collected at sites downstream from areas of low recreational use (Suk et al., 1987; Sorenson et al., 1987). The number of cysts detected in the streams ranged from 0.3 to 10.9 cysts/100 l, but the method used to detect and enumerate cysts was found to have 10 to 30% efficiency. These data indicate that intensity of human use may play a significant role in *Giardia* contamination of surface water. Fecal material from infected humans may reach streams and lakes directly or from runoff during snow melt and rains. Humans may also infect wild animals which could become a reservoir for infection and source of water contamination. Domestic animals could also be a source of infection for wild animals or a direct source of water contamination. *Giardia* cysts were also found in stream water from three of five watersheds in Rocky Mountain National Park, Colorado, where human use was high or beaver were present (Monzingo et al., 1987). No cysts were found in two watersheds characterized by low human use and poor beaver habitat.

Methods for detecting *Giardia* cysts in water were developed to assist in the investigation of suspected waterborne disease outbreaks and have also been useful for evaluating the effectiveness of drinking water treatment processes. A positive water sample even in the absence of a recognized outbreak can be important because it can spur local authorities into upgrading water treatment. However, the current state of the art in sampling and analysis is such that a negative sample does not necessarily indicate a safe drinking water supply. Little or no information is available on the efficiency, selectivity, and specificity of the methods with different waters. Thus, quantitative data on numbers of cysts in water must be interpreted with caution even when the data are from a single laboratory. When the efficiency has been determined of the ability of the current methods for sampling and enumerating *Giardia* cysts, recovery rates have generally been low. This suggests not only that the number of cysts have probably been underestimated but also that, in negative water samples, cysts could have been present and gone undetected. In addition, current technology does not permit a rapid assessment of the viability of cysts detected; viability must be determined by testing in animal models. Thus, a standard is not likely to be established in the near future for *Giardia* cysts in water. Neither should a quantitative comparison of cyst concentrations be made without considering the potential sources of error.

Giardia cysts were isolated from water samples in at least 22 outbreaks in the United States. In several outbreaks including those where water samples did not yield *Giardia*, cysts were recovered from beavers or beaver feces on the watershed. While beavers have been implicated as the source of several outbreaks, their significance in transmitting giardiasis to humans must be placed in perspective. Recent data show a higher prevalence of infection in muskrats than beaver. In Minnesota investigators found live-trapped beavers to have a *Giardia* prevalence of about 17% and live-trapped muskrats to have a prevalence of 80 to 100% (Craun and Jakubowski, 1987). Examination of stools from more than 900 kill-trapped beavers and muskrats collected in Minnesota and in four New England states, showed an overall *Giardia* prevalence of 35% in muskrats and 10% in beavers (Craun and Jakubowski, 1987). This prevalence is similar to the overall prevalence of 11% and 41% reported for kill-trapped beavers and muskrats, respectively, in a survey of 662 animals commercially trapped from 1976 in 1979 in Washington State (Frost et al., 1980). A *Giardia* survey in British Columbia, Canada, from April 1985 to July 1986 found *Giardia* positive specimens from beavers commercially trapped in all parts of the province included in the survey (Isaac-Renton et al., 1987). Overall, of 299 beaver specimens examined, 14.7% were positive for *Giardia*, and of 20 muskrats examined, 40% were positive. In southwestern New Jersey, 70% of 220 muskrat fecal specimens collected from 12 sites were found to contain *Giardia* cysts (Kirkpatrick and Benson, 1987). Because of the high prevalence of infection in muskrats and an apparent lack of variation in prevalence of infection among geographic regions for both beavers and muskrats, animal stool surveys may have little utility in assessing *Giardia* risks in water supplies.

Other watershed animals that have not routinely been included in animal surveys may also be important as reservoirs of infection. Recently a survey showed 65% of 722 fecal samples collected from small rodents in central Washington Cascade mountains were positive for *Giardia*. Water voles (*Microtus*) were found to be heavily infected; morphologically the cysts and trophozoites were of the *G. duodenalis* type (Pacha et al., 1987). Microtines and other small rodents inhabit moist alpine meadows and stream banks, and their habits lend themselves to the contamination of surface water. These populations of small rodents appear to maintain their infection throughout the year. There was no difference in the percentage of positive animals in areas receiving much, and those receiving little human use.

In addition to beavers and muskrats, *Giardia* infect a wide variety of animals. Kulda and Nohynkova (1978) list over 40 species of animals in which *Giardia* have been found. The species specificity or the infectivity of *Giardia* cysts from animals to humans is not yet entirely clear. Several investigators have reported successfully infecting a variety of animals, including dog, beaver, muskrat, gerbil, and rat, with cysts from humans, and this suggests that cysts from animals may be infective for humans (Jakubowski, 1988). Nevertheless, this wide distribution indicates that all surface water supplies, no matter how well protected from human activities, are subject to contamination with *Giardia* from animal or human sources at any time. The degree and significance of water supply contamination will vary with the number of infected animals on the watershed or with the extent of sewage contamination, as well as with dilution and die-off.

The development of methods for detection of *Giardia* cysts in water samples is relatively recent. *Giardia* cysts were first detected in a water supply during the Rome, New York, outbreak in 1974-75 (Shaw et al., 1977). A pressure sand filter was used to filter more than one million liters of surface water; the sediment from backwash was collected in 55 gallon drums. A single *Giardia* cyst was found on microscopic examination of these sediments, which were also fed to *Giardia* free beagle puppies. Two of 10 sediment aliquots produced infection in the pups indicating the presence of *Giardia* in the raw water. Previous attempts to identify *Giardia* cysts in water samples, were unsuccessful. Brady and Wolfe (1974) investigated five cases of giardiasis in Tennessee in 1973 and reported finding 'numerous trophozoites of *G. lamblia*' in water samples from an underground cistern apparently contaminated by sewage from a pit privy. However, the methods used to isolate and identify the trophozoites were not explicitly described and the findings have been questioned (Rendtorff, 1975; Wright, 1975). *Giardia* cysts were detected in sewage samples during the 1965-66 outbreak in Aspen (Moore et al., 1969), but no cysts were detected in two-liter water samples from ten sites throughout the water distribution system.

The first practical method of sample collection and examination of water samples for cysts was developed in 1976 to assist in the investigation of waterborne outbreaks (Jakubowski et al., 1978; Jakubowski and Ericksen, 1979). The sampling device weighed

TABLE 7

Major water supply deficiencies responsible for waterborne outbreaks of giardiasis and other illnesses in the United States, 1971–85

Water supply and treatment deficiencies	Percent of all waterborne outbreaks	
	Giardiasis	Other illnesses
1. Surface water source		
Chlorination only	42	7
Filtration	16	2
Untreated	13	5
2. Groundwater source		
Untreated	7	36
Chlorination only	4	21
3. Contamination of distribution systesm		
Cross-connection	6	10
Other	3	7
4. Other/insufficient data	10	13
Total	100%	100%

less than 3 kg and consisted of a blend orlon filter, garden hose, water meter, and flow limiting device. Since cysts are present in relatively low numbers in waters, concentration of water samples is necessary, and the method involves microscopic examination of large-volume concentrates for detection and identification of cysts. A volume of at least 380 liters is passed through a 1 μm nominal porosity depth filter, the retained particles are extracted by washing the filter fibers and concentrated by sedimentation or centrifugation; the cysts then are separated from the other particles, and examined by microscopy. Methods currently in use are a variation of that method, but they all consist of four basic steps: concentration, purification, detection and identification (Craun and Jakubowski, 1987). These methods are discussed in more detail in chapter 20.

6. Conclusions

Most waterborne outbreaks of giardiasis have occurred in water systems using surface water sources. In the United States 71% of the waterborne outbreaks of giardiasis reported during 1971-85 were attributed to contaminated, inadequately treated surface water systems (Table 7). Only 14% of waterborne outbreaks of other illnesses were reported in surface water systems; most (57%) waterborne outbreaks of illnesses other than giardiasis were attributed to contaminated, inadequately treated groundwater (Table 7). Although all water sources are subject to contamination, surface water sources are more likely to be contaminated with *Giardia* than are groundwater sources. Outbreaks in groundwater systems are attributed primarily to the overflow or seepage of human sewage or the entry of contaminated surface water into inadequately developed or protected wells and springs (Craun, 1985). Surface water supplies with treatment that is marginal or absent are at high risk of transmitting *Giardia* because *Giardia* cysts can survive for several months in cold waters and relatively low numbers of *Giardia* are required for human infection. In addition, watersheds can be contaminated by both human sewage and animals, such as beavers and muskrats which may serve as constant sources of *Giardia* for streams and reservoirs.

Untreated surface water should not be consumed by hikers or campers no matter how clean and clear mountain streams may appear. Approximately 154 community water systems in the United States use untreated surface water; these are small systems with an average population of 715. Although only one waterborne outbreak of giardiasis has been reported in these systems, underreporting of outbreaks is likely, and these communities are at increased risk of giardiasis.

Thirty waterborne outbreaks and 12 048 cases of giardiasis were reported since 1971 in U.S. communities where surface water was treated only with chlorine resulting in a rate of 24.4 waterborne outbreaks/1000 facilities and 38.8 cases/million person-years. In filtered water systems the waterborne giardiasis rate was found to be much lower: only 3.3 waterborne outbreaks/1000 facilities and 3.7 cases/million person-years.

Simple disinfection has been inadequate as the only treatment of surface water, and despite existing regulations for coliforms and turbidity, waterborne outbreaks have continued to occur. Currently under consideration by the Environmental Protection Agency are criteria by which state regulatory agencies will determine when filtration will be required for public water systems using surface water sources (Anonymous, 1987). Outbreaks have occurred in filtered surface water supplies but only where structural defects, inadequate pretreatment or operational problems have been identified. This emphasizes the importance of good design, conscientious operation of water treatment facilities, and surveillance.

Coliform organisms are used as an indication of fecal contamination of water supplies, and negative results have usually been interpreted as providing assurance that the water is free of enteric pathogens. Since *Giardia* cysts have been found in water supplies in the absence of coliforms, this interpretation must be reevaluated. Regulations have been established by EPA for coliforms and turbidity in drinking water, and sampling schedules have been prescribed for these constituents. Giardiasis outbreaks have occurred in water systems that have met the coliform and turbidity standards. In several outbreaks, water systems were found to exceed the standards, but this did not prompt corrective action. These standards and their applicability to the routine surveillance of water systems for the prevention of outbreaks must also be reevaluated.

Work is needed on all four basic steps of detection methodology for *Giardia* cysts in water. While a positive result from a water sample can be important in identifying water supplies which may require additional treatment or attention, a negative result cannot at this time be interpreted as meaning the water supply is *Giardia* free. Methods need to be simplified and evaluated in controlled comparative studies with a variety of waters. The sensitivity and specificity of the methodology must be established before quantitative data are meaningful.

Since animals have been implicated in the spread of *Giardia* infection to man, all surface water supplies are at risk of contamination with *Giardia*. Existing cyst detection methods or watershed animal stool surveys may be of little value in assessing the risk for the waterborne transmission of giardiasis for a specific water supply. Since surface water supplies are subject to fecal contamination from a variety of animal and human sources, water supplies must provide adequate treatment that is capable of removing and inactivating *Giardia* cysts. In all but exceptional situations, effective filtration must be provided to prevent the waterborne transmission of giardiasis. *Giardia* cysts can be inactivated by chlorine, but high concentrations of chlorine and long contact times are required. Sole reliance should not be placed on disinfection as the only barrier against waterborne transmission of *Giardia*. Properly designed and operated filtration plants can make disinfection more effective by removing turbidity and some substances that exert chlorine demand. Filtration can also remove *Giardia* and other microorganisms leaving fewer in the water for disinfection to inactivate.

References

Akin, E.W. and Jakubowski, W. (1986) Drinking water transmission of giardiasis in the United States. Water Sci. Technol. 18, 219-226.

Allison, D.J. (1984) Giardiasis: a recent investigation. Can. J. Public Health 75, 318-320.

Anderson, T., Forssell, J. and Sterner, G. (1972) Outbreak of giardiasis: effect of a new antiflagellate drug, tinidazole. Br. Med. J. 2, 449-451.

Anonymous (1978) Intestinal parasites ranging far afield in the United States. J. Am. Med. Assoc. 239, 2756.

Aust Kettis, A. and Magnius, L. (1973) *Giardia lamblia* infection in a group of students after a visit to Leningrad in March 1970. Scand. J. Infect. Dis. 5, 289-292.

Barker, W.H., Jr. (1974) Foodborne disease surveillance: Washington State. Am. J. Public Health 64, 26.

Batik, O., Craun, G.F. and Pipes, W.O. (1983) Routine coliform monitoring and waterborne disease outbreaks. J. Environ. Health 45, 227-230.

Benenson, A.S. (Ed.) (1980) Control of Communicable Diseases in Man. Am. Public Health Assoc., Washington, D.C., pp. 50-52.

Black, R.E., Dykes, A.C., Sinclair, S.P. et al. (1977) Giardiasis in day-care centers. Evidence for person to person transmission. Pediatrics 60, 485-491.

Boreham, P.F.L. and Phillips, R.E. (1986) Giardiasis in Mount Isa, northwest Queensland. Med. J. Aust. 144, 524-528.

Brady, P.G. and Wolfe, J.C. (1974) Waterborne giardiasis. Ann. Intern. Med. 81, 498-499.

Brodsky, R.E., Spencer, H.C., Jr. and Schultz, M.G. (1974) Giardiasis in American travelers to the Soviet Union. J. Infect. Dis. 130, 319-323.

CDC (1970) Giardiasis in travelers. Morbid. Mortal. Weekly Rep. 19, 455.

CDC (1974) *Giardia lamblia* infection in travelers to the Soviet Union. Morbid. Mortal. Weekly Rep. 23, 78-79.

CDC (1975) Giardiasis in Rome, New York, and in travelers to the Soviet Union. Morbid. Mortal. Weekly Rep. 24, 371.

CDC (1977) Giardiasis-California, Colorado. Morbid. Mortal. Weekly Rep. 26, 60, 92.
CDC (1978) Giardiasis-Vail, Colorado. Morbid. Mortal. Weekly Rep. 27, 155.
CDC (1980) Waterborne giardiasis-California, Colorado, Oregon, Pennsylvania. Morbid. Mortal. Weekly Rep. 29, 121-123.
CDC (1983) Outbreak of diarrheal illness associated with a natural disaster: Utah. Morbid. Mortal. Weekly Rep. 32, 662-664.
Chute, C., Smith, R. and Baron, J. (1985) Risk factors for endemic giardiasis. Am. J. Epidemiol. 122, 515.
Chute, C.G., Smith, R.P. and Baron, J.A. (1987) Risk factors for endemic giardiasis. Am. J. Public Health 77, 585-587.
Craun, G.F. and McCabe, L.J. (1973) Review of the causes of waterborne disease outbreaks. J. Am. Water Works Assoc. 65, 74-84.
Craun, G.F. (1978) Impact of the coliform standard on the transmission of disease. In: C.W. Hendricks (Ed.), Evaluation of the Microbiology Standards for Drinking Water. USEPA-570/9-78-OOC, pp. 21-35.
Craun, G.F. (1979) Waterborne Outbreaks of Giardiasis. In: W. Jakubowski and J.C. Hoff (Eds), Waterborne Transmission of Giardiasis. U.S. Environmental Protection Agency, pp. 127-149.
Craun, G.F. (1984) Waterborne outbreaks of giardiasis: current status. In: S.L. Erlandsen and E.A. Meyer (Eds), Giardia and Giardiasis. Plenum Press, New York, pp. 243-261.
Craun, G.F. (1985) A summary of waterborne illness transmitted through contaminated groundwater. J. Environ. Health 48, 122-217.
Craun, G.F. (1986a) Statistics of Waterborne Outbreaks in the U.S. (1920-80). In: G.F. Craun (Ed.), Waterborne Disease in the United States, CRC Press Inc., Boca Raton, FL, pp. 73-160.
Craun, G.F. (1986b) Water not sole source of disease transmission. J. Am. Water Works Assoc. 78, 4.
Craun, G.F. (1986c) Waterborne giardiasis in the United States 1965-84. Lancet ii, 513-514.
Craun, G.F. and Jakubowski, W. (1987) Status of Waterborne Giardiasis Outbreaks and Monitoring Methods. In: C.L. Tate Jr. (Ed.), Proceedings of the International Symposium on Water Related Health Issues. Am. Water Resources Assoc., Bethesda, MD, pp. 167-174.
Davis, C. and Ritchie, L.S. (1948) Clinical manifestations and treatment of epidemic amebiasis occurring in occupants of the Mantetsu apartment building, Tokyo, Japan. Am. J. Trop. Med. 28, 817-823.
Dykes, A.C., Juranek, D.D., Lorenz, R.A. et al. (1980) Municipal waterborne giardiasis: an epidemiologic investigation. Ann. Intern. Med. 92, 165-170.
Editorial (1980) Giardiasis and Water. Lancet i, 1176.
EPA (1987) National primary drinking water regulations; filtration and disinfection; turbidity, *Giardia lamblia*, viruses, *Legionella*, and heterotrophic bacteria; proposed rule. Fed. Reg. 52, 42178-42222.
Faubert, G.M., Belosevic, M., Walker, T.S. et al. (1983) Comparative studies on the pattern of infection with *Giardia* spp. in Mongolian gerbils. J. Parasitol. 69, 802-805.
Fiumara, N. (1973) Giardiasis in travelers to the Soviet Union. New Engl. J. Med. 288, 1410-1411.
Forssell, J., Lantrop, K and Sterner, G. (1972) Giardiasis among Swedish tourists after a visit to the Soviet Union. Lakartidningen 69, 1132-1137.
Frost, F., Plan, B. and Liechty, B. (1980) Giardia prevalence in commercially trapped mammals. J. Environ. Health 42, 245-249.
Frost, F., Harter, L., Plan, B., Fukutaki, K. and Holman, B. (1983) Giardiasis in Washington State. U.S. Environmental Protection Agency (600/1-82-016), Research Triangle Park, NC, 91 pp.
Gendel, E. (1974) Giardiasis in Russia. New Engl. J. Med. 290, 286.
Great Lakes – Upper Mississippi River Board of State Sanitary Engineers, 1976. Recommended Standards for Water Works, State of New York Department of Health, Albany, NY, 94 pp.
Harter, L., Frost, F. and Jakubowski, W. (1982) *Giardia* prevalence among 1 to 3 year old children in two Washington state counties. Am. J. Public Health 72, 386-388.
Harter, L., Frost, F., Vogt, R., Little, A.A., Hopkins, R., Gaspard, B. and Lippy, E.C. (1985) A three-state study of waterborne disease surveillance techniques. Am. J. Public Health 75, 1327-1328.
Hausler, W.J., Jr., Davis, W.E. and Moyer, N.P. (1984) Development and testing of a filter system for isolation

of *Giardia lamblia* cysts from water. App. Environ. Microbiol. 47, 1346-1347.

Hopkins, R.S., Shillam, P., Gaspard, B., Eisnach, L. and Karlin, R.J. (1985) Waterborne disease in Colorado: three years' surveillance and 18 outbreaks. Am. J. Public Health 75, 254-257.

Isaac-Renton, J.L., Moricz, M.M. and Proctor, E.M. (1987) A *Giardia* survey of fur-bearing water mammals in British Columbia, Canada. J. Environ. Health 50, 80-83.

Istre, G.R., Dunlop, T.S., Gaspard, G.B. and Hopkins, R.S. (1984) Waterborne giardiasis at a mountain resort: evidence for acquired immunity. Am. J. Public Health 74, 602-604.

Jakubowski, W. (1984) Detection of *Giardia* Cysts in Drinking Water: State-of-the-Art. In: S.L. Erlandsen and E.A. Meyer (Eds), *Giardia* and Giardiasis. Plenum Press, New York, NY, pp. 263-286.

Jakubowski, W. (1988) Purple burps and the filtration of drinking water supplies. Am. J. Public Health 78, 123-124.

Jakubowski, W., Chang, S.L., Ericksen, T.H., Lippy, E.C. and Akin, E.A. (1978) Large-Volume Sampling of Water Supplies for Microorganisms. J. Am. Water Works Assoc. 70, 702-706.

Jakubowski, W. and Ericksen, T.H. (1979) Methods for Detection of *Giardia* Cysts in Water Supplies. In: W. Jakubowski and J.C. Hoff (Eds), Waterborne Transmission of Giardiasis, U.S. Environmental Protection Agency 600-/9-79-001, Cincinnati, OH, pp. 193-210.

Jephcott, A.E., Begg, N.T. and Baker, I.A. (1986) Outbreak of giardiasis associated with mains water in the United Kingdom. Lancet i, 730-732.

Johnson, D.D. (1972) Enteritis secondary to *Giardia lamblia* in students traveling on tour in Russia. J. Am. Coll. Health Assoc. 20, 207-208.

Jokipii, L. (1972) Giardiaasia Leningradista. Duodecim (Finland) 88, 522-526.

Jokipii, L. and Jokipii, A.M.M. (1974) Giardiasis in travelers: a prospective study. J. Infect. Dis. 130, 295-299.

Kent, G.P., Greenspan, J.R., Herndon, J.L. et al. (1988) Epidemic giardiasis caused by a contaminated water supply. Am. J. Public Health 78, 139-143.

Keystone, J.S., Krajden, S. and Warren, M.R. (1978) Person-to-person transmission of *Giardia lamblia* in day-care nurseries. Can. Med. Assoc. J. 119, 241-258.

Kirkpatrick, C.E. and Benson, C.E. (1987) Presence of *Giardia* spp. and absence of *Salmonella* spp. in New Jersey muskrats. Appl. Environ. Microbiol. 53, 1790-1792.

Kirner, J.C., Littler, J.D. and Angelo, L.A. (1978) A waterborne outbreak of giardiasis in Camas, Washington. J. Am. Water Works Assoc. 70, 35-40.

Kulda, J. and Nohynkova, E. (1978) Flagellates of the human intestine and of intestines of other species. In: J.P. Kreier (Ed.), Parasitic Protozoa II. Academic Press, New York, NY, 138 pp.

Laxter, M.A. (1985) Potential exposure of Utah Army National Guard personnel to giardiasis during field training exercises: a preliminary survey. Mil. Med. 150, 23-26.

Lippy, E.C. (1978) Tracing a giardiasis outbreak at Berlin, New Hampshire. J. Am. Water Works Assoc. 70, 512-520.

Lippy, E.C. (1981) Waterborne disease: occurrence is on the upswing. J. Am. Water Works Assoc. 72, 57-62.

Logsdon, G.S., Thurman, V.C., Frindt, E.S. and Stoecker, J.G. (1985) Evaluating sedimentation and various filter media for removal of *Giardia* cysts. J. Am. Water Works Assoc. 77, 61-66.

Logsdon, G.S., Symons, J.M., Hoye, R.L., Jr. and Arozarena, M.M. (1981) Alternative filtration methods for removal of *Giardia* cysts and cyst models. J. Am. Water Works Assoc. 73, 111-118.

Lopez, C.E., Dykes, A.C., Juranek, D.D. et al. (1980) Waterborne giardiasis: a communitywide outbreak of disease and a high rate of asymptomatic infection. Am. J. Epidemiol. 112, 495-507.

Martin, J.F. and Martin, M.A. (1975) Giardiasis from Russia. Br. Med. J. 2, 89.

Meyer, W.T. (1973) Epidemic giardiasis, a continued elusive entity. Rocky Mt. Med. J. 70, 48-49.

Meyer, E.A. and Jarroll, E.L. (1980) *Giardia* and giardiasis. Am. J. Epidemiol. 111, 1-12.

McHarry, M.J. (1984) Detection of *Giardia* in sewage effluent. J. Protozool. 31, 362-364.

Monzingo, D.L., Knuckle, S.H., Stevens, D.R. and Wilson, J.T. (1987) *Giardia* in backcountry watersheds and wildlife of Rocky Mountain National Park. In: C.L. Tate Jr. (Ed.), International Symposium on Water Related Health Issues. Am. Water Resources Assoc., Bethesda, MD, pp. 153-159.

Moore, G.T., Cross, W.M., McGuire, D. et al. (1969) Epidemic giardiasis at a ski resort. New Engl. J. Med. 281, 402-407.

Neringer, R., Andersson, Y. and Baker, I.A. (1986) A waterborne outbreak of giardiasis in Sweden. Scand. J. Infect. Dis. 19, 85-90.

Osterholm, M.T., Forfang, J.C., Ristinen, T.L. et al. (1981) An outbreak of foodborne giardiasis. N. Engl. J. Med. 304, 24-28.

Pacha, R.E., Clark, G.W., Williams, A.M. et al. (1987) Small rodents and other mammals associated with mountain meadows as reservoirs of *Giardia* spp. and *Campylobacter* spp. Appl. Environ. Microbiol. 53, 1574-1579.

Rendtorff, R.C. (1954) The experimental transmission of human intestinal protozoan parasites. II. *Giardia lamblia* cysts given in capsules. Am. J. Hyg. 59, 209-220.

Rendtorff, R.C. (1975) *Giardia* in water. Ann. Intern. Med. 82, 280.

Sautter, R.L. and Knights, E.M. (1983) Muskrats and waterborne giardiasis. Lancet i, 1103.

Schmerin, M.J., Jones, T.C. and Klein, H. (1978) Giardiasis associated with homosexuality. Ann. Intern. Med. 88, 801-803.

Sealy, D.P. and Schuman, S.H. (1983) Endemic giardiasis and day care. Pediatrics 72, 154-158.

Shaw, P.K., Brodsky, R.E., Lyman, D.O., Wood, B.T., Hibler, C.P., Healy, G.R., Macleod, K.I.E., Stahl, W. and Schultz, M.G. (1977) A communitywide outbreak of giardiasis with evidence of transmission by a municipal water supply. Ann. Intern. Med. 87, 426-432.

Sorenson, S.K., Dileanis, P.D. and Riggs, J.L. (1987) Occurrence of *Giardia* cysts in streams in the Sierra Nevada, California. In: C.L. Tate Jr. (Ed.), Proceedings International Symposium on Water Related Health Issues. Am. Water Resources Assoc., Bethesda, MD, pp. 161-165.

Starko, K.M., Lippy, E.C., Dominguez, L.B. et al. (1986) Campers diarrhea outbreak traced to water-sewage link. Public Health Rpts. 101, 527-531.

Stevens, D.P. (1982) Giardiasis: host-pathogen biology. Rev. Infect. Dis. 4, 851-858.

Suk, T.J., Sorenson, S.K. and Dileanis, P.D. (1987) The relation between human presence and occurrence of *Giardia* cysts in streams in Sierra Nevada, California. J. Freshwater Ecol. 4, 71-75.

Thompson, R.G. (1983) Giardia species. Lancet i, 1327.

Veazie, L. (1969) Epidemic giardiasis. N. Engl. J. Med. 281, 853.

Veazie, L., Brownlee, I. and Sears, H.J. (1979) An outbreak of gastroenteritis associated with *Giardia lamblia*. In: W. Jakubowski and J.C. Hoff (Eds), Waterborne Transmission of Giardiasis. U.S. Environmental Protection Agency, pp. 174-191.

Walker, J.C., Conner, G., Christopher, P.J. et al. (1986) A presumed epidemic of giardiasis. Med. J. Aust. 145, 548-549.

Wallis, P.M., Zammuto, R.M. and Buchanan-Mappin, J.M. (1986) Cysts of *Giardia* spp. in mammals and surface waters in southwestern Alberta. J. Wildlife Dis. 22, 115-118.

Walzer, P.D., Wolfe, M.S. and Schultz, M.G. (1971) Giardiasis in travelers. J. Infect. Dis. 124, 235-237.

Weisman, J.B., Craun, G.F., Lawrence, D.N. et al. (1976) An epidemic of gastroenteritis traced to a contaminated public water supply. Am. J. Epidemiol. 103, 391.

Weiss, H.B., Winegar, D.A., Levy, B.S. and Washburn, J.W. (1977) Giardiasis in Minnesota, 1971-1975. Minn. Med. 60, 815-820.

Wickramanayake, G.B. (1986) Effectiveness of conventional water treatment in the prevention of waterborne giardiasis. In: C.L. Tate (Ed.), Proceedings of the International Symposium on Water Related Health Issues, Am. Water Resources Assoc., Bethesda, MD, pp. 137-144.

Wilson, H.S.P., Stauffer, S.J. and Walker, T.S. (1982) Waterborne giardiasis outbreak: Alberta. Can. Dis. Weekly Rep. 8-20, 97-98.

Wright, R.A. (1975) Giardial infection from water. Ann. Intern. Med. 82, 509-510.

Wright, R.A., Spencer, H.C., Brodsky, R.E. and Vernon, T.M. (1977) Giardiasis in Colorado: an epidemiologic study. Am. J. Epidemiol. 105, 330-336.

Giardiasis (E.A. Meyer, ed.)
© 1990 Elsevier Science Publishers B.V. (Biomedical Division)

16

Giardia among children in day care

LARRY K. PICKERING and PAUL G. ENGELKIRK

Division of Infectious Diseases, Department of Pediatrics, University of Texas Medical School at Houston and Program in Medical Technology/Cytogenetics, School of Allied Health Sciences, University of Texas Health Science Center at Houston, U.S.A.

1. Introduction	295
2. Outbreaks of disease	296
3. Excretion by asymptomatic children	297
4. Predisposing characteristics and environmental factors	299
5. Transmission of illness into families	300
6. Control of infection	301
7. Summary	301
References	302

1. Introduction

Every day millions of children are placed in day care. These children, particularly those less than three years of age, have an increased incidence of diarrhea when compared to children who do not attend day care (Bartlett et al., 1985a, 1988; Reves et al., 1988). This most likely results from greater exposure of susceptible hosts to various enteropathogens, including *Giardia*. This chapter will summarize published studies of the association between *Giardia* and children in day care. These studies have evaluated the magnitude of outbreaks and sporadic cases of diarrhea due to *Giardia*, excretion of *Giardia* by asymptomatic children, predisposing characteristics and environmental factors involved, transmission of illness into families, and control of infection.

2. Outbreaks of disease

The majority of investigations of diarrhea in children in day care centers have involved outbreaks that occurred in epidemic form. These outbreaks have been caused by many enteropathogens (Bartlett et al., 1984, 1985a; Ford-Jones, 1985; Pickering et al., 1985; Pickering, 1986; Pickering and Woodward, 1982), including *Giardia* (Bartlett et al., 1985a,b; Black et al., 1977; Brown, 1948; Keystone et al., 1978; Naiman et al., 1980; Ormiston et al., 1942; Pickering and Engelkirk, 1988; Pickering et al., 1981; Polis et al., 1986; Sealy and Schuman, 1983). Children of all ages have been affected, but the attack rate has been highest for children in diapers. In one study the incidence of diarrhea among children under three years of age in day care centers was 17 times higher than among older children (Sullivan et al., 1984).

Table 1 lists reported outbreaks of *Giardia*-associated diarrhea in day care centers. Children involved in these outbreaks were generally less than three years of age. Reported attack rates varied from 17% to 54%. In several instances, different enteropathogens were identified in children involved in the same outbreak (Bartlett et al., 1985a; Black et al., 1977; Pickering et al., 1981) indicating the propensity for spread of many enteropathogens during outbreaks and the need for thorough evaluation of children involved in an outbreak.

TABLE 1

Day care center outbreaks of diarrhea associated with *Giardia*

Reference (year)	Enteropathogen(s) identified	Age of children (years)	Attack rate (%)*	No. of centers involved
Black et al. 1977	*Shigella sonnei* and *Giardia*	1–3.5	22/51 (43) 26/48 (54)	1
	Giardia	0.5–3.5	11/36 (31)	2
Keystone et al. (1978)	*Giardia*	<1–5	89/327 (27)	2
Boreham and Shepherd (1984)	*Giardia*	<1–5	14/71 (20)	1
Pickering et al. (1981)	*Giardia*	0–3	3/18 (17)	1
	Giardia, rotavirus	0–3	48/95 (51)	4
Bartlett et al. (1985a,b)	*Giardia***	0–3	29/170 (17)	12

* Attack rates are given as the number of cases/total number of children.
** Rotavirus and *Campylobacter* also were identified in three of the centers.

Epidemic giardiasis in day care centers was reported by Black et al. in 1977. They studied three centers, with overlapping epidemics of shigellosis and giardiasis occurring in one center, where 43% of the children were infected with *Shigella sonnei* and 54% infected with *Giardia*. Although some children had dual infections, the presence of one infection was not significantly associated with the presence of the other. At the other two centers, 29% and 38% of the children had *Giardia* infection, but none had *Shigella*. This prevalence was significantly higher than the 2% prevalence of *Giardia* in 42 age-matched children not in day care centers. The prevalence was highest (57%) in the 12 to 23 month old children. Other studies have reported low prevalence rates in infants younger than one year, higher rates in toddlers and declining rates in older toilet trained children (Boreham and Shepherd, 1984; Keystone et al., 1978; Pickering et al., 1981; Sagi et al., 1983; Sealy and Schuman, 1983). Keystone et al. (1978) showed that 27% of children and 5 of 70 (7%) staff had *Giardia* in their stool specimens during outbreaks of giardiasis in two day care nurseries in Toronto. In Brisbane, Australia, 14 of 71 (20%) children in a day care center were infected with *Giardia*; 36% of these children reported symptoms consistent with the disease (Boreham and Shepherd, 1984). None of 14 staff had *Giardia* in their stool specimens.

Few studies have prospectively evaluated the occurrence of diarrhea due to *Giardia* among children in day care centers (Bartlett et al., 1985a; Pickering et al., 1981; Sullivan et al., 1984). In one investigation, nine of 20 centers studied prospectively experienced 15 outbreaks of diarrhea; one was due to *Giardia*, four were due to *Giardia* and rotavirus (Pickering et al., 1981), and the remainder were associated with *Shigella* or rotavirus. In a two year prospective study of 311 children up to 36 months of age at 22 day care centers in Arizona, 170 outbreak associated cases of diarrhea were identified (Bartlett et al., 1985a); *Giardia* was associated with 29 of these 170 (17%) outbreak cases in 12 day care centers. Of the 465 sporadic cases of diarrhea that occurred during the 7464 child-months of observation (Bartlett et al., 1985a), *Giardia* was identified in 53 (11%), rotavirus in 26 (6%), *Campylobacter* in eight (2%), and *Salmonella* and *Shigella* in one each (0.8%).

3. Excretion by asymptomatic children

The excretion of enteropathogens by asymptomatic children in day care centers has been evaluated in several studies, both during and between outbreaks of diarrhea. In prospective studies of children in day care centers, pathogens were frequently found in stool specimens from asymptomatic contacts of pathogen-positive ill children (Bartlett et al., 1985a; Pickering et al., 1981). In one study, 9% of children who were asymptomatic contacts of ill children had pathogens in their stools during outbreaks. In addition, 16% of age-matched children who were asymptomatic contacts of children with pathogen-positive sporadic diarrhea had the same pathogen in stool specimens (Bartlett et al., 1985a).

In Jerusalem 23 of 77 (30%) asymptomatic nursery children aged three months to three years had *Giardia* cysts in their stools (25) (Table 2). Woo and Paterson, (1986) surveyed asymptomatic children in day care centers in Canada for the prevalence of *Giardia*. They found *Giardia* in stool specimens from 8 of 97 (8%) children between two and five years of age in one survey, and from nine of 147 (6%) children between three and five years of age in another survey (Woo and Paterson, 1986). In 1981, 900 children from three months to 10 years of age and 146 staff in 22 day care centers in Toronto had stool specimens evaluated for parasites. Overall, 19% of children and 14% of staff had intestinal parasites; *Giardia* was found in 8% of children and 2% of staff (Keystone et al., 1984). In a 1981 survey of stool specimens from children in four day care centers in South Carolina, the prevalence of *Giardia* was 0, 17, 26 and 32% (Sealy and Schuman, 1983).

Two prevalence surveys of the excretion of *Giardia* by children in day care centers in Houston (20) identified *Giardia* cysts in stool specimens from 72 children (21%) and 67 children (26%), respectively (Table 2). Trophozoites were found in 15 children (4%) and eight children (3%), respectively. There was no correlation between the frequency of recent diarrheal episodes and the finding of *Giardia*. Stool specimens containing cysts were significantly more frequent (*P*<0.0001) for 13 to 30-month-old children than for children younger than 12 months. Children attending day care centers for longer than three months were more likely to be excreting *Giardia* than those attending for less than three months. Sixty-three of 87 (74%) children whose stools were positive for *Giardia*

TABLE 2

Prevalence surveys of excretion of *Giardia* by asymptomatic children in day care centers

Location (source)	Attack rate (%)	Number of centers	Age of children (years)
Jerusalem Sagi et al. (1983)	23/77 (30)	1	0.25–3
Ontario Woo and Paterson (1986)	8/97 (8) 9/147 (6)	not stated not stated	2–5 3–5
Toronto Keystone et al. (1984)	72/900 (8) 3/146 (2)*	22 22	0.25–10 adults
South Carolina Sealy and Schuman (1983)	22/84 (26)	4	<2–11
Houston Pickering et al. (1984)	72/339 (21) 67/261 (26)	29 26	0.5–3 0.5–3
Phoenix Bartlett et al. (1985a)	94/569 (16)	22	0–3

* Staff members.

on the first survey had positive stools five months later, suggestive of either persistent or repeated infections. In a two year prospective study of diarrheal illness in 22 day care centers in Maricopa County, Arizona, 94 of 569 (16%) asymptomatic child contacts of pathogen-positive sporadic cases of *Giardia* were identified (Bartlett et al., 1985a).

In an 18 month study at one center, cysts were detected in stool specimens from 27 of 82 (33%) children at least once (Pickering et al., 1984). Twelve of these children had cysts in weekly stool specimens for a mean of 6.2 months (range 2 to 14 months) and trophozoites for a mean of 3.3 months (Pickering et al., 1984). The number of enteric signs and symptoms reported by teachers and parents and the monthly height and weekly weight measurements did not differ significantly when infected and noninfected children were compared. Others have shown that untreated children in day care centers who excrete cysts tended to have higher height and weight percentiles than *Giardia*-negative children (Sagi et al., 1983).

Asymptomatic excretion of *Giardia* by children younger than 36 months of age is common in day care centers and appears to be well tolerated. When diarrhea occurs, these organisms may be transmitted to previously unexposed children or to family members because of close contact and lack of personal hygiene among infants and young children. The role of symptomatic excretors of *Giardia* in transmission of this organism is unknown. *Giardia* appear to be endemic in children in day care centers in Houston, Phoenix, Canada and Israel, suggesting that eradication of this parasite from the asymptomatic day care center population is not practical.

4. Predisposing characteristics and environmental factors

Day care centers and their personnel have been evaluated with regard to incidence of diarrheal illness. Various studies have examined (1) characteristics of facilities at the center, (2) procedures used when diarrhea occurs, (3) characteristics of day care staff, and (4) cultures of environmental surfaces and hands of teachers and children. In a mail survey of patients with giardiasis and age- and sex-matched controls, Chute et al. (1987) established foreign travel, day care center exposure and household care contact as risk factors of importance for giardiasis.

The association between selected characteristics of day care centers and higher rates of diarrheal illness among children and staff members was demonstrated in a prospective study of diarrhea in children enrolled at centers (Sullivan et al., 1984). The most significant characteristic associated with a high incidence of diarrhea was the presence of young, nontoilet-trained children. When these nontoilet-trained children developed diarrhea, 58% of the centers either sent them home or isolated them on the premises, 17% either sent them home or allowed them to remain without being isolated, and 25% allowed them to remain without being isolated. Since 42% of these centers permitted mixing of well and ill children, the potential for disease transmission presumably was enhanced.

In one study (Lemp et al., 1984), a significant positive correlation was found between the incidence of diarrhea among children in day care centers and each of the following variables reported by the staff of the centers: the frequency of diapering, the frequency of contact with children less than two years of age, the frequency of meal preparation, the frequency with which food was served to children, and the percentage of staff who both diapered and either served food or prepared meals daily. The results suggest that staff members may play a role in the transmission of diarrhea in day care centers via their daily activities; however, the presence of nontoilet-trained children is the most significant factor associated with higher rates of diarrhea.

The role of fomites in the transmission of diarrhea in day care centers has been evaluated (Ekanem et al., 1983). During a nine month period, inanimate objects, air, and hands of children and staff members at five Houston day care centers were cultured monthly and again during outbreaks of diarrhea. The rates of isolation of fecal coliforms from classroom objects and hands on routine sampling between outbreaks were 12% and 17%, respectively. During outbreaks of diarrhea, fecal coliforms were recovered with greater frequency from classroom objects (38%; $P < 0.001$) and from hands (32%; $P < 0.01$). Sources of cultures that were commonly positive for fecal coliforms included diaper change areas, toys, and floors (Ekanem et al., 1983).

Teachers caring for ill children (who require more diaper changes) have less time to wash their hands between contacts with different children. In one study an increased risk of diarrhea among infants and toddlers in individual day care centers was correlated with lower scores (obtained through evaluations by nurses) for hygienic aspects of handwashing, diapering, available facilities, and group separation (Bartlett et al., 1985a, 1988). A decreased rate of diarrhea was associated with smaller groups of children (Bartlett et al., 1985a). In outbreaks of diarrhea, a shorter duration of enrollment was correlated with an increased risk of illness (Bartlett et al., 1985a; Black et al., 1977); this observation suggested that turnover of children may be a risk factor for higher rates of diarrhea at day care centers. For fear of being absent from their jobs, parents of the children often conceal illness, and sick children continue to attend the centers.

In summary, it appears that contamination of hands, communal toys, and other classroom objects, as well as lack of infection control measures, play a role in the transmission of enteropathogens in outbreaks of diarrhea at day care centers. This explanation would help to explain the frequent presence of multiple pathogens among those affected.

5. Transmission of illness into families

Several reports on the occurrence of diarrhea associated with *Giardia* in family members of children during outbreaks at day care centers have been published (Black et al., 1977; Keystone et al., 1978; Pickering et al., 1981; Polis et al., 1986). Black et al. (1977)

reported that 5 of 20 (25%) family members of 14 *Giardia* positive children were infected with the parasite, whereas none of the family members of 11 *Giardia* negative children were infected. Keystone et al. (1978) reported diarrhea in 22 (12%) of 181 family contacts of 89 day care children with diarrhea due to *Giardia*. The overall secondary attack rate for gastroenteritis in studies in Houston of day care centers was 10% (34 of 331 family contacts) (Pickering et al., 1981). Secondary attack rates were significantly higher when *Shigella* (26%), *Giardia* (17%), or rotavirus (15%) was identified in outbreaks than when no enteropathogen was identified in sporadic cases at day care centers (0.6%). Polis et al. (1986) found *Giardia* in household members of 7 of 15 (47%) families of children in day care centers with *Giardia*. During initial contact of staff members with children, infection may also be prominent in adults, especially in those, such as nursing staff, in direct contact with children (Ormiston et al., 1942). The spread of enteric infection beyond the day care center into families, and then into the general community, appears to be an important public health problem that requires further evaluation.

6. Control of infection

Transmission of an enteropathogen in a day care center depends partly on the characteristics of the agent, such as infective dose, survival in the environment, and virulence. Transmission also may be affected by characteristics of the center, particularly hygienic aspects of child handling, environmental practices, and ages of children enrolled. Children infected in a day care center or elsewhere may subsequently transmit infection within the center and into their households and the community-at- large. Based upon day care studies of diarrhea and hepatitis A (Pickering and Woodward, 1982), both of which are transmitted by the fecal-oral route, measures that may prevent or limit diarrhea in centers include education of day care center employees and parents regarding hygiene practices, including hand washing (Black et al., 1981); understanding and implementation of regulations; reporting of notifiable diseases; and continued review and enforcement of infection control policies.

7. Summary

Diarrhea due to *Giardia* in day care centers primarily involves children under three years of age. Because the increase in day care center use has been most rapid in this age group, further control efforts should focus on the epidemiology and control of *Giardia* within this group. Day care staff, parents, and licensing agencies must be kept informed of modes of transmission, practical methods of prevention and control, and the costs associated with failure to address these issues.

Acknowledgements

Supported in part by grant 13021 from the National Institutes of Health.

References

Bartlett, A.V., Jarvis, B.A., Ross, V., Katz, T.M., Dalia, M.A., Englender, S.J. and Anderson, L.J. (1988) Diarrheal illness among infants and toddlers in day care centers: effects of active surveillance and staff training without subsequent monitoring. Am. J. Epidemiol. 127, 808–817.

Bartlett, A.V., Moore, M., Gary, G.W., Starko, K.M., Erben, J.J. and Meredith, B.A. (1985a) Diarrheal illness among infants and toddlers in day care centers. I. Epidemiology and pathogens. J. Pediatr. 107, 495-502.

Bartlett, A.V., Moore, M., Gary, G.W., Starko, K.M., Erben, J.J. and Meredith, B.A. (1985b) Diarrheal diseases among infants and toddlers in day care centers. II. Comparison with day care homes and households. J. Pediatr. 107, 503-509.

Bartlett, A.V., Broome, C.V., Hadler, S.C., Juranek, D.D., Tacket, C.O., Amler, R.W., Brink, E.W., Onorato, I.M., Orenstein, W.A., Bloch, A.B., Seggerson, J.J. and Snider, D.E. (1984) Public health considerations of infectious diseases in child day care centers. J. Pediatr. 105, 683-701.

Black, R.E., Dykes, A.C., Sinclair, S.P. and Wells, J.G. (1977) Giardiasis in day-care centers: evidence of person-to-person transmission. Pediatrics. 60, 486-491.

Black, R.E., Dykes, A.C., Anderson, K.E., Wells, J.G., Sinclair, S.P., Gary, Jr., W.G., Hatch, M.H. and Gangarosa, E.J. (1981) Handwashing to prevent diarrhea in day-care centers. Am. J. Epidemiol. 113, 445-451.

Boreham, P.L.F. and Shepherd, R.W. (1984) Giardiasis in child-care centers. Med. J. Aust. 141, 263 (letter).

Brown, E.H. (1948) *Giardia lamblia*. The incidence and results of infestation of children in residential nurseries. Arch. Dis. Child. 23, 119-128.

Chute, C.G., Smith, R.P. and Baron, J.A. (1987) Risk factors for endemic giardiasis. Am. J. Public Health 77, 585-587.

Ekanem, E.E., DuPont, H.L., Pickering, L.K., Selwyn, B.J. and Hawkins, C.M. (1983) Transmission dynamics of enteric bacteria in day-care centers. Am. J. Epidemiol. 118, 562-572.

Ford-Jones, E.L. (1985) Outbreak of diarrhea in a day nursery in Ontario. Can. Med. Assoc. J. 132, 1171-1172.

Keystone, J.S., Yanf, J., Grisdale, D., Harrington, M., Pillon, L., Andreychuk, R. (1984) Intestinal parasites in metropolitan Toronto day-care centers. Can. Med. Assoc. J. 131, 733-735.

Keystone, J.S., Krajden, S. and Warren, M.R. (1978) Person-to-person transmission of *Giardia lamblia* in day-care nurseries. Can. Med. Assoc. J. 119, 241-248.

Lemp, G.F., Woodward, W.E., Pickering, L.K., Sullivan, P.S. and DuPont, H.L. (1984) The relationship of staff to the incidence of diarrhea in day care centers. Am. J. Epidemiol. 120, 750-758.

Naiman, H.L., Sekla, L. and Albritton, W.L. (1980) Giardiasis and other intestinal parasitic infections in a Manitoba residential school for the mentally retarded. Can. Med. Assoc. J. 122, 185-188.

Ormiston, G., Taylor, J., Wilson, G.S. (1942) Enteritis in a nursery home associated with *Giardia lamblia*. Br. Med. J. 2, 151-154.

Pickering, L.K. and Engelkirk, P.G. (1988) *Giardia lamblia*. Pediatr. Clin. N. Am. 35, 565–577.

Pickering, L.K., Bartlett, A.V. and Woodward, W.E. (1986) Acute infectious diarrhea among children in day care: epidemiology and control. Rev. Infect. Dis. 8, 539-547.

Pickering, L.K. (1986) The day care center diarrhea dilemma. Am. J. Public Health 76, 623-624.

Pickering, L.K., Woodward, W.E., DuPont, H.L. and Sullivan, P. (1984) Occurrence of *Giardia lamblia* in children in day care centers. J. Pediatr. 104, 522-526.

Pickering, L.K. and Woodward, W.E. (1982) Diarrhea in day care centers. Pediatr. Infect. Dis. 1, 47-52.

Pickering, L.K., Evans, D.G., DuPont, H.L., Vollet, J.J. and Evans, D.J. (1981) Diarrhea caused by *Shigella*, rotavirus, and *Giardia* in day care centers: prospective study. J. Pediatr. 99, 51-56.

Polis, M.A., Tuazon, C.U., Alling, D.W. and Talmanis, E. (1986) Transmission of *Giardia lamblia* from a day care center to the community. Am. J. Public Health 76, 1142-1144.

Reves, R.R., Morrow, A.L., Bartlett, III, A.V. and Pickering, L.K. (1988) A case control study of acute diarrhea in children in a health maintenance organization (HMO): risk estimates associated with nonbreastfeeding and day care. Soc. Ped. Res. Washington, D.C., May, 1988.

Sagi, E.F., Shapiro, M. and Deckelbaum, R.J. (1983) *Giardia lamblia*: prevalence, influence on growth, and symptomatology in healthy nursery children. Isr. J. Med. Sci. 19, 815-817.

Sealy, D.P. and Schuman, S.H. (1983) Endemic giardiasis and day care. Pediatrics 72, 154-158.

Sullivan, P., Woodward, W.E., Pickering, L.K., DuPont, H.L. (1984) Longitudinal study of diarrheal disease in day care centers. Am. J. Public Health 74, 987-991.

Woo, P.T.K. and Paterson, W.B. (1986) *Giardia lamblia* in children in day-care centres in southern Ontario, Canada, and susceptibility of animals to *G. lamblia*. Trans. R. Soc. Trop. Med. Hyg. 80, 56-59.

Giardiasis (E.A. Meyer, ed.)
© 1990 Elsevier Science Publishers B.V. (Biomedical Division)

17

Giardiasis in perspective: the evidence of animals as a source of human *Giardia* infections

GEORGE R. HEALY

905 Vistavia Circle, Decatur, GA 30033, U.S.A.

1. Introduction	305
2. Human to human transmission	306
2.1. Natural	306
2.2. Experimental	306
3. Animal to human transmission	307
3.1. Natural	307
3.1.1. Domestic animals	307
3.1.2. Wild animals	309
3.2. Experimental	311
References	312

1. Introduction

As an infectious agent inhabiting the upper part of the human gastrointestinal tract, *Giardia* is one of a number of human-to-human transmitted organisms, which include viruses, bacteria, other protozoa and helminths. Because of the widespread distribution of *Giardia* among a variety of domestic and wild animals, the potential for *Giardia* to be a zoonotic agent has aroused widespread curiosity and concern. While animal to human transmission is controversial, the evidence for human-to-human spread is well known.

2. Human-to-human transmission

2.1. Natural

The evidence for person-to-person transmission of *Giardia* has accumulated from a variety of sources. Perhaps none has been as incontrovertible in the last several years, as those documenting giardiasis outbreaks in day care centers. Infections have spread through the facilities and in some cases, to family members of the children (Pickering and Engelkirk, Chapter 16 of this volume). Infections in adult male homosexuals have also disclosed person-to-person transmission in numerous cases where no other vehicle of transmission could be identified (Phillips et al., 1981).

Barnard and Jackson (1984) reviewed the evidence for the transmission of *Giardia* by fecally contaminated foods. The report of Osterholm et al. (1981) in particular, focused on an outbreak of foodborne giardiasis in which the vehicle of infection was determined to be contaminated salmon salad. A person mixing the salad had recently changed the diaper of a $1\frac{1}{2}$ year old child whose stools were found to contain *Giardia* cysts.

2.2. Experimental

The classic studies involving experimental infections of humans with human source *Giardia* cysts were conducted by Rendtorff (1954), over 35 years ago. Using cysts obtained from stools of infected prison volunteers, Rendtorff was able to infect 21 of 35 (60%) male volunteers, each of whom was given from ten to one million cysts in capsules.

No further human-to-human infection studies were done until 1987, when Nash et al. (1987) attempted to infect volunteers with two different isolates of *Giardia* (GM/S and Isr) derived from human infections. The investigators fed the volunteers trophozoites grown in axenic culture. Scrupulous sterility studies were made to insure that no contaminating viruses or bacteria were present in the inoculum. The parasites were administered by gavage, using a polyvinyl tube ascertained to be in the small intestine. Successful infections were documented by recovery of cysts/trophozoites in the volunteers' stools, as well as, in some cases, the accompanying variety of the usual symptoms of giardiasis. The original report must be read for details. Suffice it to say that Nash et al. were able to infect volunteers with only the GM/S isolate. This isolate was obtained from the stools of an NIH scientist who had previously travelled to Japan, and later camped in the Alaska wilderness about two weeks before he experienced symptoms.

Isolate Isr, obtained from stools of a year old child with diarrhea, did not infect volunteers fed the trophozoites. The authors did record positive, but transient, stool-positive ELISA test results for *Giardia* antigen in stools. They attributed the positive reactions to antigenic components of the inoculum (5×10^4 trophozoites), which were excreted and detected in the stools by the very sensitive ELISA test.

The success with isolate GM/S was the first fulfillment of Koch's postulates for human *Giardia*. An organism, recovered from a symptomatic person, was cultured, and when ingested by other individuals, produced typical symptoms with the recovery and culture of the organism from stool specimens during the infection. Strain GM/S and Isr possessed different DNA restriction endonuclease patterns, surface antigens and excretory-secretory products, (Nash et al., 1985; Nash and Keister, 1985). Further studies are certainly warranted. However, it is of interest that an isolate of human *Giardia* (Isr), from a symptomatic person, failed to establish an infection in other humans under carefully controlled conditions. Such discrepant results with the two isolates raise questions concerning the possible infection of humans from animal sources.

3. Animal-to-human transmission

3.1. Natural

3.1.1. Domestic animals

The close association between humans and domestic animals, particularly pets (dogs, cats) has been suspected as a means whereby zoonotic giardiasis occurs and may be responsible for some human infections. *Giardia* infections in dogs have been reported by several authors. Kirkpatrick and Farrell (1982) tabulated the results of 6 studies, carried out in the United States up to 1982. A total of 395 of 3523 (12%) dogs were found infected with *Giardia*. Individual surveys recorded from 1.9 to 36% infections. Studies involved necropsy findings as well as stool examinations. In recent years, Hoskins et al. (1982) found 34 of 4752 (1%) dogs infected; Baker et al. (1987) 48 of 200 (24%); Hewlett et al. (1982) 25 of 37 (68%); Stehr-Green et al. (1987) 49 of 143 (34%). Recently, in Canada's Alberta Province, Lewis (1988) found 101 of 1005 (10%) of stray dogs and 57 of 678 (8%) of dogs in animal shelters in Calgary and Edmonton, with *Giardia*.

The above studies involved puppies as well as adult animals. Prevalence rates recorded are undoubtedly lower than the number of actual infections. Most stool findings were based on the examination of a single stool specimen. The acyclic shedding of *Giardia* cysts has been noted in humans (Danciger and Lopez, 1979) and in dogs (Hewlett et al., 1982). It is probable that a single stool examination may fail to detect a patent infection in 20-50% of animals or humans. Even in successful infections of laboratory animals (gerbils) with human source *Giardia* cysts, parasites were not detected on some days, even when stools collected over a 24 h period were pooled before being examined (Visvesvara et al., 1988).

From the above studies and anecdotal information from veterinary practitioners it is apparent that dogs, especially puppies, harbor *Giardia* organisms, with the possibility that the prevalence is higher than reported. Brushing, petting, scratching of dogs, especially puppies, or allowing dogs to lick the face after anal grooming, make for fecal soiling of the person by the pet, with the possibility of infection if the dog is excreting *Giardia* cysts. Nonetheless, in spite of the close dog-human relationship, there has not been a documented report of human giardiasis from the dog. Bemrick (1984), in his cogent review of the transmission of *Giardia*, stated that over many years, handling hundreds of dog fecal samples positive for *Giardia*, without special precautions, no one in his laboratory had shown clinical symptoms of giardiasis, nor had *Giardia* cysts been demonstrated in periodic fecal examinations. While Bemrick indicated 'no special precautions' were taken, the inherent safety practised in a facility handling countless dog stools, would be far above that of a household and a pet animal. Nonetheless, a report of household giardiasis from a dog source still awaits confirmation.

Fewer studies have been carried out of cats as a source of zoonotic giardiasis. Brightman and Slonka (1976) recorded 5 cases of clinical giardiasis in cats. Davies and Hibler (1979) found 1 of 4 cats infected in their animal survey of New Mexico and Colorado. Wolf and Eckert (1979) in Germany recovered cysts in stools of 6 of 927 (0.6%) cats examined in the period 1978-1979. Kirkpatrick and Farrell (1982) tabulated the results of 3 studies on *Giardia* prevalence in cats. A total of 36 of 1195 (3%) of the cats were infected. Belosevic et al. (1984) reported a small outbreak of feline giardiasis (2 of 4 animals) in a commercial cat breeding facility.

Cases of cat-to-human transmitted giardiasis are extremely rare. Davies and Hibler (1979) cursorily stated knowledge of a family of 5 with giardiasis. A pet cat was excreting cysts. Likewise, the same authors reported two other individuals with severe giardiasis. The pet cat of one of the individuals was also shedding *Giardia* cysts. Few details of these anecdotal infections were supplied; whether the humans had infected the cats or vice-versa is an unanswered question.

Cats may be an unrecognized source of human giardiasis. They serve as zoonotic reservoirs of several human diseases, paramount among which is toxoplasmosis. The entire family of the Felidae, of which cats are the domestic member, are recognized as the primary hosts of *Toxoplasma*. Human infections arising from the ingestion of *Toxoplasma* oocysts results in a spectrum of disease from the asymptomatic to the severe. The most serious is the primary infection of a pregnant woman, with the possible severe-to-fatal infection of the fetus. The cat-pregnant woman link is well documented (Frenkel and Dubey, 1972). Although the prevalence rate of giardiasis in cats appears low, their primary epidemiologic significance may be in isolated cases in families. Reasons for the lack of cat-to-human giardiasis recognition might be: (1) *Giardia* cysts are not as resistant to environmental vagaries as are *Toxoplasma* oocysts; (2) the *Giardia* species in cats does not infect humans; (3) giardiasis in humans, recognizeable by typical signs and symptoms, is a less severe disease, easily diagnosed, and amenable to therapy and thus the cat-human transmission goes unrecognized.

Attempts to infect dogs and/or cats with human source *Giardia* organisms have produced mixed results. Davies and Hibler (1979) and Hewlett et al. (1982) were able to infect dogs with human source *Giardia* cysts. Kirkpatrick and Green (1985) found only one of 6 laboratory reared cats, which had been fed cultured human-source *Giardia* trophozoites, positive for *Giardia*. In another experiment, 2 of 8 cats fed cysts of human origin, excreted cysts. However, one animal passed cysts for just one day, the other only two days. Kirkpatrick and Green concluded that cats were probably poor (inefficient) reservoir hosts for human *Giardia*.

In a well documented paper, Woo and Patterson (1986) fed adult cats and kittens as well as adult dogs and puppies with *Giardia* cysts from humans. The organisms were obtained from the stools of clinically ill as well as asymptomatic children in day care centers. The authors were unable to infect any of the dogs or cats with cysts. In addition, kittens could not be infected with cultured trophozoites from a human strain of *Giardia*. Woo and Patterson employed rigid criteria for determining that the experimental animals were free of endogenous *Giardia* before exposure to the organisms from the childrens' stools. The authors concluded that dogs and cats are not susceptible to infection with human *Giardia*, and as such they are of no importance in the spread of giardiasis in the human population.

While *Giardia* organisms have been recovered from other domestic and semi-domestic animals such as cattle, sheep, pigs and goats, the role of such species in zoonotic giardiasis is unknown or considered very problematic. No natural human infection attributable to farm animals (sensu stricto) has been reported. With the discovery that *Giardia* was important as a cause of numerous waterborne outbreaks of diarrheal disease (Craun, Chapter 15 of this volume), the focus has shifted to wild animals as the culprit(s) in possible zoonotic giardiasis.

3.1.2. Wild animals
The first detailed report of an epidemic of giardiasis from fecally contaminated water was published by Moore et al. (1969), regarding Aspen, Colorado. An earlier note, in the form of a letter, involved Portland Oregon, was reported by Veazie (1969), but was not appreciated for its significance at the time. The final details of the outbreak were published ten years later by Veazie et al. (1979). Other waterborne outbreaks of giardiasis have been documented in the intervening years, (Craun, Chapter 15 of this volume).

It became apparent as these published and other anecdotal reports of waterborne giardiasis emerged, that not all such reports were associated with obvious human fecal pollution. Of particular interest, was the occurrence of such events in the mountainous areas of the U.S., especially the West and Northwest, in areas of sparse human habitation. Dykes et al. (1980) sounded the alarm with their report of an outbreak of giardiasis in Camas, Washington. Investigation of the watershed supplying the city, revealed no signs of human fecal contamination, but animal trappings yielded 3 *Giardia*-infected beavers. The organisms were infectious to specific pathogen-free beagle puppies. Thus the sobriquet 'beaver fever' (Jakubowski, 1988), a Canadian name for giardiasis was born.

As aquatic animals, beavers were thought to be a likely source of waterborne giardiasis. Davies and Hibler (1979), had found 46 of 244 (18%) beavers positive for *Giardia*. They concluded that beavers might be considered as important 'sentinel animals' for giardiasis. They did not find *Giardia* in 21 muskrats that they examined. Navin et al. (1985) attributed an outbreak of giardiasis in Reno, Nevada to a waterborne source from municipal water. A beaver, subsequently found to be infected with *Giardia* at necropsy, had built a lodge in a diversion pipe leading to Highland Reservoir, where water was held prior to distribution to the city. *Giardia* cysts, however, were found in raw water samples obtained upstream from the infected beaver. Cysts were also found in water from an additional reservoir – Hunter Creek – where no beaver were found.

Kent et al. (1988) recently published a report of epidemic giardiasis in Pittsfield, Massachusetts, believed to be caused by a contaminated water supply. Two reservoirs (A and B) supplied the city with chlorinated, but unfiltered, water. A third reservoir (C), was used after a dormant period of 3 years while an upgrading of reservoir A was begun. *Giardia* cysts were recovered from all 3 reservoirs; with higher concentrations in reservoir C. *Giardia* cysts from reservoir C were fed to beaver and muskrats. Trophozoites, found in the intestines of the necropsied animals, were morphologically similar to *Giardia* of human origin, not those of beavers as determined by Erlandsen and Bemrick (1988). One of 3 beavers trapped near reservoir C was found to have *Giardia*; none of 6 trapped near reservoir B was positive. Human activity was evident around reservoir C, by the presence of discarded beverage cans and graffiti – modern man's petroglyphs!

The initial interest in beavers as the source of waterborne giardiasis spurred efforts to determine the extent of infection of the animals in various areas. Frost et al. (1980) examined trapped animals in Washington State over a period of 3 trapping seasons. Nine species (beaver, muskrat, nutria, mink, racoon, river otter, bobcat, coyote and lynx) were examined. *Giardia* were only found in the beavers and muskrats. For the 3 year total, 57 of 529 (11%) beavers and 55 of 133 (41%) muskrats were infected. The finding of a high prevalence of *Giardia* in muskrats stimulated interest in this aquatic mammal as a possible source of waterborne human giardiasis. Evidence of muskrat presence is apparently harder to muster than that of beavers. Muskrat do not build lodges or dens, and are much more prolific than beavers, without giving evidence of their large numbers.

Further studies on beaver and muskrat giardiasis were forthcoming. Pacha et al. (1985) found 156 of 189 (83%) muskrats infected. Isaac-Renton et al. (1987), in British Columbia, found 44 of 299 (15%) beaver fecal samples positive and 8 of 20 (40%) muskrats infected. In their extensive survey of giardiasis in beavers and muskrats, Erlandsen and Bemrick (1988) found high prevalence rates in animals examined from two geographic areas. In the New England area, 29 of 171 (17%) beavers and all of 96 muskrats had *Giardia* trophozoites in intestinal scrapings. When fecal samples were collected from the same area from both species, cysts were found in 43 of 369 (12%) beaver stools and 143 of 432 (33%) muskrat samples. In the Minnesota area, Erlandsen and Bemrick examined fecal specimens and found 9 of 89 (10%) beavers and all of 49 muskrat stools contained *Giardia*.

The high prevalence of giardiasis among muskrats has elevated them to a greater level of suspicion in zoonotic giardiasis. The status of wild animal giardiasis continues to change. Pacha et al. (1987) examined microtine rodent fecal samples and found 469 of

722 (65%) positive for *Giardia*. Recently, Georgi et al. (1986) reported *Giardia* infection in a great blue heron in New York, thereby adding aquatic birds to the list of possible wild animal reservoirs for human waterborne infections. Erlandsen and Bemrick (1988) have added to the list with a report of *Giardia* infections in green herons and egrets. The herons and egrets can fly to various watersheds and presumably contaminate wider areas of the landscape than the earthbound beavers and muskrats! Trophozoites from these birds, examined by Erlandsen and Bemrick, possessed morphologic characters compatible with human *Giardia lamblia* organisms, i.e. claw-hammer shaped median bodies.

Erlandsen and Bemrick (1988) and Erlandsen et al. (1988) called attention to the fact that *Giardia* cysts found in microtine rodents, (muskrats and voles) contain two trophozoites, so-called binary cysts. They have determined that these cyst forms are not host dependent, but retain their specific morphology when recovered from Mongolian gerbils and mice that have been infected with the microtine rodent cysts. If these cysts from rodents do not change their binary morphologic characteristics in human infections, one would expect to have good evidence of a muskrat-vole derived outbreak of waterborne giardiasis.

Unfortunately, in the thousands of human fecal specimens examined in waterborne outbreaks of giardiasis, no laboratory has identified (or at least reported) such cysts in fecal specimens from patients. It may well be that this knowledge is too new. Hopefully, armed with the fact, laboratories involved in examining stool specimens will be cognizant of the distinct morphology and look more critically at the internal morphology of cysts.

Morphologic, biochemical and immunochemical differences between *Giardia* species obtained from various hosts are beyond the scope of this presentation. Nonetheless, until some 'marker' for identifying *Giardia* from wild animals (such as the binary cyst above) is available, the task of attributing giardiasis outbreaks to specific animals – beavers, muskrats, birds, etc., involves circumstantial evidence, albeit strong in many cases.

3.2. Experimental

Cross species transmission experiments have been attempted by various authors, using dogs, cats, beavers, muskrats, microtine rodents, mice, rats, gerbils and various wild mammals. Animals have been infected with *Giardia* cysts/trophozoites recovered from other animals or humans. The experimental animal-to-human transmission is fraught with ethical as well as scientific problems. As noted above, only two transmission experiments in humans, both using human derived *Giardia* organisms (Rendtorff, 1954; Nash et al., 1987) were undertaken.

Two, briefly described, attempts to infect humans with animal derived *Giardia* organisms were reported by Davies and Hibler (1979). In one experiment, 2 of 3 humans, given *Giardia* cysts from a beaver source, became infected, one at 6 days post exposure, the other at 11 days post exposure. Mice, rats, hamsters and guinea pigs exposed to the same source of cysts did not become infected, while 5 dogs (including one control dog) became positive for *Giardia*. In another trial, one human, fed cysts obtained from a captive mule deer, became infected with the parasite 9 days post exposure and experienced severe clinical giardiasis. Two dogs, also fed the same mule deer source of cysts were negative for *Giardia* when stools were examined for 28 days. Although not stated specifically in these human infections, the authors did indicate that most of their experimental infections involved doses of 5000 cysts. Details were lacking as to how many stools from the humans were examined prior to the ingestion of the *Giardia* cysts, to rule out an existing infection.

These two transmission attempts indicate that, apparently, humans are susceptible to *Giardia* of beaver and mule deer origin. It is of interest that Davies and Hibler (1979) in their survey of wild animals in New Mexico and Colorado found no *Giardia* organisms in fecal samples from 35 mule deer.

References

Baker, D.H., Strombeck, D.R. and Gershwin, L.J. (1987) Laboratory diagnosis of *Giardia duodenalis* infection in dogs. J. Am. Vet. Med. Assoc. 190, 53-56.

Barnard, R.J. and Jackson, G.J. (1984) *Giardia lamblia*. The transfer of human infections by food. In: S.L. Erlandsen and E.A. Meyer (Eds.), Giardia and Giardiasis, Biology, Pathogenesis and Epidemiology. Plenum Press, New York, pp. 365-378.

Belosevic, G.M., Faubert, G.M. and MacLean, J.D. (1984) Observations on natural and experimental infections with *Giardia* isolated from cats. Can. J. Comp. Med. 48, 241-244.

Bemrick, W.J. (1984) Some perspectives on the transmission of giardiasis. In: S.L. Erlandsen and E.A. Meyer (Eds.), Giardia and Giardiasis, Biology, Pathogenesis and Epidemiology. Plenum Press, New York, pp. 379-400.

Brightman, A.H. and Slonka, G.F. (1976) A review of five clinical cases of giardiasis in cats. J. Am. Anim. Hosp. Assoc. 12, 492-497.

Danciger, M. and Lopez, M. (1975) Numbers of *Giardia* in the feces of infected children. Am. J. Trop. Med. Hyg. 24, 237-242.

Davies, R.B. and Hibler, C.P. (1979) Animal reservoirs and cross-species transmission of giardiasis. In: W. Jakubowski and J.C. Hoff (Eds.), Waterborne Transmission of Giardiasis. Environmental Protection Agency, Cincinnati, Ohio, pp. 104-126.

Dykes, A.C., Juranek, D.D., Lorenz, R.A., Sinclair, S., Jakubowski, W. and Davies, R.B. (1980) Municipal waterborne giardiasis: an epidemiologic investigation. Ann. Int. Med. 92, 165-170.

Erlandsen, S.L., Sherlock, L.A., Januschka, M., Schupp, D.G., Schaefer, F.W., Jakubowski, W. and Bemrick, W.J. (1988) Cross-species transmission of *Giardia* spp. Inoculation of beavers, muskrats with cysts of human, beaver and muskrat origin. Appl. Environ. Microbiol. 54, 2777–2785.

Erlandsen, S.L. and Bemrick, W.J. (1988) Waterborne giardiasis: source of *Giardia* cysts and evidence pertaining to their implication in human infections. In: P.M. Wallis and B.R. Hammond (Eds), Advances in *Giardia* Research. Univ. of Calgary Press, pp. 227-236.

Frenkel, J.K. and Dubey, J.P. (1972) Toxoplasmosis and its prevention in cats and man. J. Infect. Dis. 126, 664-673.

Frost, F., Plan, B. and Leichty, B. (1980) *Giardia* prevalence in commercially trapped animals. J. Environ. Health 42, 245-249.

Georgi, M.E., Carlisle, M.S. and Smiley, L.E. (1986) Giardiasis in a great blue heron (Ardea herodiasis) in New York State: another potential source of waterborne giardiasis. Am. J. Epidemiol. 123, 916-917.

Hewlett, E.L., Andrews, J.S., Ruffier, J. and Schaefer, F.W. (1982) Experimental infection of mongrel dogs with *Giardia lamblia* cysts and cultured trophozoites. J. Infect. Dis. 152, 1166-1171.

Hoskins, J.D., Malone, J.B., Smith, P.H. and Uhl, S.A. (1982) Prevalence of parasitism diagnosed by fecal examination in Louisiana dogs. Am. J. Vet. Res. 43, 1106-1109.

Isaac-Renton, J.L., Moriez, M.M. and Proctor, E.M. (1987) A *Giardia* survey of fur-bearing mammals in British Columbia. J. Environ. Health. 50, 80-83.

Jakubowski, W. (1988) Purple burps and the filtration of drinking water supplies. Am. J. Public Health 78, 123-125.

Kent, G.P., Greenspan, J.R., Herndon, J.L., Mofenson, L.M., Harris, J.S., Eng, T.R. and Waskin, H.A. (1988) Epidemic giardiasis caused by a contaminated public water supply. Am. J. Public Health 78, 139-143.

Kirkpatrick, C.E. and Farrell, J.P. (1982) Giardiasia. Compend. Contin. Ed. Pract. Vet. 4, 367-377.

Kirkpatrick, C.E. and Farrell, J.P. (1984) Feline giardiasis: observations on natural and induced infections. Am. J. Vet. Res. 45, 2182-2188.

Kirkpatrick, C.E. and Green, B. (1985) Susceptibility of domestic cats to infections with *Giardia lamblia* cysts and trophozoites from human sources. J. Clin. Microbiol. 21, 678-680.

Lewis, P.D. (1988) Prevalence of *Giardia* sp. in dogs from Alberta. In: P.M. Wallis and B.R. Hammond (Eds.), Advances in *Giardia* Research. Univ. of Calgary Press, pp. 61-64.

Moore, G.T., Cross, W.M., McGuire, D., Mollahan, C.S., Gleason, N.N., Healy, G.R. and Newton, L.H. (1969) Epidemic giardiasis at a ski resort. N. Engl. J. Med. 281, 402-407.

Nash, T.E., McCutchan, T., Keister, D., Dame, J.B., Conrad, J.D. and Gillin, F.D. (1985) Restriction endonuclease analysis of DNA from 15 *Giardia* isolates obtained from humans and animals. J. Infect. Dis. 152, 64-73.

Nash, T.E. and Keister, D.B. (1985) Differences in excretory-secretory products and surface antigens among 19 isolates of *Giardia*. J. Infect. Dis. 152, 1166-1171.

Nash, T.E., Herrington, D.A., Losonsky, G.A. and Levine, M.M. (1987) Experimental human infections with *Giardia lamblia*. J. Infect. Dis. 156, 974-984.

Navin, T.R., Juranek, D.D., Ford, M., Minedew, D.J., Lippey, E.C. and Pollard, R.A. (1985) Case control study of waterborne giardiasis in Reno Nevada. Am. J. Epidemiol. 122, 269-275.

Osterholm, M.T., Forgang, J.C., Ristinen, T.L., Dean, A.G., Washburn, J.W., Godes, J.R., Rude, R.A. and McCullough, J.C. (1981) An outbreak of foodborne giardiasis. N. Engl. J. Med. 304, 24-28.

Pacha, R.E., Clark, G.W. and Williams, E.A. (1985) Occurrence of *Campylobacter jejuni* and *Giardia* species in muskrat (*Ondatra zibethica*). Appl. Environ. Microbiol. 50, 177-178.

Pacha, R.E., Clark, G.W., Williams, E.A., Carter, A.M., Scheffelmaier, J.J. and Debuschere, P. (1987) Small rodents and other mammals associated with mountain meadows as reservoirs of *Giardia* spp. and *Campylobacter* spp. Appl. Environ. Microbiol. 53, 1574-1579.

Phillips, S.C., Mildvan, D., Williams, D.C., Gelb, A.M. and White, M.C. (1981) Sexual transmission of enteric protozoa and helminths in a venereal disease clinic population. N. Engl. J. Med. 305, 603-606.

Rendtorff, R.C. (1954) The experimental transmission of human intestinal protozoan parasites. II. *Giardia lamblia* cysts given in capsules. Am. J. Hyg. 59, 209-220.

Stehr-Green, J.K., Murray, G., Schantz, P.M. and Wahlquist, S.P. (1987) Intestinal parasites in pet store puppies in Atlanta. Am. J. Public Health 11, 345–346.

Veazie, L. (1969) Epidemic giardiasis. N. Engl. J. Med. 281, 853.

Veazie, L., Brownlee, J. and Sears, H.J. (1979) An outbreak of gastroenteritis associated with *Giardia lamblia*. In: W. Jakubowski and J.C. Hoff (Eds), Waterborne Transmission of Giardiasis. Environmental Protection Agency Cincinnati, Ohio, pp. 174-180.

Visvesvara, G.S., Dickerson, J.W. and Healy, G.R. (1988) Variable infectivity of human-derived *Giardia lamblia* cysts for Mongolian gerbils (Meriones unguiculatus). J. Clin. Microbiol. 26, 837-841.

Wolff, V.K. and Eckert, J. (1979) Giardia Befall bei Hund und Katze und dessen mögliche Bedeutung für Menschen. Berl. Münch. Tierärztl. Wochenschr. 92, 479-484.

Woo, P.T.K. and Patterson, W.B. (1986) *Giardia lamblia* in children in day-care centres in southern Ontario, Canada, and susceptibility of animals to *G. lamblia*. Trans. R. Soc. Trop. Med. Hyg. 80, 56-59.

Giardiasis (E.A. Meyer, ed.)
© 1990 Elsevier Science Publishers B.V. (Biomedical Division)

18

Nitroimidazole treatment of giardiasis

LIISA JOKIPII and ANSSI M.M. JOKIPII

Vanhaväylä 37, 00830 Helsinki, Finland

1. Introduction	315
2. Nitroimidazole drugs	316
2.1. History	316
2.2. Mode of action	316
2.3. Selective toxicity	316
2.4. Pharmacokinetics	316
2.5. Antigiardial activity	317
3. Giardiasis	317
3.1. Diagnosis	317
3.2. Indications of treatment	318
4. Treatment of giardiasis	319
4.1. Metronidazole	319
4.2. Other nitroimidazoles	319
4.3. Single-dose therapy	319
4.4. Control	320
4.5. Reasons for failure	321
5. Future	321
References	322

1. Introduction

Giardia has been with us for a longer time than is directly known of any other microorganism. The objective parasitological diagnosis emerged from the examination of human feces with the first microscope over 300 years ago.

The concept of disease involves a subjective aspect, and giardiasis as a clinical diagnosis has been established gradually with improving sanitation and with fading of the role of fatal epidemic infections as the overwhelming everyday health concern.

Populations, for whom it is normal to be free of gastrointestinal symptoms and of *Giardia*, increasingly recognize the appearance of either. The old parasite seems to be causing a comparatively new disease.

2. Nitroimidazole drugs

2.1. History

Six years after the discovery of the antibiotic azomycin (Maeda et al., 1953), which is 2-nitroimidazole, and three years after the demonstration of its trichomonacidal activity (Horie, 1956) in Japan, the synthetic 5-nitroimidazole derivative, metronidazole (Fig. 1) was described (Cosar and Julou, 1959) and shown to cure human trichomoniasis (Durel et al., 1959) in France. In two more years it was *Giardia*'s turn to surrender to metronidazole treatment (Mandoul et al., 1961; Schneider, 1961), which ended the 25 years of quinacrine as the only drug against giardiasis.

2.2. Mode of action

The nitro group is crucial to the antimicrobial activity of metronidazole, which is inactive as such. After metabolic reduction of the nitro group within the target cell, metronidazole causes DNA damage (Müller, 1986; Edwards, 1986). The exact chemical nature of the active metabolite(s) and probable other molecular targets remain to be identified.

A few hundred 5-nitroimidazole compounds have been synthesized, less than 10 of which have been used in giardiasis to date. It is generally not doubted that all have the same mode of action as metronidazole.

2.3. Selective toxicity

The metabolic nitro reduction only takes place in an anaerobic microenvironment, and is prevented by e.g. oxygen. The antimicrobial activity of metronidazole is remarkably restricted to protozoa with an anaerobic metabolism, such as *Trichomonas, Giardia* and *Entamoeba*, and to obligately anaerobic bacteria. Because the active molecular species is a short-lived intermediate of the reductive metabolism of metronidazole, the end products released from target cells to the environment are inactive. This explains the lack of activity in normal (aerobic) human cells, and thus the safety and widespread use of the 5-nitroimidazoles.

2.4. Pharmacokinetics

As drugs the various 5-nitroimidazoles mainly resemble each other, and it is not known, which basic properties are responsible for the observed differences in therapeutic value. The drugs are well absorbed and systemically available after oral administration.

In patients with giardiasis the absorption and elimination of tinidazole and ornidazole (Fig. 2) are slower than those of metronidazole (Jokipii and Jokipii, 1979, 1982). Secnidazole (Fig. 3) is a 5-nitroimidazole characterized by an even longer half-life of 17 h (Videau et al., 1978).

2.5. Antigiardial activity

In vitro activity is direct evidence for the hypothesis that therapeutic efficacy is specific, i.e. based on drug effects on *Giardia*. Such evidence was initially provided using metronidazole and tinidazole (Jokipii and Jokipii, 1980b). Immobilization of trophozoites obtained from the duodenal mucus of patients with giardiasis (Jokipii and Jokipii, 1980a) was rapid and more so with tinidazole (Fig. 4). On the weight basis, a 4.4-fold concentration of metronidazole was needed to reach an arbitrarily defined end point, 100% immobilization in 24 h. The method reveals susceptibility and interdrug differences in a few hours, and concerns the patient at hand. All 5-nitroimidazole compounds tested so far have been found active against *Giardia*.

Several other methods have been devised since, using established axenic cultures, but they take days to provide a result, and the conclusion about the difference between metronidazole and tinidazole has been repeatedly confirmed.

3. Giardiasis

3.1. Diagnosis

Specific treatment should be based on a specific diagnosis, and therefore the rules of diagnosis are imperative in a discussion about treatment.

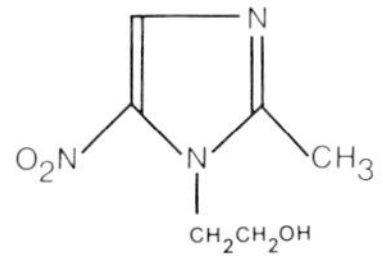

Fig. 1. Metronidazole.

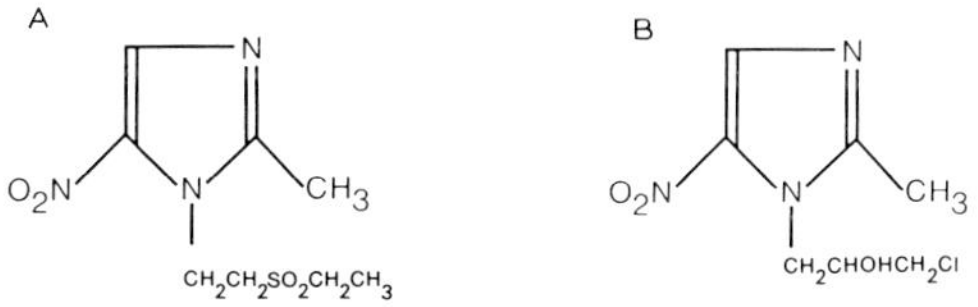

Fig. 2. Tinidazole (A) and ornidazole (B).

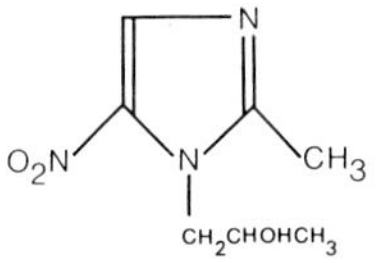

Fig. 3. Secnidazole.

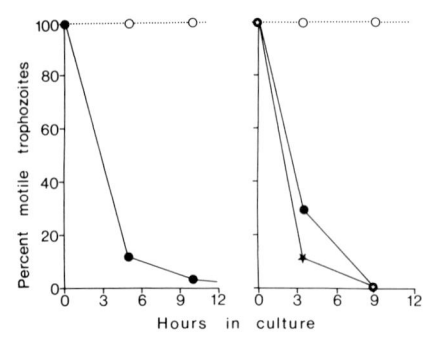

Fig. 4. Immobilization of *Giardia* from two patients in the presence of 50 µg/ml of metronidazole (•) or tinidazole (*) or in medium only (o).

The diagnosis is made parasitologically by identifying *Giardia*, usually as cysts in feces after concentration. Exceptionally, one can look for trophozoites in feces or in material from the small intestine.

There are no pathognomonic symptoms or signs (Jokipii and Jokipii, 1983), and this is equally true of traveler's giardiasis, of the more chronic endemic variety, as well as in children (Jokipii and Jokipii, 1986). Diagnoses in individual cases cannot be made by available indirect methods such as serology (Jokipii and Jokipii, 1984).

After the acquisition of *Giardia*, there is a period of prepatency (Rendtorff, 1954), and stool examinations frequently give negative results for approximately three weeks, i.e. even after the appearance of symptoms (Jokipii and Jokipii, 1977). Cyst excretion may fluctuate resulting in false negative diagnoses (Danciger and Lopez, 1975). Thus, repeated stool examinations are required before giardiasis can be considered an unlikely diagnosis in a suspected case.

Finally, to suspect giardiasis means to suspect the ingestion of fecal material. In that setting, the identification of one potential pathogen is no evidence against the simultaneous presence of another pathogen. Giardiasis is not excluded by diagnosing something else.

3.2. Indications of treatment

If giardiasis is diagnosed, the patient should be treated. The availability and official contraindications of drugs vary from one country to another, and should not be disregarded, though influenced. Since teratogenicity has not emerged despite extensive use of at least metronidazole, tinidazole and ornidazole, pregnancy should not be regarded as a contraindication at present.

In the absence of the parasitological diagnosis, the treatment of suspected giardiasis is a very common question that has no one answer. The answer obviously depends on the alternatives and the degree of suspicion, both of which are local and individual. Since nitroimidazole treatment has become such an everyday routine, its administration might save the patient and the doctor from disproportionate efforts in rare cases, but the neglect of adequate standard parasitology is never justifiable. Furthermore, as drugs have many targets besides *Giardia*, it must be understood that a relief of symptoms as such does not allow, retrospectively, the specific diagnosis of giardiasis.

A third question is that of diagnosed giardiasis in a person who has no symptoms. To begin with, the diversity of symptoms should be recognized and remembered: the presence or absence of diarrhea – or other symptoms of gastroenteritis for that matter – alone does not decide whether we are dealing with symptomatic or asymptomatic giardiasis (Jokipii and Jokipii, 1983, 1986). In addition, children may fail to reveal symptoms. All giardiasis should be treated, because it causes subclinical malabsorption, because symptoms may appear later and periodically, and because a carrier is a reservoir of *Giardia* and a risk for others. An exception to this rule might result from the fact that in some parts of the world the prevalence of giardiasis is so great that the probability of reinfection within a short time approaches 100%. In the same areas, expenses are a relevant concern, and thus the expected benefit might not be sufficient.

4. Treatment of giardiasis

4.1. Metronidazole

Schneider (1961) experienced a substantial improvement in the treatment of giardiasis, when he replaced quinacrine with 500 mg of metronidazole daily for five consecutive days. With minor modifications to increase the dose and/or the duration, the same regimen today remains among the recommended ones.

4.2. Other nitroimidazoles

Derivatives of metronidazole soon appeared, and benzoylmetronidazole (Fig. 5) was the first to be used in giardiasis (Schvartsman et al., 1964). In a decade, nimorazole (Fig. 6) (Cardoso Salles et al., 1970) and tinidazole (Andersson et al., 1972) joined the group, followed by ornidazole a little later (Gandahusada et al., 1974). However, their merits over the already satisfactory metronidazole (Levi et al., 1977) were too weak to bring a major breakthrough other than widening the choice of drug.

There is no apparent reason why several other nitroimidazoles that have been used in amebiasis or trichomoniasis or in animals would not be effective in human giardiasis, too.

4.3. Single-dose therapy

When metronidazole as a single dose was found to cure giardiasis (Khambatta, 1971), a new development began. In comparative evaluations it turned out that the single dose had to be repeated on the following day in order to achieve equal or better cure rates

Fig. 5. Benzoylmetronidazole.

Fig. 6. Nimorazole.

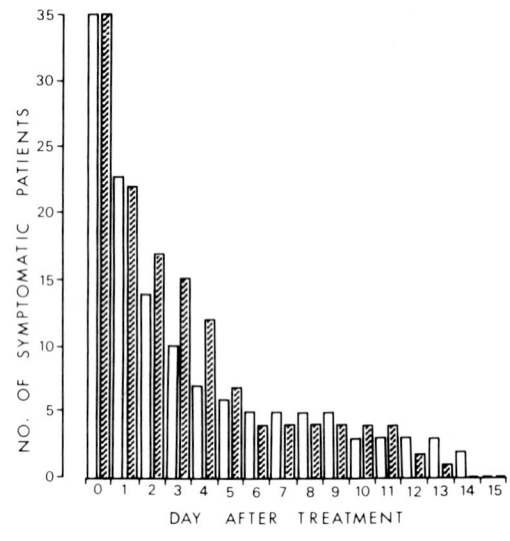

Fig. 7. Disappearance of symptoms after a single oral dose of 1.5 g of tinidazole (shaded columns) or ornidazole (white columns) in 70 patients with symptomatic giardiasis.

than with the conventional regimens (Khambatta, 1971; Jokipii and Jokipii, 1978a).

A breakthrough was roughed out in the reports of 90-100% cure rates with a single dose of 2 g of tinidazole (Farid et al., 1974; Pettersson, 1975; Schenone et al., 1975; Jokipii and Jokipii, 1976). Comparative trials established that single-dose therapy was more efficient (92 or 100%) than a week's course (Jokipii and Jokipii, 1976; Salih and Abdalla, 1977; Jokipii and Jokipii, 1978b). Ornidazole appeared to be effective as a single dose (Heimgartner and Heimgartner, 1977), and, in comparative evaluations, not different from tinidazole (Sabchareon et al., 1980; Jokipii and Jokipii, 1982). The dose of tinidazole or ornidazole could be reduced to 1.5 g, still retaining a 90% cure rate (Jokipii and Jokipii, 1982).

Both tinidazole and ornidazole as a single dose obliterate symptoms (Fig. 7) as well as *Giardia* rapidly and in most cases in a few days (Jokipii and Jokipii, 1982). Orally, 2.4 g of metronidazole is significantly less effective, and should not be used as a single dose (Jokipii and Jokipii, 1979).

4.4. Control

Schneider (1961) already emphasized the necessity of an eight-week parasitological follow-up to confirm the cure of giardiasis. His caution was justified by relevant data, when many failures after single-dose therapy were documented as late relapses (Jokipii and Jokipii, 1978a, 1978b, 1979, 1982). This demonstrated, among other things, how trials with shorter follow-up periods are not valid. The late relapses are usually both parasitological and clinical, and short-term results are misleadingly promising. It seems that the same biological facts which are responsible for prepatency also determine the reappearance of giardiasis after incomplete eradication, and therefore adequate treatment control, like diagnosis, involves repeated stool examinations.

4.5. Reasons for failure

It is not known why some patients are not easily and permanently cured. The reasons may be characteristics of the drugs, the *Giardia*, and/or the host.

In the midst of the similarities of the 5-nitroimidazoles, attention is drawn to the one exceptional major difference as regards the treatment of giardiasis, i.e. the superiority of tinidazole over metronidazole as a single dose (Jokipii and Jokipii, 1979). Therapeutic properties might be identifiable among those which differ between these two drugs.

Tinidazole is more active in immobilizing *Giardia* in vitro. Actual drug resistance is not a probable reason for treatment failures, because, if it exists at all, it is rare enough not to be found in the survey that has been carried out (Jokipii and Jokipii, 1980b). Whether the minor variability in the degree of susceptibility explains failures, remains to be studied.

Tinidazole is more slowly absorbed and eliminated than metronidazole. The therapeutic outcome in 176 patients was not related to the speed of absorption from the intestine, to the serum levels of biologically active nitroimidazole at 1 h or 24 h after administration, or to the rate of drug elimination (Jokipii and Jokipii, 1979, 1982). Thus, host characteristics affecting pharmacokinetics seem not to explain treatment failures.

Autoinfection and reinfection are associated with characteristics of the host and the society. These characteristics will not be classified as reasons for treatment failures, although even they effectively may cause the nitroimidazole effort to fail.

5. Future

Giardiasis is very common in many developing countries, and it is a factor in the five million deaths annually due to diarrheal illness in children of the third world. Giardiasis is second only to malaria in causing failure to thrive (Cole and Parkin, 1977), and the magnitude and dimensions of this problem can only be guessed. Where nutrition as such is a limiting factor, a parasite causing both diarrhea and malabsorption easily aggravates malnutrition with serious consequences. For these reasons, the biggest breakthrough we can imagine in the treatment of giardiasis would be the possibility to offer therapy to everybody. What is needed is a cheap and easy mode of (mass) therapy together with minimizing the probability of reinfection through sanitary measures.

A second major step forward would be the removal of unnecessary obstacles, which prevent the use of the best available treatments in some countries.

Not very much can be expected in the way of increasing the cure rates, which already approach 100%, or reducing the side effects, which are either harmless or rare. The 5-nitroimidazole family may well provide minor advances in these areas in the future.

References

Andersson, T., Forssell, J. and Sterner, G. (1972) Outbreak of giardiasis: effect of a new antiflagellate drug, tinidazole. Br. Med. J. 2, 449-451.
Cardoso Salles, J.M., Amaral Costa, C. and Freitas Matos, L. (1970) Avaliação da atividade da nitrimidazina na giardíase e trichomoníase genital. O Hospital 77, 257-265.
Cole, T.J. and Parkin, J.M. (1977) Infection and its effect on the growth of young children: a comparison of the Gambia and Uganda. Trans. R. Soc. Trop. Med. Hyg. 71, 196-198.
Cosar, C. and Julou, L. (1959) Activité de l'(hydroxy-2′éthyl)-1 méthyl-2 nitro-5 imidazole (8.823 R.P.) vis-à-vis des infections expérimentales a *Trichomonas vaginalis*. Ann. Inst. Pasteur 96, 238-241.
Danciger, M. and Lopez, M. (1975) Numbers of *Giardia* in the feces of infected children. Am. J. Trop. Med. Hyg. 24, 237-242.
Durel, P., Roiron, V., Siboulet, A. and Borel, L.J. (1959) Essai d'un antitrichomonas dérivé de l'imidazole (8823 R.P.). C. R. Soc. Franç. Gynécol. 29, 36-45.
Edwards, D.I. (1986) Reduction of nitroimidazoles in vitro and DNA damage. Biochem. Pharmacol. 35, 53-58.
Farid, Z., El-Masry, N.A., Miner, W.F. and Hassan, A. (1974) Tinidazole in treatment of giardiasis. Lancet 2, 721.
Gandahusada, S., Rukmono, B. and Rasad, R. (1974) Double blind trial of RO-7-0207 (Roche) and metronidazole in the treatment of intestinal giardiasis. Majalah Kedokteran Indonesia 14, 398-404.
Heimgartner, E. and Heimgartner, V. (1977) Tratamiento de la amibiasis intestinal y de la lambliasis con ornidazol. Resultados con tratamiento de breve duración (1-5 días). Invest. Méd. Int. 4, 88-94.
Horie, H. (1956) Anti-Trichomonas effect of azomycin. J. Antibiotics, Ser. A. 9, 168.
Jokipii, A.M.M. and Jokipii, L. (1977) Prepatency of giardiasis. Lancet 1, 1095-1097.
Jokipii, A.M.M. and Jokipii, L. (1978b) Comparative evaluation of two dosages of tinidazole in the treatment of giardiasis. Am. J. Trop. Med. Hyg. 27, 758-761.
Jokipii, L. and Jokipii, A.M.M. (1976) Comparison of metronidazole and tinidazole as a one-week course or as a single dose in the treatment of giardiasis. XIII International Congress of Internal Medicine, Helsinki. Abstracts, 202.
Jokipii, L. and Jokipii, A.M.M. (1978a) Comparison of four dosage schedules in the treatment of giardiasis with metronidazole. Infection 6, 92-94.
Jokipii, L. and Jokipii, A.M.M. (1979) Single-dose metronidazole and tinidazole as therapy for giardiasis: success rates, side effects, and drug absorption and elimination. J. Infect. Dis. 140, 984-988.
Jokipii, L. and Jokipii, A.M.M. (1980a) Recovery of *Giardia lamblia* from human duodenal mucus with a home-made pearl-fishing device. Ann. Trop. Med. Parasitol. 74, 93-95.
Jokipii, L. and Jokipii, A.M.M. (1980b) In vitro susceptibility of *Giardia lamblia* trophozoites to metronidazole and tinidazole. J. Infect. Dis. 141, 317-325.
Jokipii, L. and Jokipii, A.M.M. (1982) Treatment of giardiasis: comparative evaluation of ornidazole and tinidazole as a single oral dose. Gastroenterology 83, 399-404.

Jokipii, L. and Jokipii, A.M.M. (1983) Traveller's giardiasis. An analysis of clinical features. Travel Traffic Med. Intern. 1, 75-80.

Jokipii, L. and Jokipii, A.M.M. (1984) Serological diagnosis of human giardiasis. In: I. de Carneri (Ed.), Immunological Diagnosis and Other Diagnostic Methods for Parasitic Infections. Associazione Microbiologi Clinici Italiani, Milano, pp. 31-36.

Jokipii, L. and Jokipii, A.M.M. (1986) Giardiasis. In: A.I. Braude (Ed.), International Textbook of Medicine, Vol. II, Medical Microbiology and Infectious Diseases, 2nd edit., W.B. Saunders Company, Philadelphia, pp. 928-931.

Khambatta, R.B. (1971) Metronidazole in giardiasis. Ann. Trop. Med. Parasitol. 65, 487-489.

Levi, G.C., Armando de Avila, C. and Amato Neto, V. (1977) Efficacy of various drugs for treatment of giardiasis. A comparative study. Am. J. Trop. Med. Hyg. 26, 564-565.

Maeda, K., Osato, T. and Umezawa, H. (1953) A new antibiotic, azomycin. J. Antibiot. A. 6, 182.

Mandoul, R., Dargelos, R. and Millan, J. (1961) Destruction des protozoaires intestinaux de la souris par un dérivé nitré de l'imidazole. Bull. Soc. Pathol. Exot. 54, 12-16.

Müller, M. (1986) Reductive activation of nitroimidazoles in anaerobic microorganisms. Biochem. Pharmacol. 35, 37-41.

Pettersson, T. (1975) Single-dose tinidazole therapy for giardiasis. Br. Med. J. 1, 395.

Rendtorff, R.C. (1954) The experimental transmission of human intestinal protozoan parasites. II. *Giardia lamblia* cysts given in capsules. Am. J. Hyg. 59, 209-220.

Sabcharcon, A., Chongsuphajaisiddhi, T. and Attanath, P. (1980) Treatment of giardiasis in children with quinacrine, metronidazole, tinidazole and ornidazole. Southeast Asian J. Trop. Med. Public Health 11, 280-284.

Salih, S.Y. and Abdalla, R.E. (1977) Symptomatic giardiasis in Sudanese adults and its treatment with tinidazole. J. Trop. Med. Hyg. 80, 11-13.

Schenone, H., Orfali, A., Galdames, M. and Rojo, M. (1975) Tratamiento de la amibiasis y la giardiasis en niños mediante la administración oral de tinidazol, un agente antiprotozoario de amplio espectro. Bol. Chile. Parasitol. 30, 76-79.

Schneider, J. (1961) Traitement de la giardiase (lambliase) par le métronidazole. Bull. Soc. Pathol. Exot. 54, 84-93.

Schvartsman, S., Amato Neto, V., Capp, A.B. and Fiore, F.F. (1964) Nota preliminar sôbre o tratamento da giardíase por um nôvo derivado do metronidazol (9712 R.P.). O Hospital 65, 115-119.

Videau, D., Niel, G., Siboulet, A. and Catalan, F. (1978) Secnidazole. A 5-nitroimidazole derivative with a long half-life. Br. J. Vener. Dis. 54, 77-80.

Giardiasis (E.A. Meyer, ed.)
© 1990 Elsevier Science Publishers B.V. (Biomedical Division)

19

Treatment of giardiasis: the North American perspective

R.A. DAVIDSON

Department of General Medicine, University of Florida College of Medicine, Gainesville, FL 32610, U.S.A.

1. Introduction	325
2. Drugs used in the treatment of giardiasis	326
2.1. Quinacrine	326
2.2. Metronidazole	326
2.3. Furazolidone	328
2.4. Paromomycin	328
2.5. Additional drugs	328
3. Efficacy of therapy	329
4. Therapeutic recommendations	330
4.1. General population	330
4.2. Asymptomatic children	331
4.3. Asymptomatic adults	332
4.4. Pregnant patients	332
4.5. Treatment failures	332
References	333

1. Introduction

The therapy of infection with *Giardia* is somewhat controversial, at least in the United States. The 'treatment of choice' recommended by the Centers for Disease Control is quinacrine (Atabrine). Metronidazole (Flagyl) is frequently used, although not approved for this purpose by the Food and Drug Administration. Furazolidone (Furoxone) is used for treating children, and paromomycin (Humatin) has been proposed for use in pregnancy. A discussion of each drug and its risks and benefits will be followed by a critical review of efficacy trials, and recommendations for specific clinical settings.

2. Drugs used in the treatment of giardiasis

2.1. Quinacrine

Quinacrine (Atabrine), also known as mepacrine, is an acridine-yellow dye that was initially developed as an anti-malarial, and additionally has some anti-cestode activity. It is rapidly absorbed, but binds to tissues and is slowly released; around 10% of a daily dose is excreted in the urine. The drug can be detected in urine 2 months after the last dose and in hair and nails for over one year. The precise mechanism of action is unknown, but it does interfere with flavin enzymes causing depression in oxygen consumption, and it is a strong cholinesterase inhibitor. Quinacrine is an intercalating drug, and is thus incorporated into DNA. If this is its mechanism of action, it suggests that its activity may not be species-specific, but rather due to relative intra-organism concentrations (Goodman and Gilman, 1985). Pediatric and adult dosages are given in Table 1.

Quinacrine may cause frequent side effects which may hinder compliance, especially in pediatric patients. Nausea, vomiting, headache and dizziness are the most frequently reported complaints. Less frequent complaints include vertigo, excessive sweating, fever, pruritis, corneal edema, myalgias, and insomnia. Taken in large doses (such as those used for cestode infection), quinacrine may frequently cause yellow skin discoloration, or rarely cause a toxic psychosis, central nervous system stimulation or seizures. Other unusual complications of quinacrine therapy include blood dyscrasias and 'bull's eye' maculopathy with retinal pigmentation (Goodman and Gilman, 1985). The drug should be used with caution in patients with psoriasis as it may initiate or worsen existing exfoliative lesions. It should not be used in pregnancy as it easily crosses the placenta. The drug may also cause a disulfiram-like interaction with alcohol, and like other antimalarials, it may cause hemolysis in glucose-6-phosphate dehydrogenase deficient individuals.

2.2. Metronidazole.

Metronidazole is an imidazole derivative which has an easily reduced nitro group. When exposed to nitroreductase in bacterial or protozoal cells, cytotoxic compounds are produced which disrupt the helical structure of DNA (Goodman and Gilman, 1985).

TABLE 1
Pediatric and adult dosages of antigiardial drugs

Drug	Adult dose	Pediatric dose
Quinacrine*	100 mg t.i.d. × 5 d	2 mg/kg t.i.d. × 5 d**
Metronidazole	250 mg t.i.d. ×5 d	5 mg/kg t.i.d. × 5 d
Furazolidone	100 mg q.i.d. × 10 d	1.25 mg/kg q.i.d. × 10 d
Paromomycin***	10 mg/kg t.i.d. × 7 d	8-10 mg/kg t.i.d. × 7 d

* Usually given after meals; ** maximum of 300 mg/d; *** usually given with meals.

The drug is well absorbed (80% within 1 h of oral administration), and produces adequate tissue levels in bile, CSF, and subcutaneous abcesses (Rosenblatt and Edson, 1983). The normal plasma half-life is 8 to 10 h, and 10% of the drug is bound to plasma proteins (Goodman and Gilman, 1985). It appears that the drug is metabolized by the liver; plasma levels may be extremely high in hepatic failure. Most excretion takes place through the kidneys.

Metronidazole displays a broad spectrum of activity against both protozoans (*T. vaginalis, E. histolytica,* and *Giardia*) and many anaerobic cocci and bacilli, including *Bacteroides fragilis*. Pediatric and adult dosages for the treatment of giardiasis are found in Table 1.

The most frequently reported side effects are gastrointestinal, including nausea, vomiting, diarrhea, and crampy abdominal pain. Other complaints may include metallic taste, headache, dizziness, drowsiness, lassitude, paresthesias, urticaria, pruritis, and a characteristic disulfiram-like interaction with alcohol.

By far the greatest concern about the use of metronidazole is that it was found to be mutagenic in Ames *Salmonella* bacteria in serum and urine levels obtained in usual therapeutic doses (Legator et al., 1975). Later the drug (which is structurally related to azathioprine) was demonstrated to cause an increased incidence of lung and other cancers in rats and mice given continuous large dosages (Rustia and Shubik, 1979). In the face of these concerns, the following facts are reassuring.

(A) Metronidazole does not demonstrate mutagenic activity against mammalian cells in vitro (Voogd, 1981). (B) The drug is probably not teratogenic or embryotoxic, based on both human and animal studies (Morgan, 1978; Roe, 1985). (C) Several of the animal studies which demonstrated carcinogenesis have been criticized on methodologic grounds, such as not correcting for an improved survival time in one metronidazole-treated group, and not considering the effect of dietary and nutritional alterations in others (Roe, 1985). (D) An extrapolation of rodent doses to man, with several assumptions, suggests that a 'safe' dose of metronidazole might be as high as 10 g per day (Voogd, 1981). (E) Two retrospective cohort studies have demonstrated no increased incidence of malignancies among women who took metronidazole up to 16 years previously. However, one study noted an increase in lung cancers in the metronidazole group which approached significance, and both studies could reliably exclude only a large, short term risk (Beard et al., 1979; Friedman, 1980).

In summary, it is unlikely that therapeutic dosages of metronidazole will cause an increased risk of malignancies in humans, although such a possibility cannot be excluded. There is additional evidence that alternative nitroimidazoles, especially tinidazole and ornidazole, may be less mutagenic and require less drug exposure for a comparable therapeutic effect. Unfortunately, these drugs are not available in the United States, and it appears that the cost of demonstration of efficacy required by the Food and Drug Administration may prevent application for approval, given the relatively low numbers of infections and the availability of alternative therapies.

2.3. Furazolidone

Furazolidone is a synthetic nitrofuran which is minimally absorbed. Because it is marketed in a liquid preparation, it is most frequently used in pediatric populations. Its exact mechanism of action against *Giardia* is unknown; in bacteria, it inhibits certain bacterial enzyme systems (Phillips and Hailey, 1986). Other nitrofurans have been shown to form superoxides and other toxic radicals when used against trypanosomes. There is some evidence that the drug may be absorbed through damaged areas of intestine, but this is probably not a concern in giardiasis. Dosages of furazolidone in adults and children are shown in Table 1.

Side effects most frequently reported include nausea, vomiting, diarrhea and malaise. Rarely the drug may cause pruritis, urticaria, or other hypersensitivity reactions. Furazolidone, like quinacrine, can cause intravascular hemolysis in glucose-6-phosphate-dehydrogenase deficient individuals; like both quinacrine and metronidazole, it can produce a disulfiram-like syndrome with exposure to alcohol, consisting of flushing, dyspnea, fever, and nausea. Furazolidone is a monoamine oxidase inhibitor, and could conceivably provoke a hypertensive crisis on exposure to tyramine-containing foods, although this has not been reported. Lastly, furazolidone has been reported to cause cancer in rats and mice given chronic large dosages (Cohen, 1978), but as with metronidazole, the risk in humans given low dose, short-term therapy is minimal.

2.4. Paromomycin

Paromomycin is a minimally absorbed aminoglycoside with evidence of clinical efficacy against *Giardia* infection in humans (Carter et al., 1962), although this efficacy has not been seen in vitro (McIntyre et al., 1986). While its mechanism of action against *Giardia* is unknown, in one eukaryotic organism, *T. thermophila*, the drug caused depletion of polysomes with an associated decrease in lysine incorporation (Eustice and Wilhelm, 1984). Little information about its efficacy in giardiasis exists; Dobon et al. (1963) successfully treated around a third of an infected group of patients. A quarter of those treated with a 5 day course (as opposed to a 10 day course) relapsed, and 15% of all patients experienced gastrointestinal intolerance, which is the usual location of complaints. In one study in amebiasis, over 65% of treated patients developed diarrhea (Sullam et al., 1986). All other reports of efficacy in giardiasis include few patients. Serum levels considered therapeutic for other aminoglycosides cause severe renal toxicity, so the drug should not be used parenterally and should be used with caution in patients which ulcerations in the gastrointestinal tract. Recommended dosages are given in Table 1.

2.5. Additional drugs

Continuing study has shown other medications that have demonstrated antigiardial activity in vitro. Among these drugs are the tricyclic antidepressant chlorimipramine, which may act by the disruption of membrane ATPase (Weinbach et al., 1985); and bithionol, a current treatment for paragonomiasis; and two structurally similar compounds, dichlorophene and hexachlorophene, which may work by the inhibition of aerobic metabolism (Takeuchi et al., 1985). A bile salt-like antibiotic, sodium fusidate, inhibits trophozoite motility; the postulated mechanism is through inhibition of protein synthesis (Farthing and Inge, 1986).

Investigation of the metabolism of *Giardia* has revealed that, like other protozoans, the organism lacks de novo purine biosynthesis and must utilize a 'purine salvage' mechanism, using guanine and adenine phosphoribosyltransferases (Wang and Aldritt, 1983; Aldritt et al., 1985; Aldritt and Wang, 1986). Because of a unique substrate specificity, it has been proposed that a specific inhibitor might interfere with the metabolic needs of the organism. The first investigation of this approach involved the use of guanine arabinoside (Miller et al., 1987). This compound inhibited the growth in vitro of *Giardia*, and was incorporated into *Giardia* DNA in a time-dependent manner. Inhibition of synthesis of DNA, RNA, and proteins occurred with long exposures to the compound. The precise method of inhibition has not been elucidated, but this area of research holds promise for specific antigiardial chemotherapy.

3. Efficacy of therapy

The comparison of alternative therapies for any disease state is a complex issue. Evidence from rigorously designed randomized controlled clinical trials is essential, because this research design is less susceptible to bias than observational studies. Eight clinical trials were reviewed for methodologic rigor (Davidson, 1984). Although one trial included tinidazole, only trials investigating the three drugs available in the U.S. (quinacrine, metronidazole, and furazolidone) were included. Difficulties in interpreting the trials arise from lack of information concerning methods of the studies, variability in study populations, different dosages of medications studied, the appropriateness and accuracy of selected outcome measures, and inadequate sample size.

Study populations: Three trials were performed in India, and one each in the U.S., Iran, Brazil, Thailand, and Egypt. The generalizability of results from these trials to other areas is a major issue. Because cultural immunity may exist in endemic areas of infection (Stevens, 1982), response rates to drugs may be expected to vary.

Course of therapy: In four quinacrine trials, the total dose of medication given varied from 1.5 g (5 days) to 3 g (10 days). In seven trials of metronidazole, total dose ranged from 3.5 g to 5.25 g, given in 5-, 7- and 10-day courses. Six trials which evaluated furazolidone used from 2.8 g (7 days) to 4 g (10 days).

Determination of outcomes: In all cases, parasitologic cure rates were reported; some studies reported symptomatic cure rates in addition. The follow-up times in collecting stool samples varied from less than 1 week to 6 months. With long follow-up time periods in areas of high endemicity, reinfection is a frequent source of bias in determining cure rates; two studies were done on inpatients, making reinfection less likely. On the other hand, short follow-up times are also subject to bias for two reasons: patients who have been successfully treated may continue to pass non-viable cysts in the stool for up to 7 days after therapy (Martin, 1965), and recurrence may occur up to two weeks after treatment, with negative stool examinations in the interim (Kyronseppa and Pettersson, 1981).

The use of stool examination as the sole criteria for parasitologic cure can also be a source of bias. Relying on multiple stool examinations may miss as many as 30 to 50% of infected individuals (Burke, 1977). The inclusion of only patients with positive stool examinations may select those persons with heavier infections, and thus underestimate the efficacy of a drug; conversely, during follow-up, false negative stool examinations may erroneously overestimate efficacy. One of the trials utilized duodenal aspiration; all others employed multiple stool examinations.

Sample size: When there is no difference found between therapies, as was true in four of the trials, the possibility of a Type II error should be considered. Are the sample sizes large enough to be able to detect a significant therapeutic difference? As a rough rule of thumb, the detection of a therapeutic improvement of 20% with a 10% chance of a Type II error requires well over 100 patients per group. None of these trials had sample sizes that approached this number.

Summary of trials: A metanalysis of the studies, which minimizes the possibility of a Type II error, was performed to estimate the effect of the drugs with regard to cure rates and side effects. Quinacrine was investigated in four studies including 139 patients; 129 were cured (92.8%). Metronidazole, in seven studies, cured 219 of 238 persons (92%). Furazolidone, used in 6 studies, cured 150 out of 177 persons (84%). The difference between metronidazole and quinacrine was not significant, but both drugs cured significantly more patients than furazolidone ($P < 0.001$).

The reporting of side effects in the studies varied greatly, but approximately 7.1% of the metronidazole-treated patients, 9.6% of the furazolidone-treated patients, and 23% of the quinacrine-treated patients had side effects serious enough to report. Three of the four quinacrine studies disclosed enough side effects to recommend alternative therapies. Side effects due to quinacrine appeared to be most prevalent in children; in one of the studies, vomiting in children under 6 years of age was so severe that the compliance rate was only 53%.

4. Therapeutic recommendations

4.1. General population

The summary suggests that among the drugs available in the United States, metronidazole is an excellent choice of therapy, with over a 90% cure rate and the lowest rate of side effects. In adults, quinacrine is equally effective and less expensive, although it is more likely to cause side effects. Children appear especially susceptible to the side effects of quinacrine, and dosage of quinacrine and metronidazole may be difficult to measure; neither compound is readily available in liquid form for ingestion. Furazolidone, which is available in liquid form, is less effective in giardiasis than quinacrine and metronidazole. It is important to continue furazolidone therapy for a full 10 days; only a 20% cure can be expected with a five-day course (Murphy and Nelson, 1983). It is worth noting that many pharmacists can make liquid suspensions of both metronidazole and quinacrine.

There are a number of clinical settings in which clear information regarding therapy is lacking. These include asymptomatic children, especially in day care settings, asymptomatic adults, including homosexuals, pregnant patients, and the management of treatment failures.

4.2. Asymptomatic children

It is clear that person-to-person transmission of symptomatic giardiasis can occur, and that children, especially those in day care, can serve as carriers for severe infection of other children and their parents and siblings (Black et al., 1977; Keystone et al., 1978; Polis et al., 1986). The decision to treat the asymptomatic child should be based on a number of factors. In areas of high endemicity, there is some evidence that chronic giardial infection is *not* associated with malnutrition nor even with diarrhea (Walia et al., 1986; Istre et al., 1984). This suggests a similarity with the situation in animal models, which may acquire resistance to the organism, diminishing the burden of infection (Roberts-Thomson et al., 1976). This has led some to recommend withholding therapy (Goodman et al., 1984). While there are some areas of relatively high baseline infection in the U.S. (Spencer et al., 1983), many areas have infrequent and sporadic symptomatic and asymptomatic infection (Sealy and Schuman, 1983; Harter et al., 1982). In these settings it is likely that person-to-person transmission maintains the infection in the community, and may be responsible for epidemics (Polis et al., 1986). Additionally, it appears that mild symptomatology, such as anorexia, irritability and gas, may not be noted among infected children (Spencer et al., 1983). Another variable to consider would be the presence of someone in the household who would be ill-advised to contract giardiasis, such as a pregnant female or someone with immune compromise. In summary, in areas with a high underlying rate of giardiasis, in patients who are truly asymptomatic and live in a household without someone at risk, therapy could be withheld. This situation represents a small percentage of infected children; generally, in epidemic settings, in cases of questionable symptomatology or transmission within the family, asymptomatic children should be treated (Keystone et al., 1978).

4.3. Asymptomatic adults

Barrett-Connor (1984), using a Delphi technique, polled expert members of the American Society of Tropical Medicine and Hygiene concerning their opinion regarding the transmission of individual parasitic infections and the need to treat asymptomatic adult patients. About half felt there was a 1 in 10 chance that an asymptomatic *Giardia* infection would cause disease; an additional 47% estimated a 1 in 100 chance. Twenty-eight percent felt it was probable that an untreated adult would transmit a *Giardia* infection to another; 46% felt it was possible but unlikely. Sixty-three percent stated they would always treat an asymptomatic adult infected with *Giardia*; the remaining 37% said they would treat such a patient sometimes. Certainly in situations where person-to-person transmission is a major concern (primarily homosexuals, food handlers or health care workers) treating the asymptomatic adult is a reasonable plan. In the homosexual population the infection is venereal in nature and particularly endemic, and cannot be eradicated without treating sexual partners.

4.4. Pregnant patients

There is a measure of concern about the use of each of the commonly used drugs for giardiasis in pregnancy. It is clear that the most prudent approach is to avoid treatment until after delivery, especially if the patient is adequately nourished (D'Alauro et al., 1985). In emergent situations, with profound diarrhea and dehydration when therapy is deemed necessary, a reasonable approach would be the use of paromomycin, primarily because it is largely unabsorbed (Kreutner et al., 1981). Even though the failure rate is high, enough of the parasite burden may be diminished to cause a resolution of symptoms until delivery can be accomplished. Furazolidone is also poorly absorbed and would be an alternative choice.

4.5. Treatment failures

Routine follow-up for all treated patients is recommended; stool examinations should be performed at least two weeks after the completion of therapy, and in cases of clinical importance, duodenal sampling should be contemplated. Boreham et al. (1987) have listed the major possible explanations for treatment failures. These include: reinfection, poor patient compliance, variations in the pharmacokinetics of drugs, inactivation of the drug by superinfection with other organisms, and sequestration of the organism from the drug. The same investigators studied clone lines of *Giardia* strains and found that, even within stock derived from a single organism, there was tremendous variability in drug sensitivities. This raises the possibility that some organisms may survive therapy due to a natural resistance, and the offspring of these organisms may repopulate. Thus, in the absence of symptomatic family members or an obvious source of reinfection (such as in homosexuals), retreatment with an alternative drug in standard doses usually results in successful treatment. In patients with immune compromise, who may be especially difficult to treat, there is some evidence that combined chemotherapy may succeed where multiple individual drugs have failed (Taylor et al., 1987). Recent evidence regarding differing in vitro sensitivities of some *Giardia* isolates to frequently used drugs (Gordts et al., 1985; McIntyre et al., 1986) may lead to a more organized and successful approach to treatment choices in the future.

When reinfection is a plausible scenario, evaluation of family members and water supply is indicated, and may be essential (Pancorbo et al., 1985). In stable homosexual relationships, both sexual partners must be treated. Careful attention to detail in the follow-up and investigation of treatment failures may prevent local outbreaks of the infection.

References

Aldritt, S.M. and Wang, C.C. (1986) Purification and characterization of guanine phosphoribosyltransferase from *Giardia lamblia*. J. Biol. Chem. 261, 8528-8533.

Aldritt, S.M., Tien, P. and Wang, C.C. (1985) Pyrimidine salvage in *Giardia lamblia*. J. Exp. Med. 161, 437-445.

Barrett-Connor, E. (1984) Natural history of intestinal parasites in asymptomatic adults. J. Fam. Pract. 19, 635-639.

Beard, C.M., Noller, K.L., O'Fallon, W.M., Kurland, L.T. and Dockerty, M.B. (1979) Lack of evidence for cancer due to use of metronidazole. N. Engl. J. Med. 301, 519-522.

Black, R.E., Dykes, A.C. and Sinclair, S.P. (1977) Giardiasis in day-care centers: evidence of person to person transmission. Pediatrics 60, 486-491.

Boreham, P.F.L., Phillips, R.E. and Shepherd, R.W. (1987) Heterogeneity of the responses of clones of *Giardia intestinalis* to anti-giardial drugs. Trans. R. Soc. Trop. Med. Hyg. 81, 406-407.

Burke, J.A. (1977) The clinical and laboratory diagnosis of giardiasis. C.R.C. Crit. Rev. Clin. Lab. Sci. 373-391.

Carter, C.H., Bayles, A. and Thompson, P.E. (1962) Effects of paromomycin sulfate in man against *E. histolytica* and other intestinal protozoa. Am. J. Trop. Med. Hyg. 11, 4489-51, 1962.

Cohen, S.M. (1978) Toxicity and carcinogenicity of nitrofurans. In: G.T. Bryan (Ed.), Nitrofurans: Chemistry, Metabolism, Mutagenesis, and Carcinogenesis. Raven Press, New York, pp. 171-231.

Craft, J.C., Murphy, T. and Nelson, J.D. (1981) Furazolidone and quinacrine. Comparative study of therapy for giardiasis in children. Am. J. Dis. Child. 135, 164-166.

D'Alauro, F., Lee, R., Pao-In, K. and Khairallah, M. (1985) Intestinal parasites and pregnancy. Obstet. Gynecol. 66, 639-643.

Davidson, R.A. (1984) Issues in clinical parasitology: the treatment of giardiasis. Am. J. Gastroenterol. 79, 256-261.

Dobon, J.F., Cedrato, A.E. and Colom, N.M. (1963) The use of paromomycin in intestinal amoebiasis and giardiasis. El Dia Med. Jul. 11., p. 1012.

Eustice, D.C. and Wilhelm, J.M. (1984) Mechanisms of action of aminoglycoside antibiotics in eucaryotic protein synthesis. Antimicrob. Agents Chemother. 26, 53-60.

Farthing, M.J.G. and Inge, P.M.G. (1986) Antigiardial activity of the bile salt-like antibiotic sodium fusidate. J. Antimicrob. Chemother. 17, 165-171.

Friedman, G.D. (1980) Cancer after metronidazole. N. Engl. J. Med. 302, 519.

Goodman, L.S. and Gilman, A. (1985) The Pharmacological Basis of Therapeutics. McMillan, New York, pp. 1052-1057.

Goodman, R.A., Osterholm, M.T., Granoff, D.M. and Pickering, L.K. (1984) Infectious diseases and child day care. Pediatrics 74, 134-139.

Gordts, B., Hemelhof, W., Asselman, C. and Butzler, J.P. (1985) In vitro susceptibilities of 25 *Giardia lamblia* isolates of human origin to six commonly used antiprotozoal agents. Antimicrob. Agents Chemother. 28, 378-380.

Harter, L., Frost, F. and Jakubowski, W. (1982) *Giardia* prevalence among 1-to-3-year-old children in two Washington State counties. Am. J. Publ. Health. 72, 386-388.

Istre, G.R., Dunlop, T.S., Gaspard, G.B. and Hopkins, R.S. (1984) Waterborne giardiasis at a mountain resort: evidence for acquired immunity. Am. J. Publ. Health 74, 602-604.

Keystone, J.S., Krajden, S. and Warren, M.R. (1978) Person-to-person transmission of *Giardia lamblia* in day-care nurseries. Can. Med. Assoc. J. 119, 241-248.

Kreutner, A.K., Del Bene, V.E. and Amstey, M.S. (1981) Giardiasis in pregnancy. Am. J. Obstet. Gynecol. 140, 895-901.

Kyronseppa, H. and Pettersson, T. (1981) Treatment of giardiasis: relative efficacy of metronidazole as compared to tinidazole. Scand. J. Infect. Dis. 13, 311-312.

Legator, M.S., Connor, T.H. and Stoeckerl, M. (1975) Detection of mutagenic activity of metronidazole and niridazole in body fluids of humans and mice. Science 188, 1118-1125.

Martin, L.K. (1965) Randomness of particle distribution in human feces and the resulting influence on helminth egg counting. Am. J. Trop. Med. Hyg. 14, 747-759.

McIntyre, P., Boreham, P.F.L., Phillips, R.E. and Shepherd, R.W. (1986) Chemotherapy in giardiasis: clinical responses and in vitro drug sensitivity of human isolates in axenic culture. J. Pediatr. 108, 1005-1010.

Miller, R.L., Nelson, D.J., LaFon, S.W., Miller, W.H. and Krenitsky, T.A. (1987) Antigiardial activity of guanine arabinoside. Biochem. Pharmacol. 36, 2519-2525.

Morgan, I.F.K. (1978) Metronidazole treatment in pregnancy. Int. J. Gynaecol. Obstet. 15, 501-502.

Murphy, T.V. and Nelson, J.D. (1983) Five versus ten days treatment with furazolidone for giardiasis. Am. J. Dis. Child. 137, 267-270.

Pancorbo, J.M., Munoz, M.T. and Badia, J.L. (1985) Giardiasis: treatment of carriers. Lancet ii, 951.

Phillips, K.F. and Hailey, F.J. (1986) The use of furoxone: a perspective. J. Int. Med. Res. 14, 19-29.

Polis, M.A., Tuazon, C.U., Alling, D.W.S. and Talmanis, E. (1986) Transmission of *Giardia lamblia* from a day care center to the community. Am. J. Publ. Health 76, 1142-1144.

Roberts-Thomson, I.C., Stevens, D.P., Mahmoud, A.A.F. and Warren, K.S. (1976) Acquired resistance to infection in an animal model of giardiasis. J. Immunol. 117, 2036-2037.

Roe, F.J.C. (1985) Safety of nitroimidazoles. Scand. J. Infect. Dis. Suppl. 46, 72-81.

Rosenblatt, J.E. and Edson, R.S. (1983) Metronidazole. Mayo Clin. Proc. 58, 154-157.

Rustia, M. and Shubik, P. (1979) Experimental induction of hepatomas, mammary tumors, and other tumors with metronidazole in non-bred Sas:MRC(WI)BR rats. J. Natl. Cancer Inst. 63, 863-867.

Sealy, D.P. and Schuman, S.H. (1983) Endemic giardiasis and day care. Pediatrics 72, 154-158.

Spencer, M.J., Millet, V.E., Garcia, L.S., Rhee, L. and Masterson, L. (1983) Parasitic infections in a pediatric population. Ped. Infect. Dis. 2, 110-113.

Stevens, D.P. (1982) Giardiasis: host-pathogen biology. Rev. Infect. Dis. 4, 851-857.

Sullam, P.M., Slutkin, G., Gottlieb, PA-C. and Mills, J. (1986) Paromomycin therapy of endemic amebiasis in homosexual men. Sex. Transm. Dis. 3, 151-155.

Takeuchi, T., Kobayashi, S., Tanabe, M. and Fujiwara, T. (1985) In vitro inhibition of *Giardia lamblia* and *Trichomonas vaginalis* growth by bithionol, dichlorophene, and hexachlorophene. Antimicrob. Agents Chemother. 27, 65-70.

Taylor, G.D., Wenman, W.M. and Tyrell, L.J. (1987) Combined metronidazole and quinacrine hydrochloride therapy for chronic giardiasis. Can. Med. Assoc. J. 136, 1179-1180.

Voogd, C.E. (1981) On the mutagenicity of nitroimidazoles. Mutat. Res. 86, 243-277.

Walia, B.N.S., Ganguly, N.K., Mahajan, R.C., Kumar, D., Madan, I.J., Gambhir, S.K. and Kanwar, S.S. (1986) Morbidity in preschool giardia cyst excreters. Trop. Geogr. Med. 38, 367-370.

Wang, C.C. and Aldritt, S.M. (1983) Purine salvage networks in *Giardia lamblia*. J. Exp. Med. 185, 1703-1712.

Weinbach, E.C., Costa, J.L. and Weider, S.C. (1985) Antidepressant drugs suppress growth of the human pathogenic protozoan *Giardia lamblia*. Res. Comm. Chem. Pathol. Pharmacol. 47, 145-148.

20

The control of *Giardia* in water supplies

WALTER JAKUBOWSKI

Health Effects Research Laboratory, U.S. Environmental Protection Agency, Cincinnati, OH 45268, U.S.A.

1. Potential for contamination	335
2. Effectiveness of water treatment processes	338
2.1. Filtration	338
2.2. Disinfection	342
3. Drinking water guidelines and regulations	347
4. Summary	349
References	350

1. Potential for contamination

As discussed in Chapters 14–17, giardiasis is transmitted by the fecal-oral route. One vehicle for this route of transmission is contaminated drinking water. Water supplies may become contaminated by introduction of sewage into the supply or by the activity of animals on the watershed. In the absence of data on the densities of *Giardia* cysts occurring in sewage, Jakubowski and Ericksen (1979) calculated the theoretical levels of cysts that might be expected to occur in raw sewage at a specified range of infection in the population. Assuming the prevalence of infection to be between 1 and 25%, they calculated that raw sewage could contain from 9.6×10^3 cysts/l to 2.4×10^5 cysts/l, respectively. Panicker and Krishnamoorthi (1978, 1981) found *Giardia* cysts in the raw sewage of four communities in India at levels of 1.8×10^2 to 2.4×10^2 cysts/l. Sykora et al. (1987) reported finding *Giardia* cysts in raw sewage at eight Pennsylvania treatment plants at densities up to 1.4×10^3 cysts/l. These latter authors indicated that the recovery efficiency of their detection methods ranged from 6 to 14%, thus suggesting that the actual densities of cysts present may have been as high as 2.2×10^4/l of raw sewage. McHarry (1984), examining only the effluents from several sewage treatment plants in Illinois, found the highest levels of cysts to be about one per liter of effluent. She concluded that it was doubtful that this level of discharge into a stream would be a substantial threat to the quality of water for human consumption and recreation or for wildlife. However, Sykora et al. (1988) calculated that a river receiving discharges from the Pennsylvania sewage treatment plants could contain more than 8 cysts/gallon of river water even though the cyst densities in the treated sewage effluents had been reduced up to 99.8% as compared to the raw sewage.

Waterborne outbreaks of giardiasis have also occurred on water supplies having no apparent source of sewage contamination (Craun and Jakubowski, 1987). *Giardia* organisms are widely distributed in nature and infections have been reported in more than 40 species of animals (Kulda and Nohynkova, 1978). Determining species specificity, or conversely, cross-species infectivity of *Giardia*, is not easily accomplished due to a variety of factors relating to both the organisms and to the hosts (Woo, 1984). Assessing the infectivity for humans of animal source *Giardia* is even more difficult to accomplish because of inherent constraints in conducting human volunteer studies. The results of cross-species infectivity experiments must be interpreted with caution. For instance, Nash et al. (1987) inoculated two groups of human volunteers with *Giardia* isolated from two different human sources. He satisfied Koch's postulates for *Giardia* by producing infection and disease in the group of volunteers receiving the GS/M strain of *Giardia*. However, the human-source strain designated Isr failed to even establish infection in the other group of volunteers. Obviously, since the Isr strain had been isolated from a human case, one cannot conclude that it is not infective for humans. Cross-species interpretation problems notwithstanding, it does appear that *Giardia* organisms, at least of the *G. lamblia* or *G. duodenalis* type (Filice, 1952), may infect more than one species of host. In addition, there is anecdotal information that humans may become infected with cysts from mule deer and beaver (Davies and Hibler, 1979) and from muskrats (C. Hibler, personal communication).

A number of animal to animal and human to animal *Giardia* infectivity studies have been reported and these were reviewed by Woo (1984). He indicated that most of these studies were contradictory and inconclusive. He further concluded that the host specificity of *Giardia* from animals is variable and that there is evidence to suggest that dogs may be reservoirs for human *Giardia*. However, Woo and Paterson (1986) were unable to infect mice, hamsters, rats, cats and dogs with *Giardia* cysts from clinical and non-clinical patients and they interpreted their results as proving that cats and dogs are not reservoirs of *G. lamblia*. Beavers have been epidemiologically implicated as a source of infection in waterborne outbreaks in the United States but Bemrick (1984) reviewed published information on these outbreaks and concluded that the evidence is circumstantial. Controlled experiments have demonstrated that human-source *Giardia* can cause infections in beavers and in muskrats (Erlandsen and Bemrick, 1988). Several studies have shown the prevalence of *Giardia* infection to be about 15% in beavers and up to 95% in muskrats (Davies and Hibler, 1979; Frost et al., 1980; Pacha et al., 1985; Kirkpatrick and Benson, 1987; Erlandsen and Bemrick, 1988). Beavers and muskrats are logical sources of water supply contamination because of the prevalence of infection in these animals and because of their aquatic habits. However, due to our state-of-knowledge on speciation of *Giardia*, it has not yet been possible to unequivocally identify the host of origin in any waterborne outbreak.

Whether from sewage or from animal contamination, *Giardia* spp. cysts are environmentally resistant and can survive for relatively long periods in water. Although freezing is detrimental to cyst survival, Bingham et al. (1979) obtained low levels of excystation (<1%) for up to 14 days with *G. duodenalis* cysts stored at $-13°C$. Similar results were obtained by Wickramanayake et al. (1985) who reported 0.4% excystation of *G. muris* cysts after 20 days storage at $-6°C$. *Giardia* spp. cysts appear to survive best in water at temperatures of 4 to 8°C. Faubert et al. (1986) found that *G. muris* were still infective for mice when the cysts were purified and suspended in tapwater or well water for 20 days at 4°C. However, the cysts were noninfective after 3 days storage at 4°C in fecal pellets suspended in saline. This is in contrast to the results of Craft (1982) who was able to infect rats after storing cysts in liquefied feces for one year at 4°C. Wickramanayake et al. (1985), using *G. muris* cysts suspended in water, found little change in percentage excystation after 25 days storage at 5°C. Bingham et al. (1979) could induce excystation (<5%) in human source *Giardia* cysts after 77 days storage at 8°C. Above 20°C, cyst inactivation is relatively rapid. Wickramanayake et al. (1985) reported a drop in *G. muris* excystation from 98% to 7.2% after 3 days storage at 20°C and a similar decrease in excystation after only one day at 37°C. Schaefer et al. (1984) reported a thermal death point for *G. muris* cysts of 54°C and Jarroll et al. (1984) found that *Giardia* from humans were activated by exposure to 55°C for 5 min. Heating water to boiling has been reported to kill these cysts instantly (Bingham et al., 1979). Although desiccation of *Giardia* cysts is widely regarded as resulting in their inactivation, there are no published data to corroborate this opinion. Jarroll et al. (1984) have stated that, in preliminary experiments, no cyst survival (as determined by excystation) was found when *Giardia* cysts were air-dried at 4 or 21°C for as little as 24 h. In addition, they reported that human source *Giardia* cysts do not appear to survive exposure to artificial sea water at 4°C for 24 h.

The environmental resistance of *Giardia* cysts, the endemicity of the infection in humans and in a wide variety of animals, and the low infectious dose all support the potential for contamination of water supplies and the transmission of the disease by this route. Considering the uncertainty in establishing the cross-species infectivity of *Giardia* spp. and the present unavailability of methods for readily speciating the organisms, it would be prudent from a public health point of view to consider all organisms of the *Giardia duodenalis* type as potentially infectious for humans. While this may be a conservative assumption, it would provide a practical basis for developing and implementing control procedures. If this assumption is accepted, then it would follow that all surface water supplies are subject to contamination either through human or animal sources. It would be ecologically irresponsible and morally unacceptable, in addition to being practically impossible in most cases, to attempt eliminating all potential animal sources of contamination on a watershed. However, various control measures could be implemented to minimize contamination of water supplies. While beavers and muskrats have not definitely been proven to be the source of contamination in waterborne outbreaks, the extent of their activity on the watershed can be determined and trapping programs can keep populations of these animals in check. Animal control programs should be especially rigorous in areas where water supply intakes are located. If possible, provision should be made for closing water supply intakes and for using alternate supplies during periods of heavy runoff. Sanitary surveys would be useful in identifying and correcting sewage discharges and septic tank drainage areas on the watershed. All of these measures can decrease the potential for water supply contamination with *Giardia* but they cannot eliminate it. Public water supplies must therefore provide adequate treatment in order to ensure against transmission of disease.

2. Effectiveness of water treatment processes

Sixty-nine percent (62/90) of the waterborne giardiasis outbreaks occurring from 1965 through 1984 in the United States were in community water supply systems (Craun and Jakubowski, 1987). Many of the water supplies in those states reporting waterborne giardiasis outbreaks come from mountain streams or lakes not contaminated by wastewater discharges. Because the water quality of the sources is good, and because the watershed is often in a sparsely populated area that may be protected or restricted with respect to human activity, treatment of the water is frequently minimal, usually involving only disinfection. Of the community outbreaks, 74% (46/62) involved surface water supplies that were chlorinated only or inadequately treated, accounting for 91% (18 898/20 766) of the cases. Information gathered primarily within the last ten years indicates that *Giardia* cysts can be effectively removed and inactivated in water supplies by a combination of filtration and disinfection.

2.1. Filtration

Filtration of drinking water supplies means the use of a process for removing particulate matter from water by passage through porous media. A variety of filtration technologies are employed for this purpose, including diatomaceous earth (DE) filtration, slow sand filtration and coagulation-filtration. Conventional filtration, direct filtration and in-line filtration are categories of coagulation-filtration. All of these processes, when applied to an appropriate raw water, can remove 99% or more of the *Giardia* cysts, if the processes are properly operated and maintained (Logsdon, 1988). The discussion below addresses filtration technologies primarily with respect to *Giardia* cyst removal. However, selection of an appropriate technology for a given water supply must take into consideration the raw water quality and capabilities for removal of other contaminants such as bacteria, viruses, organic and inorganic turbidity and dissolved substances.

The earliest work specifically addressing *Giardia* removal by filtration was with DE filters. DE filtration is defined as a process that uses a precoat cake of DE filter media deposited on a support membrane (septum). The water is filtered through the cake on the septum and additional filter media (the body feed) is continuously added to the raw water in order to maintain filter cake permeability. Logsdon et al. (1981) reported on a series of studies involving DE filtration for the removal of 9 μm radioactive microspheres (cyst models) and *G. muris* cysts from water in a pilot plant operation. They consistently obtained removal of >99% of the microspheres or cysts and frequently achieved >99.9% removal. Effective filtration was dependent upon DE precoat thickness rather than on DE particle size (grade), with no improvement in filter performance at precoat thicknesses >1.0 kg/m^2. Filter efficiency decreased at lesser precoat thicknesses or when no body feed was used. These authors indicated that effluent turbidity was not an effective indicator of DE filtration efficiency and that reliance must be placed on proper operation and maintenance instead. Subsequent work by DeWalle et al. (1984) and by Pyper (1985) with human source *Giardia* cysts confirmed that DE filtration could remove >99% of cysts. DE filtration studies were extended by Langé et al. (1986) to address a variety of filtration rates, water temperatures and grades of diatomaceous earth for the removal of *Giardia* cysts, turbidity and bacteria. At filtration rates of 2.4-9.6 m/h, temperatures from 3.5-15°C and with four different particle sizes of diatomaceous earth, cyst removals >99% were obtained. Water temperature did not affect DE filter performance but finer particle size DE and lower filtration rates resulted in higher removals of bacteria and turbidity. DE filtration is effective for *Giardia* cyst removal, is not affected by low water temperatures, does not require a large amount of space for the treatment plant and has been used for supplies up to 6 × 10^6 liters/day (Logsdon, 1988). However, the raw water must be of high quality (low turbidity and good microbiological quality). In addition, DE filtration cannot remove dissolved substances or very fine particles without some additional treatment and there are problems in maintaining a perfect film of DE on the septum. These problems have restricted the extent to which DE filters are used for municipal purposes.

Slow sand filtration is a process whereby raw water is passed through a bed of sand at low velocity (generally less than 0.4 m/h), thus producing substantial particulate removal by physical and biological mechanisms. Bellamy et al. (1985b) describe slow sand filtration as a passive process since it is subject to very little control by an operator. There is no chemical addition or backwash involved in the process. Effective sand particle sizes range from 0.15 to 0.35 mm (with a uniformity coefficient of less than 2) and a sand bed depth ranging from 60 to 120 cm supported by graded gravel 30 to 50 cm deep. Hydraulic loading rates range from 0.04 to 0.4 m/h and filtered water is collected in drain tiles at the bottom of the support gravel. Physical removal of particles is accomplished by straining through the sand layer; biological removal occurs as the result of growth of organisms within the sand bed and gravel support. In addition, the 'schmutzdecke,' a layer of inert and biological materials, forms on the surface of the sand bed and contributes to process effectiveness. A curing time, ranging from weeks to months, is required in order for the biological population to become established and for the slow sand filter to operate at full potential. Operation and maintenance of a slow sand filter requires periodic (depending upon head loss) removal of the schmutzdecke by scraping, and replacement of sand after repeated scrapings have reduced depth in the bed to the lowest acceptable design value.

The effectiveness of slow sand filters for human source *Giardia* cyst removal has been studied by Bellamy et al. (1985a,b) and by Pyper (1985). Using a pilot plant operation, Bellamy et al. (1985a,b) studied the effect of hydraulic loading rate, water temperature, the degree of schmutzdecke formation and the maturity of the sand bed on removal of these cysts. At hydraulic loading rates of 0.04 to 0.4 m/h, cyst removals were uniformly high and averaged 99.98 to 99.99%. Temperature at the time of filtration had no discernible influence on the efficiency of removal. The authors indicated that cyst removal exceeded 98% for all operating conditions tested and they stated that, as the sand bed matures biologically, the removal improves to virtually 100% for cysts. Pyper (1985) studied a wider range of temperatures and obtained cyst removals of 99.98 to 99.99% at 7.5 to 21°C. Cyst removals ranged from 99.36 to 99.91% at 0.5 and 7.5°C but decreased to 93.7% at 0.5°C when cysts and primary unchlorinated sewage effluent were simultaneously added to the raw water. Seelaus et al. (1986) evaluated an operating community slow sand filtration plant for removal of *Giardia* cysts and other microscopic particles. They detected naturally-occurring *Giardia* cysts in 5/11 raw water influent samples but did not find any cysts in eleven effluent samples from the slow sand filter. They concluded that the treatment was effective in removing *Giardia* cysts and in providing a stable effluent quality for utilities with a low operating budget. *Giardia* cysts can be effectively removed by slow sand filters and small plants ($<1 \times 10^6$ l/day) are simple to construct, operate and maintain (Logsdon, 1988). Slow sand filters may not be appropriate for medium to large systems because of operating labor and land costs.

Coagulation-filtration is a generic term for the treatment train most commonly used for water supplies in the United States. Depending upon what treatment processes are applied prior to filtration, the treatment may be classified as conventional – employing coagulation, flocculation and sedimentation; direct – using coagulation and flocculation, but no sedimentation; or in-line – with coagulation, but no flocculation or sedimentation prior to filtration. Pretreatment or conditioning of the water involves the addition of chemicals such as alum and/or various types of polymers (anionic, cationic, nonionic). Coagulation-filtration technologies have also been referred to as rapid rate and granular media filtration. The filtration media may consist of sand, anthracite, granular activated carbon (GAC) or various combinations of these. The versatility of coagulation-filtration allows the consultant engineer considerable flexibility in designing site-specific treatment trains that can be adapted to a variety of water quality conditions. However, this same versatility makes it difficult to study and evaluate a 'typical' coagulation-filtration treatment train for *Giardia* cyst removal.

Several studies on coagulation-filtration effectiveness for *Giardia* removal have been conducted over a wide variety of conditions. Logsdon et al. (1985) investigated cyst removal by the coagulation and sedimentation process with raw waters having turbidities of 7.5 to 32 NTU and using various combinations of alum and anionic polymer. For a continuously flowing sedimentation basin, cyst removal ranged from 65 to 93% and improved as turbidity removal improved. The use of an anionic polymer and a higher dosage of alum enhanced both cyst removal and turbidity removal. Wickramanayake (1986), in reviewing this study and data obtained by Haas et al. (1985) on indicator organism removal, concluded that turbidity reduction can be considered as a surrogate for the removal of coliforms, acid-fast organisms, yeasts and *Giardia* cysts. Logsdon et al. (1981, 1985) also examined different filter media (sand, anthracite, GAC, dual media) used under varying conditions of ripening, turbidity loading and backwashing. Sand, dual media and GAC filters were generally more effective than anthracite in removing cysts, probably because the anthracite is a coarser medium having a larger particle size (about 0.9 mm). Relatively small increases in turbidity (0.2-0.3 NTU) of the filtered water resulted in less effective cyst removal. A filter-to-waste period in the beginning of a filter run just after backwashing was recommended because cyst removals may not be optimal early in the run. DeWalle et al. (1984) indicated that *Giardia* removal by direct filtration was >99% when the filtered water turbidity was <0.3 NTU. Al-Ani et al. (1986) examined the use of rapid rate filtration for low turbidity raw waters (<1 NTU) and they concluded that, with proper chemical pretreatment, removals of turbidity >70%, of bacteria >99%, and of *Giardia* >95% can be achieved. In the absence of chemical pretreatment, only 0 to 70% removal of these contaminants can be expected. Mosher and Hendricks (1986) studied rapid rate filtration of low turbidity waters at temperatures down to 0.2°C using field-scale pilot filters. They obtained >99.8% removal of *Giardia* cysts by dual-media filters when proper chemical pretreatment was applied. With no chemical coagulation, *Giardia* cyst removal was 80-91%. Logsdon (1988), in reviewing the above studies, concluded that direct filtration can remove >99.9% of the *Giardia* cysts when the raw water is properly coagulated and filtered.

The coagulation-filtration technology can be designed to remove *Giardia* cysts effectively, as well as a variety of other contaminants, and it offers a considerable degree of flexibility. However, it is a fairly sophisticated technology that requires a substantial amount of operating skill. Constant monitoring of the raw water pH, temperature and turbidity is necessary with concomitant adjustment of the operation in order to produce a high quality water.

Alternate filtration technologies include package treatment plants and cartridge filters. Package treatment plants may be used to treat community water supplies or for recreational areas, state parks, construction camps, ski resorts and other areas where potable water from a municipal supply may not be available (USEPA, 1989a). Package treatment plants could incorporate any of the filtration technologies discussed above, i.e., DE, slow sand or coagulation-filtration. They are available in capacities to treat up to 23×10^6 l/day. Horn et al. (1988) have evaluated a dual-stage packaged system for low turbidity (<1-4 NTU) waters at temperatures of 0.2 to 9°C. Greater than 99% of added *Giardia* cysts were removed when proper chemical pretreatment was applied and when the filtration rate was equal to or less than 10 gallons/min/ft^2. However, while package treatment plants can be effective in treating water, the experience has been that many have not consistently met turbidity or coliform standards in the filtered water (Morand et al., 1980; Morand and Young, 1983). Package treatment plants may require skilled operators and some minimum level of maintenance in order to produce a satisfactory water.

Cartridge filters composed of various materials (ceramics, paper, yarn-wound fibers, etc.) and with rated pore sizes down to 0.2 μm have been used for removing microbiological contaminants from water. These devices are sometimes referred to as point-of-use/point-of-entry (POU/POE) devices because they may be installed on the consumer's tap or on the service connection entering a home or building. Some cartridge filters may be impregnated with bacteriostatic compounds (e.g. silver) to prevent growth of organisms in the water remaining in the filter holder during periods of non-use. Other units (water purifiers) may incorporate a disinfectant compound for the inactivation of microorganisms in the filtered water. Long (1983) evaluated 17 commercial cartridge filters composed of various materials and with rated porosities of 0.2 to 10 μm for particulate removal. He used 5.7 μm styrene divinylbenzene microspheres as cyst models and found that 10/17 cartridge filters removed >99.99% of the microspheres. Schmidt and Meier (1984) challenged two types of cartridge filters with 5×10^4 to 1×10^5 *G. muris* cysts daily for 26 days and were unable to recover any cysts in the filtered water throughout the testing period. In an unpublished test of another cartridge filter challenged with 3×10^5 human source *Giardia* cysts, removal efficiencies ranged from 99.5% to 99.99% in five trials (USEPA, 1989a). The National Sanitation Foundation (NSF) has published a protocol for evaluating cyst removal by cartridge filter drinking water treatment units (NSF, 1982). The protocol involves challenging the filter with at least 10^4 particles of a silicate test dust in the 4 to 6 μm size range. In order to be acceptable, the filter must remove at least 99.9% of the particles. A U.S. governmental task group has developed a draft guide standard and protocol for testing microbiological water purifiers (USEPA, 1987a). The task group report accepts the NSF protocol for determining physical removal of cysts and provides procedures for evaluating inactivation of cysts by disinfectants.

Cartridge filters may provide a feasible method for small water systems to remove *Giardia* cysts. They are simple to use and do not require skilled personnel, but they should be limited to low turbidity waters since cleaning and replacement costs may be impractical with source waters having moderate or high turbidity. Cartridge filters may also be of value for emergency use in a community when a waterborne outbreak has been recognized.

2.2. Disinfection

While filtration can reduce the levels of microorganisms in water, disinfection is an additional and necessary barrier for ensuring a microbiologically safe water supply where surface water is the source. As with filtration, all of the more reliable information on the effectiveness of disinfection for inactivation of *Giardia* cysts has been developed in the last few years. As recently as 1977, the impression was still being conveyed that *Giardia* cysts could survive in 0.5% chlorinated water for two to three days (Burke, 1977). Hoff (1979) traced the probable source of this impression to a misinterpretation by one author of another investigator's work more than 60 years ago. Information gathered since 1979 demonstrates that *Giardia* cysts can indeed be inactivated, under the proper conditions, by much lower concentrations of chlorine as well as by other disinfecting agents. A detailed review of *Giardia* cyst disinfection can be found in Jarroll (1988).

Interpreting the results of studies on the inactivation of cysts by disinfectants is dependent in large part upon the measure of viability that is used. Early studies used vital staining techniques (e.g., exclusion of eosin) to determine if cysts were dead or alive and these studies have been reviewed by Jarroll et al. (1984). Several investigators have found eosin exclusion to be an unreliable indicator of cyst viability in that it consistently indicates higher levels of viability than does either in vitro excystation or animal infectivity (Bingham et al., 1979; Kasprzak and Majewska, 1983; Faubert et al., 1986). The development and improvement of excystation techniques is discussed by Schaefer in chapter 7 of this volume. Currently available excystation techniques can routinely produce >90% excystation with *G. muris,* although excystation of *G. duodenalis* cysts continues to be highly variable. The use of animal models for *G. muris* is reviewed by Stevens, and for the *G. duodenalis*-type of organism, by Faubert and Belosevic in Chapter 4. Hoff et al. (1985) compared in vitro excystation and animal infectivity as measures of *G. muris* cyst inactivation by chlorine and found that the inactivation results obtained with both techniques were comparable. They concluded that the excystation technique was simpler, less expensive and less time consuming than animal infectivity, and that excystation could be used to determine the effects of disinfectants on cyst viability. However, due to procedural limitations, the excystation technique cannot be easily used to determine levels of cyst inactivation much greater than 99% (Hoff, 1986; Hibler et al., 1987). The discussion below will address only those disinfection data obtained in studies where excystation or animal infectivity have been used as the indicator of viability since these currently appear to be the most reliable end-points.

Using in vitro excystation, Jarroll et al. (1981) studied the effect of chlorine on human source *Giardia* cysts at temperatures of 5 to 25°C, pH 6 to 8, contact times of 10 to 60 min and chlorine concentrations of 1 to 8 mg/l. This investigation showed that *Giardia* cysts were not indestructible by chlorine: >99% of the cysts were inactivated at 25°C by 1.5 mg of chlorine/l after only 10 min of contact time at pH 6, 7 and 8. However, as expected based on previously available information with other microorganisms, chlorine effectiveness decreased with decreasing temperatures and with increasing pH. At 5°C with 2 mg chlorine/l and 30 min contact time at pH 8, <30% of the cysts had been inactivated. Using a modified excystation procedure with *G. duodenalis* (human) and *G. muris* cysts exposed to 2.5 mg/l chlorine at 5°C, Rice et al. (1982) obtained comparable results. In addition, they found that *Giardia* cysts from asymptomatic and symptomatic donors behaved similarly to inactivation by chlorine. However, the *G. muris* cysts were consistently more resistant than the human source cysts at the maximum exposure times (30-60 min). This observation prompted these authors to suggest that *G. muris* may be a valid model for the human parasite in disinfection studies, apparently on the premise that inactivation results obtained with *G. muris* would be conservative and would err on the side of safety. The greater resistance of *G. muris* cysts to inactivation has subsequently been confirmed by other investigators using chlorine as well as other chemical disinfectants (Wickramanayake, 1985; Leahy et al., 1987; Rubin, 1988). Leahy et al. (1987) also found that *G. muris* cysts have a pH-dependent resistance to inactivation, with chlorine being most effective at neutral pH and slightly less so in acidic solutions. They concluded that *G. muris* cysts rank among the microorganisms that are most resistant to inactivation by free chlorine.

Faubert et al. (1986) used *G. muris* cysts and infectivity in mice to study the effects of chlorination practices at a Canadian drinking water treatment plant. They concluded that the routine chlorination procedures, as performed in this modern water treatment plant, had no cysticidal effect. However, their experimental design did not allow a determination of the degree of cyst inactivation obtained. Animals were inoculated with 1000 cysts from the chlorinated water and it is possible that infection could have occurred even though 99.9% of the cysts had been inactivated.

Hibler et al. (1987) conducted an extensive quantitative animal infectivity study to evaluate chlorine effects on human-source *Giardia* cysts. They used more than 3700 gerbils to investigate the inactivation of *Giardia* at temperatures of 0.5 to 5°C, pH 6 to 8, chlorine concentrations of 0.3 mg to 2.5 mg/l and different contact times. They selected temperatures of 0.5 to 5°C because many of the water supplies in U.S. communities experiencing waterborne outbreaks of giardiasis have source waters within this range. They calculated C·t values (referred to also as CT or C × T) for their data, where C is the chlorine concentration in mg/l and t is the contact time in minutes. Using C·t values provides a means for comparing biocidal inactivation data obtained under a variety of experimental conditions (Hoff, 1986). The mean predicted C·t values obtained by Hibler et al. (1987) for 99.9 to 99.99% inactivation are shown in Table 1. The higher the C·t value, the less effective is the disinfection. For example, a C·t value of 200 would require twice as much chlorine or twice the contact time to achieve the same level of inactivation attainable at a C·t of 100. As reported previously by other investigators, chlorination was less effective at lower temperatures and at higher pH. Hibler et al. (1987) also reported that results with chlorine concentrations above 2.5 mg/l were erratic and they suggested that C·t's calculated with higher concentrations than this may not be reliable.

Hoff (1986) calculated C·t values for 99% inactivation of cysts by chlorine from published and unpublished data from a variety of sources. The mean C·t values for human *Giardia* and for *G. muris* are presented in Tables 2 and 3, respectively. The effectiveness of chlorination increases considerably at temperatures of 15 to 25°C as compared to 5°C. In addition to the temperature and pH effects, the greater resistance of *G. muris* to inactivation can be seen, especially at 25°C.

A variety of other disinfectants and disinfecting processes may be used by the water

TABLE 1

C · t values for 99.9 to 99.99% inactivation of *Giardia duodenalis* (*lamblia*) cysts by free chlorine[a]

Temperature (°C)	pH	Mean C · t
0.5	6	185
	7	289
	8	342
2.5	6	142
	7	252
	8	268
5.0	6	146
	7	161
	8	280

[a] Hibler et al., 1987.

TABLE 2

C · t values for 99% inactivation of human-source *Giardia* cysts by free chlorine[a]

Temperature (°C)	pH	Chlorine (mg/l)	Contact Time (min)	Mean C · t
5	6	1.0–8.0	6–84	65–75
	7	2.0–8.0	7–152	97–118
	8	2.0–8.0	57–164	110–142
15	6	2.5–3.0	7	20
	7	2.5–3.0	6–18	32
	8	2.5 3.0	7–21	37
25	6	1.5	<6	<9
	7	1.5	<7	<10
	8	1.5	<8	<12

[a] Adapted from Hoff, 1986.

supply industry including chlorine dioxide, chloramines, ozone and ultraviolet irradiation. Data on the effectiveness of these disinfectants are very limited. Leahy (1985) evaluated chlorine dioxide for inactivation of *G. muris* cysts using excystation as an indicator of viability. His results indicated that chlorine dioxide effectiveness increased as the pH was raised from 5 to 9, in contrast to results previously reported for chlorine but consistent with the effect of pH on chlorine dioxide efficiency reported for viruses and bacteria. Chlorine dioxide was about an order of magnitude more effective than free chlorine at 25°C and about two orders of magnitude more effective at pH 9. Rubin (1988) found that C·t values for *G. muris* inactivation by preformed monochloramine

TABLE 3

C · t values for 99% inactivation of *Giardia muris* cysts by free chlorine[a]

Temperature (°C)	pH	Chlorine (mg/l)	Contact Time (min)	Mean C · t
3	6.5	0.24–1.1	37–297	68
	7.5	0.24–1.0	150–770	140
5	7	0.41–2.73	236–467	360
25	5	4.4–13	4–16	66
	7	2.9–7.1	4–16	29
	9	11.6–72.6	3–16	206

[a] Adapted from Hoff, 1986.

were substantially higher than those for chlorine at pH 7 and at 5°C. He ranked the chemical disinfectants in decreasing order of effectiveness for inactivating *G. muris* cysts as follows: ozone, chlorine dioxide, elemental iodine, free chlorine and monochloramine. A study of the inactivation of *G. muris* cysts by chloramines as they are being formed has also been reported (Meyer et al., 1988). The C·t values produced were lower than those reported by Rubin (1988) with preformed monochloramines, but they were higher than those obtained with free chlorine. Wickramanayake et al. (1984, 1985) studied ozone inactivation of human *Giardia* and *G. muris* cysts and found ozone to be more effective than chlorine and less affected by temperature from 5 to 25°C. Rice and Hoff (1981) evaluated ultraviolet (UV) irradiation for inactivation of human source *Giardia* cysts. They obtained a 99.9% reduction in *Escherichia coli* at a dose of 3000 μW-s/cm^2 but only less than a one-logarithm$_{(10)}$ reduction in cyst viability at doses up to 63 000 μW-s/cm^2. They suggested that UV irradiation is not a viable disinfection method for *Giardia* in water, since commercial systems are designed to operate at a dose range of 25 000-35 000 μW-s/cm^2. Carlson et al. (1985) evaluated UV irradiation with *G. muris* cysts and concluded that the cysts were significantly more resistant to inactivation than *E. coli* and were more resistant than *Yersinia* sp.

The previous discussion has been directed to treatment techniques for removal or inactivation of *Giardia* in public water supplies. However, giardiasis is also known as 'backpacker's disease', striking unwary individuals in their pursuit of recreational activities. The clarity or remoteness of a stream, spring or lake is not an indication of its microbiological purity. Kahn and Visscher (1975), prompted by their experience with giardiasis after drinking untreated water from a partly frozen mountain stream, proposed a method using saturated iodine solution to disinfect water for travelers and hikers. They had not, however, determined the effectiveness of this method for inactivating *Giardia* cysts. Jarroll et al. (1980) evaluated the Kahn and Visscher method, and five other small quantity halogen disinfection methods, with clear and cloudy water at temperatures of 3 and 20°C and contact times of 15 to 40 min using excystation of human source *Giardia*.

The other five methods included commercially available organic iodine and chlorine, tincture of iodine and chlorine bleach. The disinfectants were used as recommended by the manufacturers or by the authors of the articles in which the method was proposed. Jarroll et al. (1980) found that all of the methods were completely effective at 20°C in cloudy and clear water. However, the Kahn and Visscher method was less than completely effective in cloudy and clear water at 3°C. Three other methods failed to destroy all of the cysts in clear water at 3°C. The failure to inactivate cysts in clear, cold water was apparently related to the lower concentrations of the disinfectants recommended for treating clear water. The authors stressed the importance of water temperature when using halogen disinfection methods. Marchin et al. (1983, 1986) evaluated organic resin triiodide and pentaiodide compounds for cyst removal in water purifier devices. They found the pentaiodide to be a more effective disinfectant than the triiodide for bacteria, viruses, *G. duodenalis* (human) and *G. muris* cysts. However, there is a delay between resin treatment and devitalization of the cysts and an adequate contact period must be allowed before consumption of the water. In a brochure prepared at Idaho State University (Brock and Brock, 1987) some sound advice is offered to recreational users of wilderness areas: the simplest way to ensure that the water you drink is safe is to carry water obtained from a known safe source; the most reliable method for treating a water of unknown purity is by boiling.

3. Drinking water guidelines and regulations

There are presently no numerical standards for *Giardia* cysts in drinking water. Part of the reason for this lack of numerical standards is our state of knowledge on speciation of the organisms and the unavailability of suitable methods to monitor water for satisfying a standard. Methods now being used to detect *Giardia* cysts in water rely on microscopic examination of purified concentrates obtained from large-volume (usually >100 gallon) samples (Craun and Jakubowski, 1987). Cyst identification in the concentrate is based on size, shape and internal morphological characteristics of detected objects or on fluorescent antibody reactions. However, current techniques cannot differentiate *G. muris* from *G. duodenalis*-type cysts, nor can they provide information on the viability of the cysts. Cysts that have been inactivated by natural means or by chemical disinfectants may be detected as well as viable cysts. There is no public health significance related to inactivated microorganisms in drinking water and any meaningful numerical standard should be based on viable *Giardia* cysts. In addition, present detection methods are still tedious, expensive and time-consuming. If a standard is to be effective in preventing disease transmission, results of sample analysis should be available before treated drinking water is distributed to consumers, and not one or two days later by which time a significant proportion of the population may have been exposed.

Although numerical standards have not been established, efforts have been made to develop recommendations, guidelines and regulations addressing *Giardia* in drinking water supplies. Benenson (1985), in the 14th edition of his volume on the control of communicable diseases, recommends two preventive control measures for drinking water supplies with respect to *Giardia*: protecting water supplies against human or animal fecal contamination, and the filtration of water supplies that are at risk of such contamination. The World Health Organization (WHO, 1984) developed guidelines for drinking water quality intended to supersede previously established European and international standards, to be used by countries as a basis for developing their own standards for ensuring the safety of drinking water supplies. The WHO guidelines address organisms, chemical and physical aspects and radioactive materials in drinking water. Concerning *Giardia*, the WHO guidelines state that drinking water should not contain any pathogenic intestinal protozoa and that drinking water sources not subject to fecal contamination should be used where possible. Routine monitoring was not recommended because of detection method limitations. The WHO further recommends that, where fecal contamination is likely or unavoidable, effective filtration should be used, and attempts should be made to identify and remove sources of contamination and to correct deficiencies in the treatment and distribution systems. Drinking water quality guidelines developed for Canada (CCREM, 1987) state that 'No watershed can be effectively quarantined from *Giardia*' and that all surface water supplies should receive disinfection as a minimum treatment. The Canadian guidelines indicate that effective treatment must be provided when water supplies are obtained from polluted sources. The guidelines suggest that several levels of raw water coliform or fecal coliform densities, measured over a 30-day period, should be used to determine the degree of treatment required. Disinfection is required if any raw water sample contains fecal coliforms or if more than 5% of samples exceed 10 total coliforms/100 ml. If more than 10% of the raw water samples have fecal coliforms in the range of 10-100/100 ml, or total coliforms between 100-1000/100 ml, partial treatment (a combination of coagulation-flocculation, sedimentation and filtration, or equivalent advanced forms of treatment) followed by disinfection is recommended. When the raw water fecal coliform density is >100/100 ml, or when the total coliform density is >1000/100 ml in more than 10% of the samples, complete treatment (coagulation-flocculation, sedimentation, filtration and disinfection) should be provided. The Canadian guidelines also recommend that auxiliary treatment (prechlorination, presedimentation, or equivalent, and postchlorination) should be used when the total coliforms exceed 5000/100 ml in more than 10% of the raw water samples.

In the United States, as many as 21 million people may be at risk of giardiasis from their drinking water because their water comes from unfiltered surface water supplies (USEPA, 1987b). Drinking water regulations in the U.S. are based on the Safe Drinking Water Act (SDWA) of 1974, as amended (SDWA, 1986). This law requires establishing maximum contaminant levels in drinking water for those contaminants that may have an adverse effect on health. When monitoring methods for the contaminant are not technologically or economically feasible, then treatment regulations must be developed to reduce the levels of that contaminant in the water. *Giardia* is a drinking water contaminant that may have an adverse effect on health but, as previously mentioned, suitable methods to monitor for the organism in order to satisfy a standard are not available. Since a maximum contaminant level could not be established, the U.S. Environmental Protection Agency (USEPA) solicited comments on a proposal to require filtration for all surface water supplies (USEPA, 1985). This proposal was superseded by the U.S. Congress in 1986 when it amended the SDWA to address filtration and disinfection of water supplies. The amendments required the USEPA to establish criteria to be used by the states in deciding which surface water supplies must install filtration. Responding to this mandate, the USEPA (1987b) published a proposed rule or regulation addressing surface water treatment for *Giardia*, viruses, *Legionella*, plate count bacteria and turbidity. The final regulation was published in June 1989 (USEPA, 1989).

The regulation indicates that surface water supplies must install filtration if they fail to meet source water quality criteria for total or fecal coliforms and turbidity, and site-specific criteria concerning disinfectant levels, watershed management programs, monitoring, waterborne disease outbreak history and compliance with regulations for coliforms and trihalomethanes. Existing filtered water supplies, as well as those installing filtration under the regulation, must meet turbidity performance requirements and must maintain a disinfectant residual within the distribution system. For *Giardia*, all water systems will be required to provide treatment (disinfection or a combination of filtration and disinfection) capable of removing or inactivating at least 99.9% of the cysts. Unfiltered water supplies that can satisfy the source water quality and site-specific criteria do not have to install filtration but must achieve the same reductions in *Giardia* densities as water supplies using filtration. C·t tables are supplied for the various chemical disinfectants and requirements are given for ensuring effective operation of a variety of filtration technologies. Because the states must develop their own regulations for implementing the federal criteria and time will be necessary to allow installation or upgrading of the treatment, it may be four or more years (1993 or later) before full implementation is achieved. Only then can the effectiveness of the regulation in reducing the number of waterborne giardiasis outbreaks be evaluated.

4. Summary

All surface water supplies are subject to *Giardia* cyst contamination from human or animal sources. *Giardia* cysts can survive well in water, especially at lower temperatures (<20°C). Considering our state of knowledge on speciation of *Giardia* and on the infectivity of animal-source cysts for humans, it may be prudent public health policy to regard all cysts of the *G. duodenalis* type as potentially infective for humans.

Filtration technologies (diatomaceous earth, slow sand, coagulation-filtration) commonly used by the water supply industry can be designed and operated to remove 99% or more of *Giardia* cysts. Chemical disinfectants (chlorine, chlorine dioxide, chloramine, ozone) can further reduce cyst densities in drinking water but careful attention must be given to several factors – pH, temperature, demand-causing turbidity, disinfectant concentration and contact time – that can affect the efficiency of inactivation by these disinfectants. A multiple barrier approach utilizing a combination of filtration and disinfection appears to be the most appropriate way for ensuring the safety of a water supply with respect to *Giardia* cysts.

There are no numerical standards for *Giardia* cysts in drinking water due to monitoring method limitations. Guidelines, recommendations and regulations for controlling *Giardia* in water supplies have been developed or proposed by national and international organizations.

Disclaimer This document has been reviewed in accordance with U.S. Environmental Protection Agency policy and approved for publication. Mention of trade names or commercial products does not constitute endorsement or recommendation for use.

References

Al-Ani, M.Y., Hendricks, D.W., Logsdon, G.S. and Hibler, C.P. (1986) Removing *Giardia* cysts from low turbidity waters by rapid rate filtration. J. Am. Water Works Assoc. 78(5), 66-73.

Bellamy, W.D., Hendricks, D.W. and Logsdon, G.S. (1985a) Slow sand filtration: influences of selected process variables. J. Am. Water Works Assoc. 77(12), 62-66.

Bellamy, W.D., Silverman, G.P., Hendricks, D.W. and Logsdon, G.S. (1985b) Removing *Giardia* cysts with slow sand filtration. J. Am. Water Works Assoc. 77(2), 52-60.

Bemrick, W.J. (1984) Some perspectives on the transmission of giardiasis. In: S.L. Erlandsen and E.A. Meyer (Eds), *Giardia* and Giardiasis. Plenum, New York, pp. 379-400.

Benenson, A.S. (1985) Control of communicable diseases in man. American Public Health Association, Washington, D.C.

Bingham, A.K., Jarroll, E.L., Jr. and Meyer, E.A. (1979) *Giardia* sp.: physical factors of excystation in vitro, and excystation vs eosin exclusion as determinants of viability. Exp. Parasitol. 47, 284-291.

Brock, J.T. and Brock, R.M. (1987) Backcountry water – *Giardia* and other potential health hazards. Dept. of Biological Sciences, Idaho State University, Pocatello, Idaho (brochure).

Burke, J.A. (1977) The clinical and laboratory diagnosis of giardiasis. CRC Critical Reviews in Clin. Lab. Sci. 7, 373-391.

Carlson, D.A., Seabloom, R.W., DeWalle, F.B., Wetzler, T.F., Engeset, J., Butler, R., Wangsuphachart, S. and Wang, S. (1985) Ultraviolet disinfection of water for small water supplies. EPA-600/2-85-092, U.S. Environmental Protection Agency, Cincinnati, Ohio.

CCREM (1987) Canadian Water Quality Guidelines. Prepared by the Task Force on Water Quality Guidelines of the Canadian Council of Resource and Environment Ministers, Ottawa, Ontario.

Craft, J.C. (1982) Experimental infection with *Giardia lamblia* in rats. J. Infect. Dis. 145, 495-498.

Craun, G.C. and Jakubowski, W. (1987) Status of waterborne giardiasis outbreaks and monitoring methods. In: C.L. Tate, Jr. (Ed.), International Symposium on Water-Related Health Issues Proceedings. Am. Water Resources Association, TPS87-3, Bethesda, Maryland.

Davies, R.B. and Hibler, C.P. (1979) Animal Reservoirs and cross-species transmission of *Giardia*. In: W. Jakubowski and J.C. Hoff (Eds), Waterborne Transmission of Giardiasis. EPA-600/9-79-001, U.S. Environmental Protection Agency, Cincinnati, Ohio, pp. 104-126.

DeWalle, F.F., Engeset, J. and Lawrence, W. (1984) Removal of *Giardia lamblia* cysts by drinking water treatment plants. EPA-600/2-84-069, U.S. Environmental Protection Agency, Cincinnati, Ohio.

Erlandsen, S.L. and Bemrick, W.J. (1988) Waterborne giardiasis: sources of *Giardia* cysts and evidence pertaining to their implication in human infection. In: P.M. Wallis and B.R. Hammond (Eds), Advances in *Giardia* Research, University of Calgary Press, Calgary, Alberta, pp. 227–236.

Faubert, G.M., Leziy, S.S., Bourassa, A. and MacLean, J.D. (1986) Effects of environmental conditions and standard chlorination practices on the infectivity of *Giardia* cysts. Dis. Aquat. Org. 2, 1-5.

Filice, F.P. (1952) Studies on the cytology and life history of a *Giardia* from the laboratory rat. Univ. Calif. Publ. Zool. 57, 53-143.

Frost, F., Plan, B. and Liechty, B. (1980) *Giardia* prevalence in commercially trapped mammals. J. Environ. Health 42, 245-249.

Haas, C.N., Severin, B.F., Roy, D., Engelbrecht, R.S. and Lalchandani, A. (1985) Removal of new indicators by coagulation and filtration. J. Am. Water Works Assoc. 77(2), 67-71.

Hibler, C.P., Hancock, C.M., Perger, L.M., Wegrzya, J.G. and Swabby, K.D. (1987) Inactivation of *Giardia* cysts with chlorine at 0.5°C to 5.0°C. Am. Water Works Assoc. Research Foundation, Denver, Colorado.

Hoff, J.C. (1979) Disinfection resistance of *Giardia* cysts: origins of current concepts and research in progress. In: W. Jakubowski and J.C. Hoff (Eds), Waterborne Transmission of Giardiasis. EPA-600/9-79-001, U.S. Environmental Protection Agency, Cincinnati, Ohio, pp. 231- 239.

Hoff, J.C. (1986) Inactivation of microbial agents by chemical disinfectants. EPA-600/2-86-067, U.S. Environmental Protection Agency, Cincinnati, Ohio.

Hoff, J.C., Rice, E.W. and Schaefer, F.W., III. (1985) Comparison of animal infectivity and excystation as measures of *Giardia muris* cyst inactivation by chlorine. Appl. Environ. Microbiol. 50, 1115-1117.

Horn, J.B., Hendricks, D.W., Scanlan, J.M., Rozelle, L.T. and Trnka, W.C. (1988) Removing *Giardia* cysts and other particles from low turbidity water using dual-stage filtration. J. Am. Water Works Association 80(2), 68-77.

Jakubowski, W. and Ericksen, T.H. (1979) Methods for detection of *Giardia* cysts in water supplies. In: W. Jakubowski and J.C. Hoff (Eds.), Waterborne Transmission of Giardiasis. EPA-600/9-79-001, U.S. Environmental Protection Agency, Cincinnati, Ohio, pp. 193-210.

Jarroll, E.L. (1988) Effect of disinfectants on *Giardia* cysts. CRC Crit. Rev. Environ. Control 18, 1-28.

Jarroll, E.L., Bingham, A.K. and Meyer, E.A. (1980) *Giardia* cyst destruction: effectiveness of six small-quantity water disinfection methods. Am. J. Trop. Med. Hyg. 29, 8-11.

Jarroll, E.L., Bingham, A.K. and Meyer, E.A. (1981) Effect of chlorine on *Giardia lamblia* cyst viability. Appl. Environ. Microbiol. 41, 483-487.

Jarroll, E.L., Hoff, J.C. and Meyer, E.A. (1984) Resistance of cysts to disinfection agents. In: S.L. Erlandsen and E.A. Meyer (Eds), *Giardia* and Giardiasis. Plenum, New York, pp. 311-328.

Kahn, F.H. and Visscher, B.R. (1975) Water disinfection in the wilderness – a simple, effective method of iodination. West. J. Med. 122, 450-453.

Kasprzak, W. and Majewska, A.C. (1983) Infectivity of *Giardia* sp. cysts in relation to eosin exclusion and excystation in vitro. Tropenmed. Parasitol. 34, 70-72.

Kasprzak, W. and Majewska, A.C. (1987) Efficacy of methods for assessing *Giardia* cyst viability. Wiado. Parazytol. 33, 147-155.

Kirkpatrick, C.E. and Benson, C.E. (1987) Presence of *Giardia* spp. and absence of *Salmonella* spp. in New Jersey muskrats (*Ondatra zibethicus*). Appl. Environ. Microbiol. 53, 1790-1792.

Kulda, J. and Nohynkova, E. (1978) Flagellates of the human intestine and of intestines of other species. In: J.P. Kreier (Ed.), Parasitic Protozoa II. Academic Press, New York, pp. 1-138.

Langé, K.P., Bellamy, W.D., Hendricks, D.W. and Logsdon, G.S. (1986) Diatomaceous earth filtration of *Giardia* cysts and other substances. J. Am. Water Works Assoc. 78(1), 76-84.

Leahy, J.G. (1985) Inactivation of *Giardia muris* cysts by chlorine and chlorine dioxide. Master's Thesis, Ohio State University, Dept. of Civil Engineering, Columbus, Ohio.

Leahy, J.G., Rubin, A.J. and Sproul, O.J. (1987) Inactivation of *Giardia muris* cysts by free chlorine. Appl.

Environ. Microbiol. 53, 1448–1453.

Logsdon, G.S. (1988) Comparison of some filtration processes appropriate for *Giardia* cyst removal. In: P.M. Wallis and B.R. Hammond (Eds), Advances in *Giardia* Research. Univ. of Calgary Press, Calgary, Alberta, pp. 95–102.

Logsdon, G.S., Symons, J.M., Hoye, R.L., Jr. and Arozarena, M.M. (1981) Alternative filtration methods for removal of *Giardia* cysts and cyst models. J. Am. Water Works Assoc. 73(2), 111-118.

Logsdon, G.S., Thurman, V.C., Frindt, E.S. and Stoecker, J.G. (1985) Evaluating sedimentation and various filter media for removal of *Giardia* cysts. J. Am. Water Works Assoc. 77(2), 61-66.

Long, W.R. (1983) Evaluation of cartridge filters for the removal of *Giardia lamblia* cyst models from drinking water systems. J. Environ. Health 45, 220-225.

Marchin, G.L., Fina, L.R. and Lambert, J.L. (1986) The biocidal properties of the pentacide/demand-type resin -I_5. In: Technology Conference Proceedings – Advances in Water Analysis and Treatment, Am. Water Works Assoc., Denver, Colorado, pp. 461-472.

Marchin, G.L., Fina, L.R., Lambert, J.L. and Fina, G.T. (1983) Effect of resin disinfectants -I_3 and -I_5 on *Giardia muris* and *Giardia lamblia*. Appl. Environ. Microbiol. 46, 965-969.

McHarry, M.J. (1984) Detection of *Giardia* in sewage effluent. J. Protozool. 31, 362-364.

Meyer, E.A., Glicker, J., Bingham, A.K. and Edwards, R. (1988) Inactivation of *G. muris* cysts by chloramines. Water Res. Bull. 25, 335–340.

Morand, J.M., Cobb, C.R., Clark, R.M. and Richard, G.S. (1980) Package water treatment plants, volume 1, a performance evaluation. EPA-600/2-80-008a, U.S. Environmental Protection Agency, Cincinnati, Ohio.

Morand, J.M. and Young, M.J. (1983) Performance characteristics of package water treatment plants, project summary. EPA-600/S2-82-101, U.S. Environmental Protection Agency, Cincinnati, Ohio.

Mosher, R.R. and Hendricks, D.W. (1986) Rapid rate filtration of low turbidity water using field-scale pilot filters. J. Am. Water Works Assoc. 78(12), 42-51.

Nash, T.E., Herrington, D.A., Losonsky, G.A. and Levine, M.M. (1987) Experimental human infections with *Giardia lamblia*. J. Infect. Dis. 156, 974-984.

NSF (1982) Drinking Water Treatment Units, Health Effects, Standard Number 53. National Sanitation Foundation, Ann Arbor, Michigan.

Pacha, R.E., Clark, G.W. and Williams, E.A. (1985) Occurrence of *Campylobacter jejuni* and *Giardia* species in muskrat (*Ondatra zibethicus*). Appl. Environ. Microbiol. 50, 177-178.

Panicker, P.V.R.C. and Krishnamoorthi, K.P. (1978) Studies on intestinal helminthic eggs and protozoan cysts in sewage. Environ. Health (Indian) 20, 75-78.

Panicker, P.V.R.C. and Krishnamoorthi, K.P. (1981) Parasite egg and cyst reduction in oxidation ditches and aerated lagoons. J. Water Pollut. Control Fed. 53, 1413-1419.

Pyper, G.R. (1985) Slow sand filter and package treatment plant evaluation: operating costs and removal of bacteria, *Giardia* and trihalomethanes. EPA-600/2-85-052, U.S. Environmental Protection Agency, Cincinnati, Ohio.

Rice, E.W. and Hoff, J.C. (1981) Inactivation of *Giardia lamblia* cysts by ultraviolet irradiation. Appl. Environ. Microbiol. 42, 546-547.

Rice, E.W., Hoff, J.C. and Schaefer, F.W., III. (1982) Inactivation of *Giardia* cysts by chlorine. Appl. Environ. Microbiol. 43, 250-251.

Rubin, A.J. (1988) Factors affecting the inactivation of *Giardia* cysts by monochloramine and comparison with other disinfectants. In: Proceedings: Conference on Current Research in Drinking Water Treatment, U.S. Environmental Protection Agency/American Water Works Association Research Foundation. U.S. Environmental Protection Agency, Cincinnati, Ohio.

Schaefer, F.W., III, Rice, E.W. and Hoff, J.C. (1984) Factors promoting in vitro excystation of *Giardia muris* cysts. Trans. R. Soc. Trop. Med. Hyg. 78, 795-800.

Schmidt, S.D. and Meier, P.G. (1984) Evaluation of *Giardia* cyst removal via portable water filtration devices. J. Freshwater Ecol. 2, 435-439.

SDWA (1986) The Safe Drinking Water Act as amended by the Safe Drinking Water Act Amendments of

1986. Public Law 99-339, June, 19, 1986, GPO, Washington, D.C.

Seelaus, T.J., Hendricks, D.W. and Janonis, B.A. (1986) Design and operation of a slow sand filter. J. Am. Water Works Assoc. 78(12), 35-41.

Sykora, J.L., Bancroft, W.D., States, S.J., Shapiro, M.A., Boutros, S.N., Keleti, G., Turzai, M. and Conley, L.F. (1988) *Giardia* cysts in raw and treated sewage. In: G.S. Logsdon (Ed.), Controlling Waterborne Giardiasis: A State of the Art Review. Environmental Engineering Division, Am. Soc. Civil Engineers, New York, NY, pp. 22–33.

Sykora, J.L., States, S.J., Bancroft, W.D., Boutros, S.N., Shapiro, M.A. and Conley, L.F. (1987) Monitoring of water and wastewater for *Giardia*. In: Technology Conference Proceedings, Advances in Water Analysis and Treatment, WQTC-14, 1986. Am. Water Works Association, Denver, Colorado, pp. 1043-1054.

USEPA (1985) National Primary Drinking Water Regulations, Synthetic Organic Chemicals and Microorganisms; Proposed Rule. Federal Register, Nov. 13, 1985, 50(219), 46936-47022.

USEPA (1987a) Draft Guide Standard and Protocol for Testing Microbiological Water Purifiers: Report of Task Force, revised April, 1987. U.S. Environmental Protection Agency, Office of Pesticides Programs and Office of Drinking Water, Washington, D.C.

USEPA (1987b) National Primary Drinking Water Regulations; Filtration, Disinfection, Turbidity, *Giardia lamblia*, Viruses, *Legionella*, and Heterotrophic Bacteria; Proposed Rule. Federal Register, Nov. 3, 1987; 52(212), 42177-42222.

USEPA (1989a) Guidance Manual for Compliance with the Filtration and Disinfection Requirements for Public Water Systems Using Surface Water Sources. Criteria and Standards Division, Office of Water, U.S. Environmental Protection Agency, Washington, D.C., in press.

USEPA (1989b) National Primary Drinking Water Regulations: Filtration, Disinfection, Turbidity, *Giardia lamblia*, Viruses, Legionella, and Heterotropic Bacteria: Final Rule. Federal Register, June 29, 1989; 54(124), 27486-27541.

WHO (1984) Guidelines for Drinking Water Quality. Volume 1, Recommendations. World Health Organization, Geneva.

Wickramanayake, G.B. (1986) Effectiveness of conventional water treatment in the prevention of waterborne giardiasis. In: C.L. Tate, Jr. (Ed.), International Symposium on Water-Related Health Issues Proceedings. TPS87-3, Am. Water Resources Assoc., Bethesda, Maryland, pp. 137-144.

Wickramanayake, G.B., Rubin, A.J. and Sproul, O.J. (1984) Inactivation of *Giardia lamblia* cysts with ozone. Appl. Environ. Microbiol. 48, 671-672.

Wickramanayake, G.B., Rubin, A.J. and Sproul, O.J. (1985) Effects of ozone and storage temperature on *Giardia* cysts. Jour. Am. Water Works Assoc. 77(8), 74-77.

Woo, P.K. (1984) Evidence for animal reservoirs and transmission of *Giardia* infection between animal species. In: S.L. Erlandsen and E.A. Meyer (Eds), *Giardia* and Giardiasis. Plenum, New York, pp. 341-359.

Woo, P.T.K. and Paterson, W.B. (1986) *Giardia lamblia* in children in day-care centres in southern Ontario, Canada, and susceptibility of animals to *G. lamblia*. Trans. R. Soc. Trop. Med. Hyg. 80, 56-59.

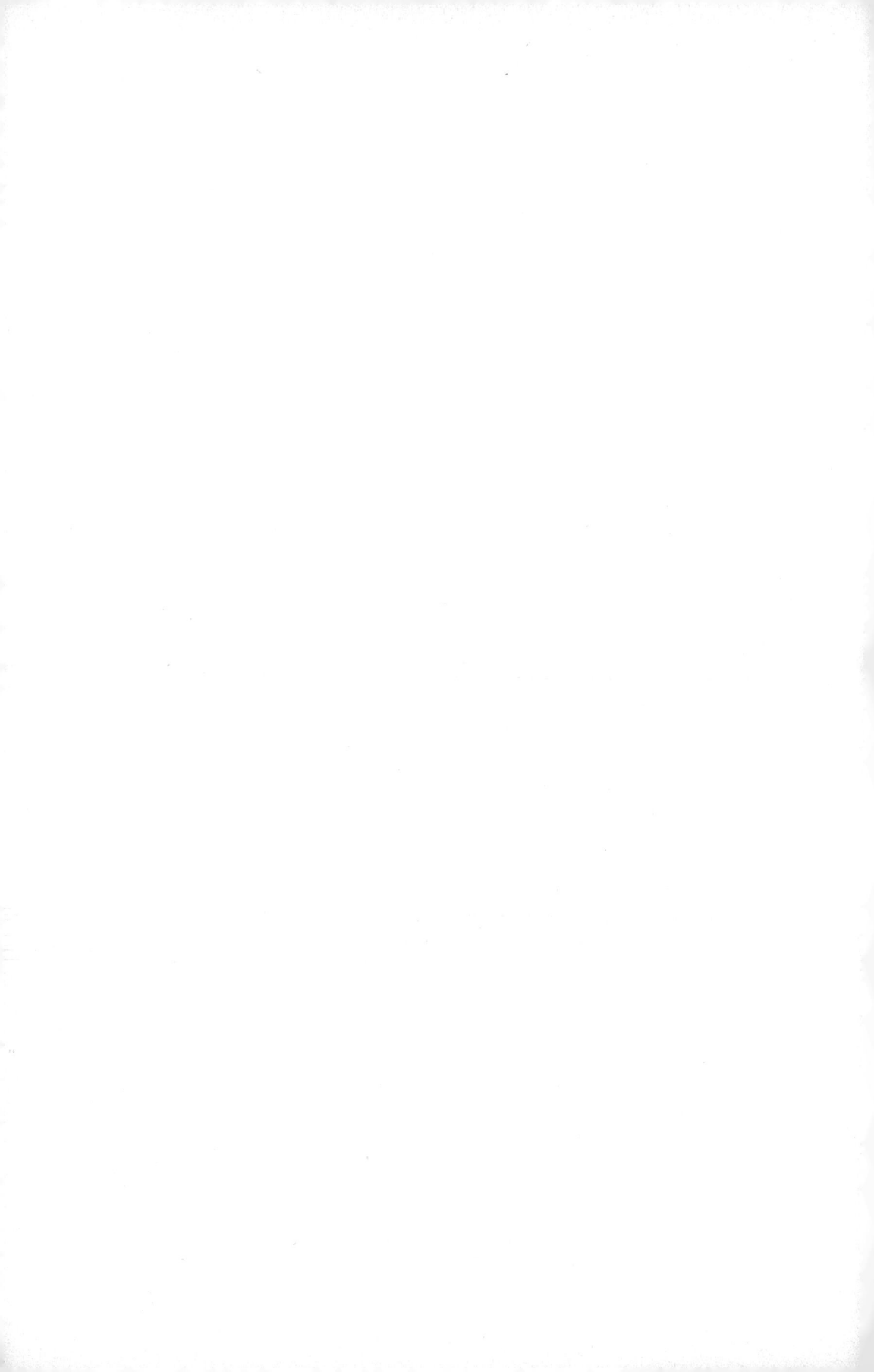

21

Prospects and future goals

E.A. MEYER

Department of Microbiology and Immunology, Oregon Health Sciences University, Portland, OR 97201-3098, U.S.A.

Ideally, the control of an infectious disease proceeds simultaneously along two different lines. On the one hand, measures are directed against the disease itself, employing whatever medical interventions (including chemotherapy and improvement of sanitation) are afforded by our knowledge at the time. On the other hand, research proceeds on the disease and the pathogenic parasite that causes it, research, the aim of which is the development of methods, including vaccines and improved chemotherapy, to facilitate disease control or eradication.

Sadly, when one considers the prospects for present-day disease control in developing countries, the outlook is less than bright. There exist simply too many important infectious diseases, and an insufficiency of trained personnel and money to address them.

To remedy this situation, a strategy has emerged, the objective of which is the most effective use of the limited resources available to resolve these problems. This strategy involves setting disease priorities, priorities based on prevalence, morbidity, mortality and feasibility of control of each disease. The end result of such an exercise is the ranking of diseases into groups. Control of those diseases which receive a high priority might best be addressed by primary health care measures, the first disease-control measure mentioned above. Other diseases, held to the same criteria, may receive a low priority; control of such diseases via primary health care is not deemed practicable at this time. Rather, it is suggested that the most cost effective approach to their eventual control is via research.

Walsh and Warren conducted such an assessment of diseases in developing countries, and reported their recommendations in 1979. Malaria and schistosomiasis were among those diseases which received a high priority. Interestingly, giardiasis and amebiasis were among those diseases that received a low priority, principally on the basis of difficulty of control. Controlling these diseases would require providing high levels of economic development, which in turn involves improvements in water purification, food handling and sanitation. We are faced, in both instances, which situations involving significant infection, disease, and morbidity rates in which noticeable progress in disease control at present will probably only result from advances that accompany economic development of the type seen in more developed countries. Given this situation, Walsh and Warren argue, we would be better advised to expend our limited resources on research that will reduce the ultimate cost of controlling this disease. It is to be hoped that the recent spectacular advances in biotechnology shortly will be applied to this problem, and provide measures that will permit control of giardiasis in developing countries, even before high levels of economic development are achieved.

Many of the authors who have contributed to this volume have indicated in their respective chapters the gaps which presently remain in our knowledge, which problems remain to be solved, and what our future goals should be. Many of these points, summarized in the following discussion, were also made in reports generated by the World Health Organization in 1980, 1986 and 1987.

High on a wish-list of contributions that would improve our understanding of *Giardia* infection in humans would be the development of improved methods of diagnosing *Giardia* infections. A procedure is needed that is sensitive, specific and noninvasive, and which will rapidly reveal those infections which are now difficult to diagnose. Only when we have such a test can we accurately accumulate other much-needed data, including: (a) Determining the prevalence of giardiasis and *Giardia* infection in developed and developing countries. Much of the data now available were collected on selected populations and hence are not representative. Even now, we can only roughly estimate the magnitude of the problem. The data of Walsh and Warren (1979) clearly must be considered estimates. (b) Determining the ratio of symptomatic to asymptomatic infections in developing, and developed, countries. (c) Determining the impact of *Giardia* infection and disease on growth, development and nutrition (Latham, 1982; Solomons, 1982).

With the above information in hand, we will be better able to understand the magnitude of this problem. The true incidence of infection and the nutritional impact of the disease are necessary prerequisites to formulating the most cost effective strategy for attacking it.

Despite impressive contributions to our knowledge of the interaction of the *Giardia* trophozoite and its host, we still do not completely understand the pathogenesis and pathophysiology of giardiasis, including the mechanism of absorptive dysfunction. Continued research is needed in these areas.

The role of wild and domestic animals in human giardiasis remains to be elucidated. It has been established that drinking water can at times be the source of epidemics of giardiasis in humans. It is suspected, based largely on circumstantial evidence, that the cysts in the water were excreted by lower animals. Presently, the beaver and the muskrat are considered the two most likely animal sources of *Giardia*. A recent cross-transmission study by Erlandsen et al. (1988) suggests that these two animals must be considered as possible sources of human *Giardia* infection; nevertheless, a great variety of other *Giardia*-infected mammals and birds cannot be excluded as possible reservoirs of human infection. Further, no animal, other than humans can be assigned a major role as a reservoir of *Giardia* infection of humans at this time. Clearly, much remains to be learned about the epidemiology of this infection.

Consideration should be given to the development of a protective vaccine against *Giardia* (Stevens, 1985). Observations made to date indicate a role for immunity in this disease, and justify efforts to develop such a vaccine. An effective vaccine to protect against this organism could result in reduction of disease, even before the introduction of the much-needed (but more expensive) improvements in sanitation.

The existing therapeutic agents for treating these infections need to be thoroughly evaluated (Davidson, 1984). Other imidazoles that are more effective and less carcinogenic than metronidazole should be considered for release in the United States.

With respect to the organism itself, what problems deserve attention? Agreement should be reached with respect to the taxonomy and nomenclature of the genus *Giardia*. Particular attention should be paid to that group of *Giardia* which have median bodies of the type described by Filice as '*duodenalis*-type'. This is so, because (a) this is the only type that has been shown to infect humans, and (b) this same type occurs in a great variety of *Giardia* that infect other mammals (including beaver and muskrat). *Giardia* from humans has been variously described as *Giardia lamblia*, *Giardia intestinalis*, and *Giardia duodenalis*. Cross-transmission studies, which indicate that a number of *Giardia* are *not* highly host specific, argue against using the animal host (e.g., the human) as the criterion for naming its *Giardia* (*G. lamblia*). Ultimately, the classification of these organisms may well involve characterization of *Giardia* proteins (including isoenzymes) and nucleic acids; it may additionally involve cross-transmission studies. In any event, it would be highly desirable to reach a consensus regarding *Giardia* nomenclature; such consensus would eliminate much literature confusion.

Improved methods are needed for culturing these organisms. Presently, it is only possible to culture a relatively small minority of the *Giardia* isolated from humans, in addition to strains from a few lower animals. Until we can culture most, if not all, of these protozoa, we will only have a limited knowledge of the diversity of strains that exist.

In addition to improving methods of culture of *Giardia* of the *duodenalis*-type, efforts should be made to grow *Giardia* of other median-body types, particularly *G. muris*. None of these organisms has yet been cultured; they fail to grow on media which support *duodenalis*-type *Giardia*. *Giardia* in the mouse is now a widely used and highly useful animal model; the availability of these same protozoa in axenic culture would expand the usefulness of this model.

We need improved methods of (1) detecting *Giardia* in drinking water supplies and (2) differentiating *duodenalis*-type organisms (if not those *Giardia* capable of causing human disease) from other *Giardia*. Such information is valuable in assessing the safety of drinking water supplies.

In recent decades, we have learned a great deal about *Giardia*. Nevertheless, it can be seen that much remains to be done before it can be removed from the WHO list of the 10 major parasites of humans.

References

Davidson, R.A. (1984) Issues in clinical parasitology: the treatment of giardiasis. Am. J. Gastroenterol. 79, 256-261.

Erlandsen, S.L., Sherlock, L.A., Januschka, M., Schupp, D.G., Schaefer, F.W., Jakubowski, W. and Bemrick, W.J. (1988) Cross-species transmission of *Giardia* spp.: inoculation of beavers and muskrats with cysts of human, beaver, mouse, and muskrat origin. Appl. Environ. Microbiol. 54, 2777–2785.

Latham, M.C. (1982) Needed research on the interactions of certain parasitic diseases and nutrition in humans. Rev. Infect. Dis. 4, 896-900.

Solomons, N.W. (1982) Giardiasis: nutritional implications. Rev. Infect. Dis. 4, 859-870.

Stevens, D.P. (1985) Selective primary health care: strategies for control of disease in the developing world. XIX. Giardiasis. Rev. Infect. Dis. 7, 530-535.

Walsh, J.A. and Warren, K.S. (1979) Selective primary health care: an interim strategy for disease control in developing countries. N. Engl. J. Med. 301, 967-974.

World Health Organization (1980) Parasite-related diarrhoeas. Report of a WHO Scientific Working Group. Bull. WHO 58, 819-830.

World Health Organization (1986) Major parasitic infections: a global review. WHO. Hlth. Statist. Quart. 39, 145-160.

World Health Organization (1989) Prevention and control of intestinal parasitic infections. Report of a WHO Expert Committee. WHO Tech. Rep. Series 749.

Subject Index

Acid phosphatase, 34, 38, 61, 114
Actin, see *Giardia*, contractile proteins
Age distribution of *Giardia* infection, 237–241
    and antibodies to *Giardia*, 238
AIDS, 159
Alpha-actinin, see *Giardia*, contractile proteins
Amebiasis, 159
Animal incidence of infection, 307–312
    beaver, 309
    cats, 308–309
    dogs, 307–309
    muskrat, 310
Animal infectivity and cyst viability, 132–133
Animal models, 7, 57, 77–88, 91–96, 132–133, 143–144
Animal reservoirs, evidence for, 305–312
Antibody, 55, 166, 188–196, 220–224, 244–245
Antibody-independent killing, 202
Antigenic variation, 217
Anti-*Giardia* antibodies, 170–190
    G. muris, 170
    human milk, 190, 202, 220 221, 224
    intestinal secretions, 190
    saliva, 190
    serum, 188–190, 221
Atabrine, see Quinacrine
Attachment to substrates, 12, 43–47

Beaver, 104–105, 113, 142, 256, 279, 286, 309, 310, 336
Benzoylmetronidazole, 319, 320
Bile salts, 139, 202–204, 209, 216
Bile salt stimulated lipase (BSL), 202–204, 206, 243–244
Bile stimulates *Giardia* encystation, 142–143
Bile stimulates *Giardia* growth, 6, 103
Bithionol, 329
Boiling water, 347
Bovine serum albumin, 209

Candida, 6, 100, 206, 217
Carbohydrate metabolism, 62–65
Cartridge filters, 341–342
Cats, 308–309
Cellular immune responses, 93, 218–219, 224
Chemotaxonomy, 54–57
Chemotherapy, 7–8, 318–322, 325–333, 357
Chitin, 38, 73–75, 151–152
Chloramines, 345–346
Chlorimipramine, 328
Chlorine disinfection, 28, 120, 278–283, 288–290, 343–345, 347
Chlorine dioxide, 345–346
Cholecystitis, 179
Classification, 51–58
Clinical features, 175–179
    of the acute stage of the disease, 176–177
    asymptomatic cyst-passing stage, 179
    incidence, summarized, 177
    incubation and prepatent periods, 176
    post-*Giardia* lactose intolerance, 180
    of the subacute and chronic stages, 177–179
Coagulation-filtration, 340–341, 401
Colchicine, 161
Coliforms, failure as a predictor of outbreaks, 276, 277, 280, 283
Complement, 170, 220
Corticosteroids, 166–168
Cortisone, 85, 160, 165
Control measures, 257–258
Counterimmunoelectrophoresis (CIE), 192–194
Cryptosporidiosis, 176
Ct values, 344–346, 349
Cultivation of trophozoites, 6–7, 99–108
    future prospects, 357
    G. agilis type, 6–7
    G. duodenalis type, 6
    G. muris type, 6–7, 128
    inoculum preparation, 105–107

Karapetyan's methods, 100
TPS-1 medium, 6, 101–104
TYI-S-33 medium, 6, 88, 101–105, 108
Culture initiation, 99–105
Culture management, 108
Cyclosporin, 166
Cysteine, essential for *Giardia* growth, 6, 103
Cyst maturation, 124, 130
Cyst morphology, ultrastructure, 34–38
Cyst production in infection, 160
types of excreters, 181, 244
Cysts,
axonemes, 38
carbohydrate analysis, 151
chitin, 38, 73–75, 151–152
comparison, in vitro and in vivo, 145–146
concentration and purification, 88, 92, 106–107
detection, 286, 288, 347
disinfection, 342–347
excystation, 103, 104, 107, 111–133
excretion, 78–83, 87–88, 92–93, 95, 181, 244, 297–299
filtration, 258, 280–282, 290, 338
identification, 347
infectiousness for humans, 337, 349
maturation, 124, 130
median body, 144
morphology, 34–38, 144–146, 311
N-acetylgalactosamine, 38, 152
N-acetylglucosamine, 38, 73–74, 151
numbers required to produce animal infections, 132
presence in sewage, 285
survival in cold water, 14, 285, 337
thermal death point, 337
transmission, 254–258, 268–270, 284, 300–301
viability, 12, 103–104, 130–134, 140, 343
Cyst wall components, identity, 37–38 148–152
carbohydrate analysis, 151
isotope incorporation, 152
and Western blots, 148–150
Cytokinesis, 112, 114, 116
Cytoskeletal proteins, 21–29
dorsal ribbons, 21–23
giardin, 23–26
microtubules, 26–29
ribbon proteins, 23–26
tubulin, 26–29

Day care centers, 258, 295–301

asymptomatic children, 297–299
contamination of hands, 300
fomites, 300
infection control, 301
nontoilet-trained children, 299–300
outbreaks, summarized, 296
predisposing characteristics for diarrhea, 299
prevalence of *Giardia*, summarized, 298
transmission to family members, 300–301
Delayed type hypersensitivity (DTH), 164, 166–167, 170
Detection of *Giardia* cysts in water, 288–290
Diagnosis, 175–196, 318, 356
by biopsy, 180, 182
counterimmunoelectrophoresis, 192–194
detection of antigen in clinical specimens, 191–195
differential, 180
ELISA, 188
empiric treatment in the absence of diagnosis, 183
examination of intestinal fluid, 181–182, 318
examination of stools, 180–181, 318
gastrointestinal radiology, 183, 187–191
hemagglutination, 188
immunodiffusion, 188
immunofluorescence, 188, 191–192
multiple stool specimens, 181
serologic tests, 183, 188–190, 318
small intestinal biopsy, 182
stool preservation kits, 181
Dichlorophene, 329
Disaccharidase deficiency, 86, 159, 161, 168, 170, 250, 252
Disinfectants, methods of comparing effects on cysts,
animal infectivity, 132–133, 343–344
eosin exclusion, 130, 343
excystation, 130, 343, 345
fluorescent staining, 130–131
vital stains, 131, 343
Disinfection of cysts, 338, 342–347
DNA restriction endonuclease, 307
Dobell, 1–3
Dogs, 105, 113, 118, 307–308
Drinking water, 112, 267–290, 335–350
Canadian guidelines, 348
effectiveness of treatment processes, 338
Giardia contamination potential, 335–338
guidelines and regulations, 347–349

treatment by boiling, 347
treatment by disinfection, 342–347
treatment in developing countries, 258
treatment by filtration, 338–342
United States guidelines, 348–349
WHO guidelines, 348

Ectosymbionts, 39–42
Encystation in vitro, 137–152
  cyst morphology, 144–146
  cyst viability, 146–148
  evidence for cyst wall formation, 148–151
  induction, 138–145
Endosymbionts, 38–42
Entamoeba histolytica, 68, 99, 102–104, 217, 269, 327
Enterotest, 118–182
Enzyme-linked immunoabsorbent assay (ELISA), 188–190, 194–195, 306
Eosin exclusion as criterion of cyst viability, 103–104, 130
Eosinophils, 157, 179–180, 183
Epidemiology, 83–84, 216–218, 235–312
Excystation,
  comparison of *G. duodenalis* and *G. muris*, 113–114, 128–130, 343–344
  factors employed, 118–128
  induction for culture initiation, 107–108
  in vivo, 112–113
  method of Bingham and Meyer, 103–104, 107, 113, 120, 125
    effect of pH, 7, 104, 120
    exposure time, 104
    gastric juice components, 104
    incubation medium, 120, 122–123
    postacid solutions, 104
    temperature, 104
  method of Chochillon et al., 123
  method of Feely, 126, 127
  method of Gonzalez-Castro, 126
  method of Kasprzak and Majewska, 122
  method of Rice and Schaefer, 120, 122, 125
    effect of storage temperature, 120
    results with *G. duodenalis* cysts, 120
    results with *G. muris* cysts, 120
  method of Sauch, 123, 124
  quantitation, 114, 118
  ultrastructure, 113–120
Experimental infections in humans, 306–307

Failure to thrive, 178, 302, 322
Fasigyn, see Tinidazole
Ferritin, 33, 61
Fever, 177–178, 249–250
Filice, 4–6, 53–54
Filtration of *Giardia* cysts in drinking water, 258, 280–282, 290, 338–342
  cartridge filters, 341–342
  coagulation-filtration, 340–341
  diatomaceous earth (DE) filtration, 338–339
  microspheres as cyst models, 339
  types of *Giardia* used in filtration studies, 339
  granular media filters, 340
  package treatment plants, 341
  slow sand filters, 338–340
Flagella, 12–16, 26, 30–31
  and paraflagellar rods, 30–31
Flagyl, see Metronidazole
Fluorescent staining, 130–131
Food and *Giardia* transmission, 112, 255, 306
Funis, 26–27, 30
Furazolidone, 7, 325, 328, 330
Furoxone, see Furazolidone
Fusidate, sodium, 329

G. agilis, 5, 6, 57
Gallbladder, 156
Gastric acidity, 243
G. duodenalis, 5, 11, 12
G. enterica, 6
Geographical distribution, summarized, 237
Gerbil, see Mongolian gerbil
G. intestinalis, 6
G. lamblia, 6
G. microti, 40, 41
G. ondatrae, 41
G. psittaci, 5
G. muris, see *Giardia* species
Giardia,
  adhesive disc, see ventral disc below
  antibodies, prevalence summarized, 222–223
  antigens, 191–196, 225–227, 307
    detection procedures summarized, 192
  attachment, 43–47
    Erlandsen's theory, 45
    Feely's theory, 43
    Holberton's theory, 43, 45
    lectins, 45
    Mueller's theory, 43
  axonemes, 12, 26, 27, 130, 132

contractile proteins, 21, 30–31, 43–45
culture management, 108
cyst morphology, 34–38
cyst survival, 337
cytokinesis, 112, 114, 116
disc cytoskeleton, 17–20
DNA restriction endonuclease patterns, 307
dorsal ribbons, 21–23
ectosymbionts, 39–41
endosymbionts,
    bacterial, 38–42
    viral, 42
excretion by asymptomatic host, 297–299
extraintestinal, 156–157
fatty acid analysis, 65
flagella, 12–16, 26, 30–31
giardin, 23–26
Golgi, 34
host specificity, 4, 57, 305–312, 336
in hypogammaglobulinemia, summarized, 221, 224
infectiousness for humans, 337
intestinal distribution, 82–83, 92, 156–157
isoenzymes, 54–56
lateral crest, 15–16, 19, 45, 46
lateral shield, 45
Leeuwenhoek's description, 1–2
life cycle, 12
lipid composition of cysts and trophozoites, 65–66
lysosomes, 34
median body, 12, 14, 26–27, 53–54
metabolism, 61–75
    carbohydrate, 62, 65
    of cysts and trophozoites, 63
    electron transport, 64–65
    EMP pathway, 62–63, 74
    energy, 62–63
    enzymes, 63–65
    evolution of carbon dioxide from glucose, 62
    flavin, 64, 74
    HM pathway, 62, 74
    hydrolases, 72–75
    inhibitors 62, 67–70, 329
    lipid, 65–66
    nucleic acid, 67–72
    pathways, 64–65
    purine, 70–72, 329
    pyrimidine, 67–70

    synthetases, 72–74
microribbons, 17, 19
microtubules, 17 19, 26–29
mitochondria, 33
nomenclature, 4–6
nonspecific defenses against, 199–211
nucleus, 52
parabasal body, 12
pathogenicity question, 3, 169–171, 215
plasma membrane, 32–33, 73
respiration, 62–64
ribbon proteins, 23–26
sensitivity to lipid hydrolysis products, summarized, 205
speciation (morphologic groups), 52–54
striated disc, see ventral disc below
taxonomy, 4–6
trophozoite morphology, 12–34
tubulin, 26–29, 33
ventral disc, 12, 14–17, 19–23, 43–45, 52
ventrolateral flange, 20–21
Giardia species, 52–56
    antigenic comparisons, 54–56
    biochemical characterization, 54–57
    chemotaxonomy, 54–57
    criteria for characterization, 52–58
    definitions, 53–54
    DNA analysis, 55–56
    Filice's recommendations, 53–54
    host specificity, 57
        cross-transmission studies, 57, 307–311
        Giardia-free animals, establishment and maintenance, 88
    immunologic characterization, 54–56
    isozyme determination, 54–56
    morphologic characterization, 53–54, 57–58
    morphometric characterization, 54
    restriction endonuclease analysis, 56
Giardiasis
    AIDS, 159, 222
    animal models, 77–88, 91–96, 132–133
    animal reservoirs, 305–312
    asymptomatic, 179, 215–218, 221, 297–298
    athymic mice, 219
    blood group A association, 242
    cellular immune responses, 218–220
        granulocytes, 226
        lymphocyte proliferation, 219
        mononuclear leukocytes, 218
    complement fixation, 220–221

counterimmunoelectrophoresis test, 192–194
day care center spread, 216, 295–301
developing countries, 216–218, 235–259
diagnosis, 175–196, 318
distribution,
    age, 237–239
    in Bangladesh, 237–240
    geographical, 237
    rural, 239
    summarized, 237
    urban, 239
efficacy of therapy, 329–330
ELISA, 188, 192, 194–195, 226–227, 306
epidemic outbreaks, 267–290, 297
failure to thrive, 322
foodborne, 255, 306
genetic studies, 94–95, 220
gerbil model for *G. muris* type, 83–84
histologic changes, 157–159, 218–219
host specificity, 305–312
humoral responses, 220–224
    antibody titers, 221–224
    ELISA, 188, 192, 224–227
    IgA, 170, 221, 224
    IgG, 222–223
    IgM, 220, 223
    indirect immunofluorescence test, 192
hypothymic mice, 220
immune response, 214–228
    during infection, 226–228
    in homosexual men, 224
    in hypogammaglobulinemia, 221
    in mice, 220
    macrophages, 219
    T cell defect, 220
immunodiffusion test, 188
immunoelectrophoresis, 192, 225
immunofluorescent test, 188
immunoglobulin level, 221–224
impact on child health, 252–254
incubation period, 176
interference with growth and development, 252–254
intestinal pathology,
    humans, 156–159
    mice, 159–171
lactose intolerance, 180
model for *G. duodenalis* type, 77–88
    cats, 81
    dogs, 81
    Mongolian gerbil, 81–83, 132, 307
    mice, 80–81, 102
    prerequisites, 78–79
    rabbits, 81
    rats, 79
mouse model for *G. muris* type, 91–96, 132, 159
murine model, 91–96, 159
nonspecific defenses, 195–211
nude mice, 93–94, 164–166, 220
and nutritional deprivation, synergistic, 179–180, 242–243, 248
pathogenesis, 155–171
pathology, 155–171
person to person transmission, 306
prepatent period, 176
prevalence by age, 237–239, 297
prevalence in developing countries, 236–240
    summarized, 237
protection via normal human milk, 202–206
reportable disease, 275
risk factors, 299
seasonality, 239–240
serologic diagnosis, 183, 188–190
stool characteristics, summarized, 178
susceptibility, 240–245
symptomatic and asymptomatic, 214–218, 246–248
symptoms,
    acute stage, 176–177
    chronic stage, 177–179
    summarized, 177
therapy, 315–333
    comparison of alternatives, 329–330
    drug dosages, summarized, 326
transmission of *Giardia*,
    animal feeding experiments, 4, 256, 311–312
    current and future status 311–312
    day care centers, 295–301
    drinking water, 267–290
    fecal–oral, 254, 268, 301
    by food, 255, 306
    homosexual transmission, 268, 306
    outbreaks of foodborne giardiasis, 255, 306
    perspectives, 305–312
    role of the beaver, 309–311
    waterborne outbreaks, 267–290
    waterborne transmission, 254–255, 267–290
Giardin, 23–26, 31
    amino acid sequence, 25

Golgi body, 33
Graft versus host reaction (GvHR), 166–167, 170
Guanine arabinoside, 329

Hexachlorophene, 329
Hexamita, 163
Hoechst 33258 staining, 40–42
Host–parasite biology, 216–218
Host specificity, 4, 268, 305–313, 349
   beaver, 256, 309–311
   cattle, 257, 309
   cats, 256, 308–309
   coyote, 310
   dogs, 256, 307–309
   egrets, 311
   herons, 217, 311
   mule deer, 312
   muskrat, 310–311
   voles, 311
Humatin, see Paromomycin
Humoral immune responses, 220–224, 244
Hydrolases, 72–75
Hypogammaglobulinemia, 158–159, 218, 220–222, 228

Immune responses, 93–95, 218–228
Immunity, cellular and humoral, 93–95, 214–228, 244–245
   G. duodenalis trophozoite antigens, 225–227
   introduction, 214–215
Immunity in mice,
   cellular, 93
   genetic control, 94
   humoral, 93
   and macrophage role, 95
   passive transfer, 95
   thymus-mediated, 93
   and *Trichinella* infection, 94–95, 168
Immunodeficiency and giardiasis, 158–159
Immunofluorescence, 21, 102, 148–191
Immunoglobulin levels, 222–223
   animal model studies, 80, 93, 170, 220
   human studies, 222–223
Immunoglobulins in giardiasis,
   anti-Giardia antibody, 220–221
   IgA class, 158, 162, 167, 170, 190–191, 120, 221–224
   IgE class, 94, 158, 162–163, 170
   IgG class, 158, 162, 170, 222–223
   IgM class, 158, 162, 170, 223–224

Induction of excystation, 107–108
Infection and disease, 246–248
Infection in infant-mother pairs, 256
Infection and malnutrition, 248–250
Inoculum, preparation for culture, 105–108
Interference reflexion microscopy, 45
Intestinal fluid and killing of *Giardia* trophozoites, 206–211
   effect of bile salts, 209
   effect of bovine serum albumin, 209
   effect of mucus, 209
   mechanism, 206–209
Intestinal mucosal changes in giardiasis, 156–171
   human giardiasis, 156–159
      changes in lamina propria plasma cells and secretory antibodies, 158
      histologic changes in immune-deficient patients, 158–159
      histologic changes in patients without immunodeficiency, 156–158
      intraepithelial lymphocyte (IEL) counts, 158
      jejunal disaccharidases, 161, 252
      lamina propria plasma cells, 158
      mucosal ultrastructure, 157–158
   murine giardiasis, 159–171
      crypt cell production rate, 163
      disaccharidase content, 159, 161, 170
      distribution of trophozoites, 160–161
      intestinal mucosa, 161–163
      intraepithelial lymphocyte (IEL) counts, 161–163, 165, 167, 170
      lamina propria plasma cells, 79, 162–163
      mucosal architecture, 79, 161
      small intestinal mucosa, 161–163
      time course of infection, 160
Intestinal protection of *Giardia*, 209–211
   bile salts, 209
   bovine serum albumin, 209
   mucus, 209–211
In vitro culture,
   axenic, 6, 101–108
   G. agilis, 6, 7
   G. duodenalis, 100–105
   G. muris, 6, 7, 127
   media, 100–103
Iodine compounds, 346–347
Iron malabsorption, 251
Isoelectric focusing (IEF), 23, 26
Isozymes (isoenzymes), 34, 55–56
Isolation of trophozoites and cysts, 105–107

cyst isolation methods, 92, 106–107
    sucrose density gradient centrifugation, 107
trophozoite isolation methods, 105–107

Jirds, see Mongolian gerbils

Karyokinesis, 112
Koch's postulates, 307, 336

Lambl, 2–5
Lectins and trophozoite attachment, 34–43, 45, 226
Life cycle, 12
Lipid metabolism and composition, 65–66
Lysosomes, 34

Macrophage, 94–95, 219–220, 226
Malabsorption, 79–80, 92, 156, 158–159, 179–180, 222, 225, 251, 319
    data, summarized, 250
Malnutrition, 80, 179–180, 243, 248, 250, 253, 331
Meadow voles, 105, 113
Median bodies, types, 5, 53–54
Mepacrine, see Quinacrine
Metabolism, 61–75, 329
Metronidazole, 7, 64, 253, 257, 316–321, 325–327
    mechanism of action, 326
    side effects, 327, 330
    teratogenicity, 327
Microtubules, 26–29
Microvillous border, 12, 45, 182
    disaccharidases, 86, 168
    lesions of, 85, 92, 95, 157–163, 168–171
Milk, 95, 202–206, 243–244
    breast feeding and cyst excretion, 95
    killing of *Giardia* by normal human milk, 202–206, 244
    and presence of maternal antibody, 256
    secretory IgA in breast milk, 221, 224, 244–245
Mitochondria, 33, 61, 113
Mongolian gerbil (*Meriones unguiculatus*), 7, 57, 81–88, 102, 104–105, 113, 128, 132, 133, 147
Morphology and cyst viability, 131–132
Mouse model for *G. muris*, 91–96, 159–171
    BALB/c mice, 93–95, 161–163, 220
    CBA mice, 160–161
    CF-1 mice, 81, 92, 161
    C3H/He mice, 94–95
    genetic studies, 94

hypothymic mice, 93–95, 165
immunologic studies, 93–95
mast-cell deficient mice, 94
nude mice, 93–95, 165, 168–169
SJL/J mice, 170
Mucosal architecture, 161
Mucus, 209–211
Muskrat, 42, 58, 142–148, 279, 286, 310, 336
Myosin, see *Giardia*, contractile proteins

Nimorazole, 319
Nippostrongylus brasiliensis, 168
Nitroimidazoles, 7, 315–322, 326–327
    efficacy vs. *Giardia*, 317
    history, 316
    mode of action, 316
    pharmacokinetics, 317
    single dose therapy, 320
    susceptible organisms, 317
    teratogenicity, 318–319, 327
Nomenclature, 4–6
Nonspecific defenses against *Giardia*, 199–211
Nucleic acid metabolism, 67–72
Nutrient intake and *Giardia* infection, 249

Opsonization, 221, 224
Ornidazole, 317, 319, 320–321
Ozone, 345–346

Package treatment plants (water filtration), 341–342
Pancreatitis, 179
Parabasal body, 12
Paromomycin, 325, 328, 332
Pattern of cyst release, 87
Peyer's patches, 93, 218–219
Phagocytosis of trophozoites by macrophages, 219–221
Plasma membrane, 32–33
Point of use/Point of entry (POU/POE) devices, 342
Pregnancy, 245, 319, 332
    and cyst excretion, 245
Prepatent period, 164, 318, 321
Prospects for control, 355–357
Purine metabolism, 70–72, 329
Pyrimidine metabolism, 67–70

Quinacrine, 7, 316, 319, 325–326
    mechanism of action, 326
    side effects, 326, 330

Reservoirs, 255–257, 288–290, 301–312
Resistance of cysts to disinfection, 338, 342–350
  animal infectivity as a measure of cyst viability, 343–344
  effect of
    boiling, 337
    chemical agents, 343–347
    desiccation, 337
    pH, 343–346
    temperature, 337, 343–347
    ultraviolet radiation, 345–346
  excystation as a measure of cyst viability, 343
  thermal death point, 337
  vital stain exclusion as a measure of cyst viability, 103, 343
Restriction endonuclease analysis, 56, 225
Risk factors, 299, 343

Saccharomyces cerevisiae, 6, 100
Salvage pathways for pyrimidines, 6
Schmutzdecke, 340
SDS-PAGE, 23, 33, 225
Secnidazole, 317
Serodiagnosis of giardiasis, 187–191
  procedures, summarized, 188
Small bowel biopsy, 159, 182
Small intestine,
  B cells, 93, 219
  biopsy, 158–159, 182
  and cell-mediated hypersensitivity, 169
  crypt cell production, 156–157, 163, 165
  disaccharidases, 85, 86, 159, 161, 167–168, 170
  eosinophils, 157, 170
  histological changes, 157
  host-related factors in pathogenesis, 169
  intraepithelial lymphocyte, 158–159, 161–170
  lamina propria, 79, 157–158, 164, 218, 219
  lymphocytes, 93, 166, 219
  lymphokines, 164
  M cell, 218
  macrophages, 94, 95, 219–221
  mast cells, 94
  microvillous border, 45, 157
  mucosal architecture, 80, 92, 158–159, 165, 167, 218
  mucosal damage in giardiasis, 155–171
  parasite-related factors in pathogenesis, 169
  secretory IgA, 220–224
  T cells, 164, 166, 168, 170, 219
  trophozoite distribution, 156–157

villus atrophy, 92, 156–159, 168, 170, 218
villus:crypt ratio, 79, 84, 86, 161, 163, 168
vitamin B12 malabsorption, 156
Speciation, 52–58
  see also *Giardia* species
Staining
  fluorescent, 40, 46, 112, 130–132
  fluorescein diacetate (FDA), 131, 147
  fluorogenic dyes, 145–147
  Giemsa, 182
  Hoechst, 33258, 40–42
  immunolabelling, 30, 32, 145, 146
  iron hematoxylin, 12, 14, 38, 182
  propidium iodide (PI), 131, 147
  trichrome, 182
  vital, 130
Steatorrhea, 179, 252
Stool examination, 181, 330
Stool preservation for examination
  merthiolate-iodine-formalin (MIF), 181
  polyvinyl alcohol, (PVA), 181
Sucrose density gradient centrifugation, 65, 88, 92, 107
Susceptibility to *Giardia* infection, 240–245
  age, 240–241
  behavior, 241
  diet, 243
  environmental factors, 241
  gastric acidity, 242
  nutritional factors, 242–243
  occupation, 242
  pregnancy, 245
  sex, 241
  socioeconomic factors, 241
Symbionts, 38–42, 56
  bacterial, 38–42, 56
  viral, 42, 56
Symptomatology and traditional diagnosis, 175–183, 246–248

Taxonomy, 4–6, 357
Tinidazole, 7, 317–321
  single dose therapy, 320
  superiority over metronidazole, 320–321
Transmission between animal species, 4, 57, 79, 83, 132, 256–257, 268, 279, 287, 311–312, 336
Transmission person to person, 3, 217, 306, 336
Transmission via the fecal–oral route, 254–255
  day care centers, 255, 295–301, 306
  food, 255, 306

food handlers, 332
host factors, 241–245
person to person, 3, 255–256, 306
pets, possible role, 307–309
venereal transmission and male homosexuals, 216, 218, 254, 268, 306, 332
waterborne, 254, 267–290
Travelers' diarrhea, 176, 245, 318
Treatment, 318–322, 325–333, 357
of asymptomatic cyst passers, 257–258, 319, 331–332
bithionol, 329
chlorimipramine, 328
dichlorophene, 329
drugs unavailable in the US, 325
empirical, 319
failure, 321–322, 332–333
follow-up, 320–322, 332
Furazolidone (Furoxone), 7, 325–328
homosexual partners, 333
immune compromised patients, 332
indications, 318
Metronidazole (Flagyl), 7, 316, 319–320, 325–327
Ornidazole, 320
Paromomycin (Humatin), 325, 328, 332
and posttreatment considerations, 321
in pregnancy, 319, 325, 332
Quinacrine (Atabrine), 7, 316, 325–326
regimens, 326
relapses, 320
sodium fusidate, 329
Tinidazole, 320
Trichinella spiralis, 94–95, 168
Trophozoite attachment, see also *Giardia*, attachment
contractile proteins, 43–45
and lectins, 45
as a means of concentration, 108
mechanism, 17–21, 43–46
hydrodynamic model, 43
role of flagellar activity, 43
role of microtubular coiling and uncoiling, 43
studied by interference-reflexion microscopy, 45
temperature, 107
Trophozoite concentration methods, 105–107
Trophozoite detachment, 107
Trophozoite metabolism, 61–75

energy and carbohydrate metabolism, 62–65
enzymes, 62–65
metabolic end-products, 62, 64
metabolic pathways, 62–65
respiration, 62–64
hydrolases, 72–74
lipid metabolism
cellular lipids, 65
fatty acid analysis, 65
incorporation of labelled precursors, 66
lipid composition, 65–66
uptake of lipids and lipid precursors, 66
nucleic acid metabolism, 67–72
purines, 70–72
pyrimidines, 67, 69
salvage pathway, 67–68, 70–71
Trophozoite morphology, ultrastructure, 12–34
axonemes, 17, 19
cytoskeletal proteins, 21–29
disc cytoskeleton, 17–20
flagella, 17, 26, 30–31
general, 12–16
lateral crest, 15, 19
median body, 12, 14, 26–27
microtubules, 17, 26–29
plasma membrane, 19, 32–33
symbionts,
bacterial and viral, 38–42
ectosymbionts, 39
endosymbionts, 38–42
tubulin, 26–29, 33
vacuolar system, 33–34
ventral disc, 15, 17–21
ventrolateral flange (VLF), 20–21
vesicles, 17
Trophozoite-substrate interaction, 19, 43–46
Tropomyosin, see *Giardia*, contractile proteins
Tubulin, 21–23, 26–29, 33

Ultrastructure, 16–38
Ultraviolet radiation, 345–346
Urinary tract, 156

Vaccine, 258–259, 357
Vacuolar system, 33–34
Viability method for cysts, compared, 130–134, 146–148, 343
Viruses, 42
Vital staining, 130, 156, 343
Vitamin A, 179, 250–251

Vitamin B12, 156, 179, 183, 250–251

Waterborne outbreaks of giardiasis, 267–290, 336, 338
  Arizona, 282
  Aspen, Colorado, 254, 269, 287, 309
  Aspen Highlands, Colorado, 281
  Australia, 284
  beaver implicated as the source, 279, 281, 284, 286, 309–310
  Berlin, New Hampshire, 281
  Bradford, Pennsylvania, 227–228
  Camas, Washington, 281, 309
  Canada, 283–284
  Colorado, 271, 274–276
  community and noncommunity water systems, 274
  Egypt, 254
  Leningrad, 254, 270
  location, in United States, 273
  Madeira, 270
  Minnesota, 271
  muskrat implicated as the source, 279, 310–311
  New Hampshire, 271
  Pennsylvania, 274, 281
  Pittsfield, Massachusetts, 278–279, 310
  Portland, Oregon, 269, 309
  Reno, Nevada, 310
  Rome, New York, 277, 287
  seasonal distribution, 276–277
  shallow wells, 272
  Soviet Union, 254, 270
  and surface waters, 273, 276–278
  Sweden, 283
  Tennessee, 287
  in travelers, 270–271
  and treatment, 273
  Tokyo, 254, 269
  types of water systems, 272, 274, 278
  United Kingdom, 283
  United States statistics, summarized, 268, 272–273
  Utah, 271–272, 282
  Vail, Colorado, 281
  Vermont, 275–276
  Washington state, 271, 275–276
  and water system deficiencies, 269, 279, 281–283, 288
Water examination for cysts, 287–288
Water voles, 287

Zinc sulfate flotation, 181
Zoonosis, 7, 256, 268, 305, 308, 310
Zymodemes, 56